HEALTH AND HUMAN BEHAVIOUR

THIRD EDITION

KEN JONES   DEBRA CREEDY

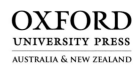

OXFORD
UNIVERSITY PRESS
AUSTRALIA & NEW ZEALAND

OXFORD
UNIVERSITY PRESS

Oxford University Press is a department of the University of Oxford.

It furthers the University's objective of excellence in research, scholarship, and education by publishing worldwide. Oxford is a registered trademark of Oxford University Press in the UK and in certain other countries.

Published in Australia by
Oxford University Press
253 Normanby Road, South Melbourne, Victoria 3205, Australia
© Ken Jones and Debra Creedy 2012

The moral rights of the authors have been asserted.

First published 2003
Second edition published 2008
Third edition published 2012
Reprinted 2013

National Library of Australia Cataloguing-in-Publication data

Author:	Jones, K. V.
Title:	Health and human behaviour / Ken Jones, Debra Creedy.
Edition:	3rd ed.
ISBN	978 0 19 557725 9 (pbk.)
Notes:	Includes bibliographical references and index.
Subjects:	Clinical health psychology.
	Health behavior.
Other Authors/Contributors:	
	Creedy, Debra Kay.
Dewey Number:	616.0019

Reproduction and communication for educational purposes

Edited and proofread by Pete Cruttenden
Typeset by diacriTech, Chennai, India
Indexed by Russell Brooks
Cover image: Corbis/Daniel Smith
Printed by Markono Print Media Pte Ltd

This book is dedicated to our families.

To my wife Aileen and children Caroline and Michael, without whom I never would have tried to write it, and to my extended family who give me added inspiration to keep up to date.

Ken

To my husband Mark for his patient support and to my children Ben, Alison and Joe, who are a great source of joy and encouragement to me.

Debra

CONTENTS

PREFACE

Each of us experiences health and illness as essential conditions of life. Our experience of health and illness affects our physical status as well as our feelings, thoughts and actions. We see constant evidence of the impact of health and illness on individuals, their families, institutions of health care and the wider community through the media and personal and fictional accounts. As the biomedical sciences have increased our knowledge about what regulates health at a biological level, individuals have become more interested in maximising their own health as well as reducing illness. We are also learning that health and illness involve much more than just the biological machine. Psychological, cultural and family issues are also intimately involved, and are frequently more important than the biological components of illness and health. The treatment of illness and the maintenance of health consume an ever-increasing portion of personal and public expenditure. As a result, health and illness have become central social and political concerns. For those training in health professions, biomedical sciences and other health-related disciplines, all of these personal and social issues need to be understood and addressed.

THE AIM OF THIS BOOK

Health and Human Behaviour has been written with entry-level students in the health professions, biomedical sciences and other health-related disciplines in mind. It is based on over 40 years of experience teaching students in these areas. The topics in the book have been carefully selected to cover the range of relevant psychological, physiological and sociological concepts, without trying to be comprehensive or detailed in the coverage of those concepts.

Its aim is to introduce concepts that students will need in a form that they will find usable. The book is intended to attract readers without a background in health, psychology and sociology to that material, and to provide enough information for readers, without overwhelming them with details of those disciplines. Readers who already have a background in these disciplines may be able to skip over sections of the material to focus on areas that are new to them.

CONTENT OF THE BOOK

In writing this book, we have tried to group ideas together in an order that will make sense to the reader. Part 1 has five chapters that focus on the foundations of health and behaviour. Chapter 1 is designed to provide an understanding of illness and disease on the one hand, and health and well-being on the other. Ways in which health and illness are measured are discussed and different models of thinking about them are presented. Our understanding of health and illness changes as we grow and develop. Chapter 2 draws on major theorists who influenced our understanding of healthy child and adolescent development. In addition to physical growth, childhood and adolescence are times of tremendous cognitive, social and emotional development. This chapter considers how children of different ages might understand illness. As a person grows from childhood to adulthood, they develop many habitual ways of behaving, responding and thinking. During adulthood, these habitual patterns of response begin to exert an influence on the person's health. Gradually, as the years pass, capabilities are lost. Although this is often thought of as a consequence of age itself, it is usually due to disease processes that happen coincidentally with ageing. Adulthood and ageing are considered in Chapter 3. Health and illness are not purely biological states, but, more importantly, personal and social events. Because of this, individuals react in a variety of ways to the experience of illness. Commonalities in these reactions and how these relate to individual experience are dealt with in Chapter 4. Perceptions about the cause, symptoms and meaning of illness play a major role in reactions to illness, so a section discussing perception is included in this chapter. Responses to acute illness can differ significantly from the experience of living with a chronic condition that is permanent, incurable and irreversible. Chapter 5 describes common reactions to chronic conditions and factors that may influence coping.

Part 2 has four chapters. Having looked at the impact of health on behaviour, Chapter 6 considers the other side of the coin: how behaviour impacts on health. The focus is on how behaviours develop and are maintained, and on the theories that can help us understand these processes. Chapter 7 introduces the concept of 'agency' and explores the effects of beliefs and attitudes on behaviour. It includes sections on health belief models, expectations and the very important concept of 'placebo'. The role that reasoning plays in moderating decisions about health is also discussed. Based on an understanding of how behaviours develop and are maintained, Chapter 8 begins to examine ways in which those behaviours can be changed to produce improvements in protective behaviours and reductions in risky ones, with the aim of producing better outcomes to health and well-being. Chapter 9 looks at a specific but highly complex example of health related behaviour. In recent years, overweight and obesity have overtaken smoking as the single most important modifiable behavioural risk to health. Given the enormous interest in the media about issues of weight and activity, this edition has added a new chapter completely devoted to providing an evidence-based look at this area.

So far, the focus of this book has largely been on behavioural and cognitive factors as they impact on health. The four chapters in Part 3 explore the critical role of emotion in health and illness, what it is and how it works. Chapter 10 examines interactions between mind and body. An integrated perspective is vital in contemporary health care and this chapter investigates the role of emotions in mental illnesses, such as anxiety and depression, as well as the effect of emotional states on the body, such as immune and cardiovascular functioning. As we did in Part 2 of the book, a complex but vital topic has been chosen as an example of how the basic concepts and principles can be applied to understanding health and well-being. Chapter 11 examines the physiological, emotional and cognitive basis and consequences of pain. The diagnosis and management of pain constitutes a large part of health care, but is often completely misunderstood. The remaining chapters in this section address another issue—stress—which is receiving much popular attention, often without the necessary evidence base for it to be fully understood. Chapter 12 explores how our appraisal of situations and our capacity to meet those demands can be experienced as stressful. Fortunately, stress is neither inevitable nor irresistible. Chapter 13 looks in more detail at stress management, examining a variety of coping behaviours, and how they can help to reduce the health impact of stressful events.

A person's beliefs, attitudes and behaviours cannot explain all that needs to be known about agency. Agents exist outside the individual as well and these are examined in Part 4 of this book. Social agents include family, friends, communities, organisations, cultures, governments and so on. Ignoring the importance of these factors on health can lead to placing too much responsibility on the individual—that is, blaming the victim. Chapter 14 explores how social factors such as culture, social class and education can influence a person's experience of the world, and their access to health care, health information and a healthy environment. The notion of a person's ability to understand health information in order to make informed decisions is known as health literacy. This edition introduces a new chapter devoted to health literacy. Chapter 15 explores factors that influence a person's capacity to obtain, understand and apply health information in their life. Understanding that people possess different levels of literacy and learn about health in various ways has important implications for promoting healthy behaviour as well as treating and preventing illness. Finally, Chapter 16 explores the different systems for supplying health care and methods of empowering individuals to care for their own health. Individuals can be helped to change, but so can families, social systems, communities and governments.

THE CASE STUDIES

Each chapter includes case studies that illustrate issues arising in that chapter. One type of case study is distributed throughout the chapter, revisiting an individual several times to look at different issues in their experience. These studies are intended to give readers the opportunity to test their grasp of those concepts before moving on to the next section. The other kind is the long case at the end of the chapter. The intention is to give students a deeper understanding of a case and the concepts addressed in the chapter. The case studies are not intended to cover every kind of health problem, but merely to illustrate the experiences of those who are ill or who want to protect their current wellness. As in real life, the case studies are about individuals, each of whom experiences health and illness differently. Some may vary from standard presentations for a condition in order to make points more clearly. Again, this parallels real life.

We would encourage readers to go beyond these simple cases and to look at the real experience of individuals of their own acquaintance in the light of the material in this book. There is no better way to understand the interaction of health and human behaviour. Nearly all students in health-related courses are required to carry out a case study of an individual with a chronic condition or medical illness as part of their course work. The first concern that many students have is that they will not be able to find such a person. Soon they come to realise that chronic conditions and medical illness are extremely common. The search for a suitable case rapidly becomes a problem of selection rather than identification. Common conditions, such as asthma, arthritis and depression, have a very high incidence among otherwise healthy individuals. However, it is also true that rare conditions—due to the very large numbers of them—are also common in spite of the small number of individuals suffering from each one.

The difficulty with much of the traditional study of the person in health and illness is that it has usually been compartmentalised into biological, psychological and sociological specialities. These compartments are usually taught by discipline specialists with little interest in a whole-person perspective. The available books are also specialised, with each presenting more detail within the speciality than most readers will need at the introductory level. Basing the study of health and illness on the experience of the individual by the use of interactive cases overcomes this compartmentalisation and increases the interest of the material for the reader. The cases chosen raise issues that we can all relate to, without including biomedical detail that most first year students would find difficult to understand.

THE SELF TESTS

Each chapter includes a small number of multiple-choice questions that are intended to enable the reader to determine whether they have understood some of the essential points of the chapter. Many of these questions are clinical, in the sense that readers are asked to think about where the information in the chapter would lead, rather than simply knowing the material. This is only the roughest of guidelines to understanding, however; thinking beyond the conceptual and factual content of the book is desirable. For this reason, a number of 'Pause and Reflect' activities are also included throughout each chapter. These are intended to encourage the extension of knowledge and deeper thought about concepts being addressed.

ADDITIONAL READING AND WEB RESOURCES

Each chapter also provides the titles of additional materials that may be of interest to readers. The materials aim to expand your knowledge by exploring related concepts or reading about the findings of current research in the area. The reader may also wish to visit some of the websites listed or watch a recorded segment on the internet to gain further insights into particular health conditions and illness responses, or access the latest facts and figures presented on government and health websites. YouTube is a useful resource, but these clips have a tendency to come and go at unpredictable times. Therefore, we have preferred to cite institutional or governmental resources, which tend to be more stable, but students are encouraged to follow their interests widely—but critically—across a variety of sources.

Miller (1990), a prominent educator in the health professions, identified levels of performance with regard to the content of education: *knows*, *knows how*, *shows how* and *does*. Our aim in teaching this material to students in the health professions and biomedical sciences is to have an impact on what they actually do in their professional activities. The self-test material can provide only an indication of what you *know*, and what you *know how* to do. Looking in depth at an individual can provide an indication of whether you can demonstrate an ability to use the material; that you can *show how* to use it. We will never know whether readers have learnt how to put their knowledge from this book into practice—how to do something in a better way—but it is our hope that this book will have prompted some positive changes in your eventual professional behaviour.

ACKNOWLEDGMENTS

This third edition of *Health and Human Behaviour* has taken several months to prepare and would not have been completed without the support of a few special people. We give heartfelt thanks to our employers, the School of Psychology and Psychiatry, the School of Primary Health Care and the Department of Medical Imaging and Radiation Science at Monash University and the School of Psychology at the University of Queensland, who supported us with time and resources to write.

Our sincere thanks to the editorial staff at OUP—Debra James and Shari Serjeant—and our editor, Pete Cruttenden, for turning our writing into a book.

PART 1

FOUNDATIONS OF HEALTH AND BEHAVIOUR

Behaviour has a central role in health, but many of the things that are needed to maintain health and avoid illness are beyond our ability to control. Sometimes this is because of our individual physical and/or psychological characteristics, and sometimes it is because of social factors and barriers. In fact, the more progress the biomedical sciences make in explaining the biological processes of the body, the clearer it becomes that there are psychological and social processes that we need to understand in order to make sense of being sick and being well. Part 1 of this book begins with an examination of these understandings.

The connections between health and behaviour are complex. It is well understood by most people that our habits affect health. The media are full of information about links between obesity and disease, and warnings about the dangers of smoking, the sun and too much alcohol. But it is equally important to recognise that health and illness affect our behaviour. The most fundamental place to begin the examination of the connections between health and behaviour is with an understanding of what health, illness and disease are—what it means to be sick or well. These concepts are not absolute values of something, but social constructs or ideas that we share with the people around us.

Chapter 1 defines some key terms and describes some of the ways in which health and illness can be measured and understood. We then explore how our understanding of health and illness changes across the lifespan. Chapter 2 draws on major developmental theorists such as Piaget, Erikson and Vygotsky who offered important observations and concepts to consider in our thinking of healthy child and adolescent development. In addition to physical growth, childhood and adolescence are times of tremendous cognitive, social and emotional development. It is also interesting to consider how children of different ages might understand illness. A child younger than 2 years might know illness as something associated with a feeling that may evoke tears. A 5-year-old might explain being sick as when you 'throw up'. A 9-year old may associate illness with particular behaviours and consequences such as staying in bed. It is interesting to note that children's understanding of health may not be as limited as once thought. Vygotsky suggested that even the youngest child can seek, understand, evaluate and use information to appreciate health and illness, especially if health resources are presented in ways that are age appropriate, culturally relevant and supported by the community in which the child lives.

During adulthood, age can affect an individual's behaviour in different ways. As individuals progress from childhood to adulthood, they develop many habitual ways of behaving, responding and thinking. During adulthood, these habitual patterns of response begin to exert an influence on the individual's health. Gradually, as the years pass, capabilities are lost. Although this is often thought of as a consequence of age itself, it is usually due to disease processes that happen coincidentally with ageing. Adulthood and ageing are considered in Chapter 3.

Chapter 4 focuses on how people react to being sick and looks at the influence that illness has on how individuals feel, think and respond. These reactions, of course, will be different for different people, which can be explained by the vulnerabilities and capabilities that the individual brings to the experience. Most episodes of illness are short, or acute; however, there are many individuals who suffer from ongoing or recurrent health problems and some of the important issues are different when illness is chronic. Chapter 5 examines reactions to living with a chronic condition.

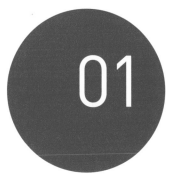

01

WHO IS SICK?
DEFINING AND MEASURING
ILLNESS, DISEASE AND HEALTH

CHAPTER OBJECTIVES

By the end of your study of this chapter, you should be able to:

- understand the importance of health and illness to the individual person
- know how concepts of health, illness and disease depend on the experience of the sick person and on the interpretations of others, particularly health professionals
- describe and compare health, illness and related concepts
- understand how health and illness are measured, and how these measures may vary according to the purposes for which they are used
- understand the medical model and the biopsychosocial model of health and illness, and the differences between them.

KEYWORDS

appraisal
attitudes
biopsychosocial model
disease
epidemiology
health
illness
incidence
medical model
morbidity
mortality
negative definition of health
prevalence
well-being

HEALTH AND ILLNESS

Health: a concept that can vary over time, and can differ between social groups, cultures, countries, families and individuals.

Illness: a subjective feeling on the part of an individual that something is not right with their health.

CROSS-REFERENCE
These differences about the meaning of health are discussed in Chapter 6.

Health and **illness** are important concepts. They have a significant impact on how an individual thinks, feels and acts. A 'sick' person is different from a 'well' person in many ways—in their own eyes, and in the eyes of others. Think, for example, about how we greet one another. Although we say 'How are you?' we rarely expect to receive a detailed explanation. We tend to assume that the other person is among the well, and that they are going to answer 'Fine'. When we greet someone who we know to be sick, we say the same thing—'How are you?'—but in this case we expect to get specific information.

Because most people tend to be reasonably well most of the time, health does not normally occupy a large place in our thoughts. However, when we do become sick, it moves right to the top of our priorities. The importance of health to our quality of life only becomes obvious to us when we are sick or in other dramatic circumstances. In the face of a major disaster in life, for example, it is not uncommon for someone to try to put the event into perspective by saying, 'At least I've got my health.'

It is not always clear exactly what being well and being sick mean. Many, if not most, people who consider themselves to be well actually have a number of symptoms or ongoing health problems but do not consider themselves to be sick. People with major disabilities may also think of themselves as well, in spite of living with pain or disability that would make most of us feel very ill indeed. Older individuals also live as well people, in spite of decreases in the sensitivity of their vision and hearing, or limitations on their movement or activity. Clearly, the meaning of health can vary over the course of a person's life, and can differ between social groups, cultures, countries, families and individuals.

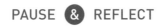

PAUSE & REFLECT

Do you consider yourself to be well or sick right at this moment? Why? Defining what health and illness are is an important first step in looking at their importance for the person.

WHO IS SICK?

Being sick is not a fact: it is a social definition. The problem of defining who is sick has significance not just for the individual but also for those around the individual. It even has a moral dimension. Many people believe, for example, that smokers deserve less medical care than, say, innocent accident victims because smokers contribute to their own illness. Others see this attitude as an example of blaming the victim for their illness.

There are basically two definitions that are commonly used to decide whether someone is really sick: the illness definition and the disease definition.

CASE STUDY

MARSHA JOHNSON AND BREAST CANCER

The aim of this case is to get you to think about what happens when an individual becomes ill in their own eyes, and the behaviours that follow from that decision.

Consider the situation of Marsha Johnson. She is 55 years old, married to a 58-year-old electrical engineer, and has two daughters now aged 30 and 33. As a young girl, Marsha emigrated with her parents and two brothers from the United Kingdom to Australia. Her parents are elderly but in good health. Marsha completed high school and works as an administrative officer with the Department of Social Services. Marsha tries to maintain her weight through the occasional diet and exercise about three times a week for around 40 minutes. She is post-menopausal. While having a shower one day, Marsha notices a lump in her left breast.

1   Is Marsha ill? Could you defend your answer using the illness definition below?

2   What might be some of the considerations Marsha takes into account when assessing her state of health?

DEFINITION 1:
THE SICK ARE THOSE WHO HAVE SYMPTOMS
(THE ILLNESS DEFINITION)

We are all familiar with the experience of feeling unwell. This personal, or subjective, feeling that something is not quite right for us is the most important indicator of illness we have. This feeling may be based on having symptoms that we do not usually have, or a symptom that we do usually have but that is worse than usual. It may also be based on what we believe to be normal for the groups that we belong to. If we have a symptom that others around us do not have, or that they consider abnormal, we feel that we are ill. Even if others do not know about or recognise our feeling, we can still feel ill and find it difficult to deal with the demands of the world around us.

CROSS-REFERENCE
Health beliefs are discussed in Chapter 7.

Each of us wants to live in a world that is understandable and obeys some rules. Whenever we are feeling not quite right, it is reasonable that we will want to understand why—and that we will look for a cause or an explanation. The kinds of causes that we accept as reasonable will depend on our own personal view of how the world works. Imagine, for example, trying to explain having the symptoms of a cold to one of your ancestors from several centuries in the past. They would never have heard of germs and would not be able to make sense out of your explanation that a cold was caused by something called a virus. Depending on where your ancestors came from, they might believe that colds were caused by mists rising from marshes, or by bad air, or even by a curse cast on them by a neighbour. They could feel ill, but draw very different conclusions about why they feel ill and (equally importantly) what to do about it.

The situation is less extreme when we deal with those living around us—such as our family and friends—because we tend to be exposed to similar information and similar experiences. It is still possible for us to differ in our beliefs about illness. Some individuals experience illness in the absence of a clear physical cause. Occasionally, the people around those individuals may feel that they are not really sick, or even believe that they are faking illness or are crazy. None of this makes the illness any less real to the person experiencing it.

CROSS-REFERENCE
This kind of disagreement about whether someone is sick is discussed again in Chapter 8.

Although for many years, the notion of illness as 'the presence of disease' has been a dominant view (Manderscheid et al. 2010), some have noted important problems with a definition of illness based on the presence of symptoms. According to Armstrong (1980: 5) we need to think more broadly about what it means to be ill for the following reasons.

• *Symptoms are very common.* It is quite likely that you will have had a potentially treatable symptom in the past few days, or more than one—a headache, muscle soreness, a cough or runny nose, anxiety or a cut or scrape. Do you consider yourself to be a sick person? Most will not. Children and older people are even more likely to have symptoms but not think of themselves as sick.

- *Most symptoms are trivial and easily forgotten.* If you woke up with a cough this morning but it got better in a couple of hours, you would probably not even remember it tomorrow. Many people live with regular symptoms—such as a runny nose or chronic pain—but have adapted to the symptoms. The symptoms have been shifted into the background level of health that they experience, so they do not consider themselves to be sick unless the symptoms are greater than, or different from, their normal experience. Even in the presence of a variety of recurrent or constant symptoms the vast majority of the elderly, for example, consider their health to be good or excellent (Trentini et al. 2011).
- *It is usually not the symptom (or even its severity or persistence) that matters to the individual.* What matters is the meaning of the symptom. A person who experiences a perceptual distortion, such as blurred vision, or a lump or pain that is unexpected or new, may be far more worried by it than the person with diabetes who experiences the symptoms of low blood sugar, or the arthritis sufferer who has swelling and severe persistent pain in their joints.
- *Even for a given individual and symptom, perception of meaning will vary according to the mood of the individual, the context of the symptom, the individual's level of knowledge and experience, their usual coping strategies and many other factors.* A symptom that looks serious to an individual may suddenly lose all significance when the individual is given a satisfactory explanation for it. Imagine finding a strange crusty lump in the middle of your back. You might have panicky thoughts of skin cancer, and because you cannot actually examine the lump, might find yourself preoccupied with thoughts of the lump, severely disrupting your daily activities. You would probably experience great relief if told that it was only a scab and that you had probably run into something or scratched an insect bite without being particularly aware of having done so.

CROSS-REFERENCE
Strategies for dealing with illness are discussed in Chapter 7, and strategies for coping with stress in Chapter 13.

Sometimes an individual may not perceive that they have a symptom. People who are suffering from the psychological condition known as mania may have never felt better in their lives. They may—in their own eyes—have great plans that only they can carry out. In the eyes of other observers, those plans may be unrealistic and impossible to carry out. The individual can require treatment even in the absence of any sense that something is wrong.

CASE STUDY

MARSHA (CONT.)

Marsha may experience different responses when she discovers the lump in her breast. If Marsha has felt a lump before, or knows or believes that the cause is trivial, she may ignore the lump and experience no change in her concept of herself as a well person. If the lump is new, has changed in size or shape, or represents to her the possibility of serious disease, she will be likely to start thinking about whether she is ill—she will begin to have a feeling that something is not quite right.

In this case, Marsha had found lumps in her breasts when she was younger. A lump would occasionally appear around the time of her menstrual period. However, Marsha has not menstruated for two years. She is also worried about the lump because her mother was diagnosed with breast cancer in her early sixties. Marsha decides that something is not right and goes to see her doctor to get a medical view of her lump. Her doctor performs some tests to confirm the nature of the lump. These tests indicate that there is about a four in ten chance that she does not have cancer.

When Marsha's mother was diagnosed with breast cancer, she had also been in good health. Marsha recalls that her mother had received a reminder for her annual breast screening and a lump was found. Within a matter of weeks, her mother had a biopsy, surgery and was having radiotherapy on the affected breast and lymph tissue. This was a very worrying time for everyone and her mother broke down and cried several times with Marsha. Her mother felt sick from the treatment, and for years afterwards needed to protect her arm on the affected side from injury and infection. Marsha found herself thinking often about her mother's experience and wondered how she would cope if she had breast cancer.

1   Does Marsha have a disease? Could you defend your answer based on the disease definition below?

2   Marsha witnessed her mother's experience of breast cancer. How might this experience influence Marsha's response to her situation?

DEFINITION 2:
THE SICK ARE THOSE WHO HAVE BEEN GIVEN A DIAGNOSIS BY A HEALTH PROFESSIONAL (THE DISEASE DEFINITION)

In Western society it is generally assumed that illness arises from pathological changes in the physical body. In most cases, these changes can—at least potentially—be observed and substantiated by health professionals. We have the means to measure high blood pressure, to observe viruses and bacteria, and to create x-ray or other images of abnormalities or injuries deep inside the body. This objective classification of pathology underlies the concept of **disease**— that there is something biomedically wrong.

Disease: an abnormal state of the body or mind of a person as identified by a qualified observer.

It is important to recognise that definitions of what is pathology can change over time and from place to place. HIV/AIDS, for example, was not originally identified by pathology. A number of people, with similar signs and symptoms, went to see their doctors feeling ill, and only then did medical scientists start looking for a common cause. Unusual numbers of a rare condition were observed and it took some time for the cause to be pinned down.

The definition of disease can change over time as well. The most commonly cited example of this in medical textbooks is homosexuality. Once considered in many societies to be a disease requiring treatment, it is now recognised as a sexual preference. So, the disease definition of who is sick also has some problems.

• *Health professionals tend to accept a patient's definition that they are sick.* Many readers will have seen news stories in which doctors were accused of giving people certificates for time off work even when the symptoms cited were minor, difficult to classify as disease or easily faked. Such media reporting is unfair, as doctors and other health professionals tend to respond to the patient's feelings as true expressions of subjective illness, such as feeling unwell, tired or stressed, or even being fed up with work. It would be far more worrying news if health professionals regarded large numbers of their patients as wasting their time, or malingering (lying). Help-seeking is seen by health professionals in most cases as justifying the giving of help, and it would be hard to argue that this is unreasonable.

- *The diagnosis and treatment of medical conditions varies from time to time and place to place.* Not long ago, a child with tonsillitis living in one state in Australia was twice as likely to have surgery as a child with tonsillitis in another state. Caesarean deliveries are more common in women with private health insurance, and it could be argued that this high rate does not reflect real medical need for them to take place. Diagnoses may even be influenced by political or religious beliefs. In the former Soviet Union, disagreeing with state policy was regarded as the first symptom of a serious mental illness.
- *Diagnosis and treatment depend on concepts of normality.* These concepts may be cultural, subcultural or even family-based. There is a tribal group in Africa in which a particular skin disorder—causing white blotches on the skin—is common. It is so common, in fact, that individuals without it are rare. As a result, these people are considered to have a disease and are treated for their unblotched skin. In an example closer to home, the definition of alcoholism varies considerably between different groups within the population. What is regarded as a symptom of alcoholism in one group—say, drinking every day of the week— may be seen as normal in another. Part of the problem in dealing with alcohol abuse in Indigenous communities is defining exactly what that term means. There may also be differences in beliefs between religious groups, locations, and men and women.

CASE STUDY

MARSHA (CONT.)

Deciding whether someone has a disease sometimes means deciding what to do next. In Marsha's case, the consequences of doing nothing to treat her symptom could be very severe. If her breast lump is cancerous, the probability of her dying could be greatly increased by inaction. Conversely, doing something about the symptom could save her life. It is likely in this case that the doctor would do everything possible to persuade Marsha that she had a disease worth treating, and that treatment of that disease should begin as soon as possible.

Marsha talked over the initial results with her husband, Peter, who was keen for Marsha to have further tests and treatment. Her daughters also thought it was a good idea for their mother to be fully tested and treated. Marsha felt in a dilemma. She wanted to have further testing to be reassured that everything was okay, but she was also worried about the possibility of having cancer. She kept thinking about her mother's experience and the long-term consequences of treatment. She was worried about losing part or all of her breast. She and Peter still had an active sex life and Marsha was worried that Peter may not find her attractive any more if she was disfigured.

After several nights of talking things through, Marsha and her husband had an appointment with her doctor. They agreed that her lump should be removed and examined to determine whether it was cancerous. During the appointment, the doctor informed her that with appropriate treatment—even if the lump was cancerous—her chance of long-term survival was good, and that she should be well.

1　Will treatment make Marsha healthy again?

2　How might this experience affect Marsha's view of her health in the short and long term?

HOW DO ILLNESS AND DISEASE COMPARE?

Usually, disease and illness go together—we feel unwell because we have a disease. However, this is not always the case, and problems may arise for the individual when disease and illness do not go together. High blood pressure (hypertension), for instance, is a measurable example of physical pathology. Having high blood pressure is dangerous; people with high blood pressure are at increased risk of stroke and heart attack. Yet most people who have undiagnosed high blood pressure are probably not even aware of the fact—they do not feel ill at all. The vast majority of those who do have the diagnosed disease of high blood pressure found out because a health professional tested for it during a routine examination. An individual who experiences no symptoms is less likely to accept treatment, and any doctor would have difficulty in persuading some of their patients to take their high blood pressure seriously—because, they say, they feel perfectly well.

PAUSE & REFLECT

The definitions presented in this chapter suggest that high blood pressure would be considered a disease, not an illness. How might this affect whether or not a patient diagnosed with high blood pressure would treat it as a serious health problem?

Is it possible to have an illness without having a disease? Again, the answer is yes. Think about a young man who notices that his hair is falling out. He feels that something is not right, and fears the consequences for his future—he does not want to be bald. When he goes to his doctor, however, he is told that there is nothing wrong with him, and that he simply is displaying normal male pattern baldness, which is largely determined by his genes. Some men are satisfied with this definition of themselves as being well and adapt to the change in their appearance. They consider themselves normal and bald. Others are dissatisfied and may pursue treatment with drugs, or even with surgery, to avoid being bald.

If the individual's need to define baldness as a disease is strong enough, they will find professionals who will agree that they need treatment. Because the larger community does not think of baldness as a disease, they will probably have to pay for that treatment out of their own pocket. The ways in which communities decide who is well or ill is discussed in Chapter 14. Briefly, though, the decision involves cultural and social values, religious beliefs and a variety of other factors.

Other cosmetic illnesses are also not considered diseases in most societies. Take the woman who considers her breasts to be too small and wants implants, or the person with crooked or discoloured but otherwise healthy teeth. The boundaries become very unclear in some instances. Is male circumcision a procedure that doctors should conduct? If there is a medical need—for example, the foreskin is too tight or chronic infections occur—then there is likely to be a high degree of agreement that they should. The United States is currently the only Western nation where male circumcision is routinely performed; the procedure is rarely performed in Western Europe and New Zealand (Masem 2012). After an exhaustive review of the evidence, the Royal Australasian College of Physicians (2010) found that circumcision did not provide significant protection against sexually transmitted illnesses (STIs) and HIV, and concluded there was no medical case for neonatal circumcision. If it is for religious purposes, then the level of agreement will differ from place to place depending on the religious mix of the community and the proportion of male babies who have the procedure. In most societies, female circumcision would be considered to be mutilation, and almost never justifiable. Most of us would be horrified to discover that a health professional in our community was involved in performing this procedure. Yet there are other societies where it is considered not only acceptable but desirable.

CROSS-REFERENCE
Stress and its
management
are discussed in
Chapters 12 and 13.

Confusion about whether illness equals disease is common in the early stages of symptoms, before a cause has been established. There are some conditions where the disease classification has had to catch up with the illness (such as HIV/AIDS), but a number of others feature in the media. For example, there is still disagreement as to whether chronic fatigue syndrome should be reclassified as post-viral syndrome (Gibson, Smith & Ward 2011). Stress leads to a great deal of illness and many lost days of work, yet is notoriously difficult to classify in terms of specific physical signs. Anxiety and depression are still in the grey area where identification of the consequences is much easier than identification of a physical pathology.

As medical science progresses, the classification of disease becomes clearer. More causes are identified and the links between causes and symptoms are better understood. Sometimes, because of new evidence, we find that we have to go back to ideas that have previously been rejected by medical science. Some herbal treatments have been accepted back into orthodox Western medicine, and the recently established medical effectiveness of meditation and relaxation has lead to a re-evaluation of the links between mind and body. We revisit some of these issues in Chapters 8 and 9.

HEALTH

Negative definition of
health: the absence of
symptoms of illness and
signs of disease.

It is not uncommon for us to think of health as the normal state, experienced whenever we are not actually ill. The more one thinks about this **negative definition of health**—the absence of disease—the less useful it appears to be. How useful is a definition that would classify whole groups or even populations as sick? Do the members of those groups consider themselves to lack health? One of the main reasons why they do not is that we all tend to measure our health against those around us. Elderly people are highly likely to suffer from sensory problems (hearing or vision), limitations on movement, or chronic health problems such as hypertension (high blood pressure), arthritis and diabetes. And yet a recent study with elderly women (Requena et al. 2010) found that physical well-being was not as important as the mental and social dimensions of life in relation to health. People in developing countries where parasites are common may see themselves as well in spite of having a condition that would be considered a serious health problem for most people in a developed country.

The World Health Organization (WHO 1946) has attempted to promote a positive definition of health that is more flexible than just the absence of disease or infirmity. Health is considered by WHO to be 'a state of complete physical, social and mental well-being' that is consistent with living a full and satisfying life. This definition is intended to be useful in all countries—in spite of the differences in economies and the scope of health care available—and responsive to local needs. While this is broadly applicable, it is also clear that problems are going to arise with the differences in health from one place to another. As an example, if all the children in a locality are suffering from brain damage as a result of early malnutrition, they may all find satisfactory lives within their society, but we would still want to do something urgently about the malnutrition.

Another way of thinking about health is in terms of what it enables the individual to do. The *Ottawa Charter for Health Promotion* (WHO 1986) talks about health as being a 'resource for everyday life, not the objective of living'. Health allows individuals to tackle their ongoing activities, while disease and illness produce barriers to those activities. Individuals have 'enough' health when it is not a particular concern for them.

WELL-BEING

The concept of **well-being**—included in the WHO definition of health given in the previous section— entered the discussion of what health means in the 1960s (Evans 1965). To some extent, it could be said that health is the opposite of disease, while well-being represents the opposite of illness; that is, a subjective sense that there is basically nothing wrong. Like illness, well-being can be completely independent of our objectively measured health or disease status.

Individuals who have capabilities and coping strategies that allow them to manage their lives without much difficulty (who have an excess of resources over demands, a concept discussed in Chapter 14) tend to find that their disease is irrelevant to their sense of being intact as a person and in control of their life. Similarly, individuals may have a sense of personal well-being in very deprived circumstances, while dealing with chronic or acute disease, and even in the face of very stressful events. It is useful to keep in mind that an individual's **appraisal** of their situation is critically important. It will affect how they think and feel about health, and what behaviours they carry out.

MEASUREMENT OF HEALTH AND ILLNESS

Decisions about what diseases exist, which ones are common or serious, and which ones should attract special attention by health professionals are usually made by the community on the basis of information about the occurrence of disease within that community. In earlier days, these decisions were often made on the basis of common knowledge or on cultural or religious grounds. In most communities now, these decisions are made on the basis of more objective measurements of health and illness within the community. The science of **epidemiology** has taken over the measurement task. Its aim is to inform the decision makers within a community about the health status of that community, or a segment of that community.

The health of a population is usually measured by looking at two characteristics: **morbidity** (amount of sickness) and **mortality** (number of deaths). It is possible to imagine a case where these two do not go together, but it is far more common for them to be closely associated. Where people are sick a lot, they tend not to live as long.

There are two aspects of morbidity that are of particular interest. First, how many people are suffering from a particular disease over a period of time? For example, how many cases of arthritis there were in a community in a year (called the **prevalence** of that disease). Second, how many new cases were observed over a period of time? For example, how many people were first diagnosed as having arthritis in a community during a year (called the **incidence** of that disease). The fact that these can differ is quite significant. The Chernobyl power station in Ukraine became the scene of the world's worst nuclear accident in 1986, and the prevalence of radiation sickness in the area was very high at that time. The incidence is low now because of clean-ups, and because there are few unaffected individuals left to develop the condition. In the same way, if the incidence of HIV infection suddenly becomes low among new-born babies because of new treatments for infected mothers, this will only affect the prevalence among children over time.

Well-being: a state of complete physical, social and mental health that is consistent with living a full and satisfying life.

Appraisal: the cognitions that an individual has about the situation they are in at a given time.

Epidemiology: the science of measuring the health status of a community.

Morbidity: the amount of disease observed within a group.

Mortality: the number of deaths observed within a group.

Prevalence: the number of existing and new cases of a specific disease present in a given population at a certain time.

Incidence: the rate at which new cases of a specific disease occur in a population during a specified period.

PAUSE & REFLECT

Following a change in the kinds of pesticides used on farms in a particular area, it is observed that a large number of babies are born with birth defects. How would the concepts of prevalence and incidence help you to understand this observation?

One very good reason for keeping a watch on the incidence and prevalence of disease in the community is that changes can help us to identify new problems or changed health conditions. An increase in the incidence of polio in parts of the USA alerted experts that the number of children receiving vaccine against it had dropped to the point that there was danger of a polio epidemic for the first time in decades.

More recently, in the Indian state of Uttar Pradesh there was a dramatic increase in polio cases (from 268 in 2001 to 1600 in 2002). An investigation by health authorities learnt that the resistance to polio vaccination came from within the marginalised, largely Muslim communities who were influenced by rumours that the polio vaccine was a Western ploy to sterilise Muslims. The investigation revealed that more than 80 per cent of the children infected in the 2002 outbreak were Muslim boys under two years old. A grassroots campaign was developed to counter these misconceptions. Larson and Ghinai (2011) describe how community members were trained and deployed as local 'champions' for polio eradication, in order to counter resistance to vaccination from within their communities. The significant decline in polio cases is evidence of the close relationship formed between the local champions and the families within these communities. The state of Uttar Pradesh has not seen a case of polio for more than a year.

Monitoring of a population also enables other trends to be predicted. The ageing of the population in Western societies has led to an increase in the prevalence of problems of ageing that will affect health care funding and decisions about the number of doctors, hospitals and nursing homes that will be needed in the near future. In Australia, this has recently led to large increases in the number of training places for health professionals within our universities, either by increasing the number of students in existing institutions or by increasing the number of institutions training particular health professionals.

We also learn a lot about health and illness in a society from looking at the causes of death. One problem with mortality measurement is that eventually everyone dies. This means that if fewer people die from, say, infections during the first year of life, more people must eventually die of other causes later in life. If we look back at statistics taken from death certificates over hundreds of years, it would appear that we are in the midst of cancer and heart disease epidemics—much larger proportions of people are dying of these conditions than ever before. If we look at the age at which people die of these causes, however, they are much older than the people dying from other causes, such as childbirth and infectious diseases. This means that we need to look at premature deaths rather than absolute numbers of deaths to tell us when immediate action is needed to improve health. Unfortunately, this can also lead us to make some unwarranted decisions about health care. Focusing all of our attention on causes of death among children will ensure some individuals will live for many more years. However, if we do not look at the quality of life experienced by those individuals, we may actually be increasing morbidity (sickness) and suffering among this group.

On the other hand, simple interventions with health-related behaviours such as diet and smoking among young people may only slightly increase the lifespan of the people concerned, but at the same time greatly improve the quality of life of those people over many years.

Interventions with the elderly may not increase length of life very significantly for anyone, but may still increase quality of life by a small but important amount for large numbers of people. As a result, when looking at what can be done to improve health it is important that we do not focus simply on adding years to life, but that we also look at adding health to life, adding quality to life, and adding life to years.

MODELS OF HEALTH AND ILLNESS

There is a variety of different ways to think about the human being in health and illness. One traditional way that has often dominated the thinking of health professionals has been called the **medical model** (Engel 1977). This model considers the individual as a case or a patient, primarily the host for some sort of disease or malfunctioning organ. The solution to the individual's disease is to return the biological function to its healthy state by chemical or surgical means, or both. It is a powerful model, because it has led to huge improvements in the development of diagnostic and treatment procedures, and because it is easy to understand.

However, if health professionals rely too heavily on the medical model, it can lead to serious problems in diagnosis and management. These may include:

• failure to consider the whole person—including feelings, needs and socioeconomic factors— as well as the physical machinery
• overlooking the well person that exists between illnesses
• failure to consider the past history of a particular episode of illness.

We live in an age when many of the major threats to health are linked to lifestyle and emotions, so adopting a disease-centred view of people can have grave consequences for their treatment.

The **biopsychosocial model** considers the individual as a whole person in a social setting; someone who may or may not be ill at any given moment (Engel 1977). This involves adding a variety of psychological and social factors to the biological ones. These include behaviours, **attitudes** and beliefs; dispositional factors such as personality; and strategies, sources of support and events in the life of the individual (Engel 1977). These factors form the major themes of this book, and are discussed in detail in later chapters.

Some advantages of taking a biopsychosocial approach are that it:

• recognises that the values of the patient and the health professional must be taken into account
• puts the focus of thinking about health and illness on the interactions between physical, psychological, social and other factors
• allows consideration to be given to the broader context of the individual and the illness, including familial, cultural and financial factors.

The biopsychosocial model is not without its problems (Schwartz 2007). By emphasising the role of lifestyle, this model may lead health professionals to overestimate the individual's control over—and therefore, their responsibility for—their own health. This may lead to less tolerance for those who do not behave in a healthy way and even victim-blaming. The emphasis on the ill person being an active participant in their own care may create an unacceptable burden on someone whose resources are already limited.

Medical model: a model that considers the individual as a case or patient, and primarily the host for some sort of disease or malfunctioning organ.

Biopsychosocial model: a model of health that considers the individual as a whole person, who may or may not be ill at any given moment.

Attitudes: the thoughts, feelings and readiness to act that an individual has about any object, person or event.

CROSS-REFERENCE
Victim-blaming is discussed in more detail in Chapter 16.

CROSS-REFERENCE
The impact of illness on the individual is discussed in Chapter 8.

PAUSE **&** REFLECT

How would the medical and biopsychosocial models differ in thinking about the causes and management of obesity?

CASE STUDY

GEOFF MITCHELL AND SLEEP APNOEA

The aim of this case is to get you to think about what happens when an individual may not be ill but is affected by changes to their well-being. Consider the impact on the individual, their family and their functioning in society.

Geoff is 58 years old and works for a logistics company as a section manager. He considers himself to be an easy-going person and is well liked by his colleagues at work. Geoff is currently experiencing difficulties in his marriage of 27 years to Sue. Their three children are young adults and living independently. Sue complains that Geoff works too much. Now that the children have left home, Sue would like to spend more leisure time with Geoff. She also complains about Geoff's snoring, which wakes her several times each night. Sue complains that she can't go back to sleep because of the noise. Geoff says that his snoring isn't that bad, and that most men his age snore. But Sue is worried that the snoring is not normal. At night in bed, she feels distressed watching Geoff stop breathing for long periods and then snort or snore while gasping for air. About two months ago, Sue told Geoff to sleep in the spare bedroom, and this move has added to the tension in their relationship.

Geoff has been steadily gaining weight for some years, but in the last year he gained 10 kilograms. He currently weighs 115 kilograms and constantly feels hungry. He tries to walk one or two mornings a week, but feels increasingly tired during the day. Recently while he was helping out at work on the fork lift, he dosed off and drove into one of the warehouse racks, which are 10 metres high. Although the rack was shaken, it remained standing and stock items didn't fall, but the forklift was damaged and it was a close call that no one was hurt. The accident frightened Geoff and he decided to see his doctor about his constant tiredness. He thought he might have a virus or perhaps be depressed or stressed.

The doctor took Geoff's history and then some measurements of his weight and blood pressure, as well as his neck, waist and hip circumference. Given Geoff's complaints of daytime tiredness, along with his age and weight, the doctor thought he may have sleep apnoea. The doctor explained that sleep apnoea occurs when the airway is obstructed (usually above the larynx) for around 10 seconds (an apnoeic event). Apnoeas end by the person rousing from their sleep (usually for 1–5 seconds) and opening the airway with a dramatic snore, snorting and gasping for air. People with severe obstructive sleep apnoea (known as OSA) may spend more of their time asleep in apnoea than they do breathing. Geoff now understood that his body wasn't getting quality rest and was being starved of oxygen at night. He was referred to a sleep clinic for further testing.

1 What might be some areas of concern for Geoff and Sue according to the biopsychosocial model of health?

2 What might be some areas of concern for Geoff according to the medical model of health?

3 Given that Geoff has been given a medical diagnosis, would he perceive himself to be ill?

4   To what extent does Geoff's lifestyle contribute to the development of obstructive sleep apnoea?

5   Do most people who complain of daytime tiredness have OSA?

6   What is the prevalence OSA in Australia?

7   Geoff had an accident at work due to his sleepiness. What may be some other consequences of OSA?

Points to consider

The person's own approach to wellness is recognised as one, if not the most, significant factor determining health status. Recognising that a symptom is not normal, or noticing the negative impact of lifestyle on well-being, often motivates a person to act or seek more information. It is estimated that around 40 per cent of middle-aged people have sleep-disordered breathing, although prevalence figures vary. This is due in large part because there is no standard agreement about the criteria for a diagnosis or how to grade its severity. Those at risk include men who are obese and hypertensive (high blood pressure), postmenopausal woman, people who complain of daytime sleepiness, and those who snore. It is estimated that 2–4 per cent of overweight adult males and 1–2 per cent of postmenopausal women require treatment for OSA. Conservative estimates of a prevalence of the general adult population rank OSA as twice as common as severe asthma and as common as type 1 diabetes.

OSA is associated with significant morbidity and mortality. Motor vehicle accidents, lost working days, increased use of health care services, poor quality of life, cognitive deficits and fatal accidents have been associated with OSA. The treatment of choice for OSA is continuous positive airway pressure (CPAP). A machine blows air at a constant pressure through the nose and into the lungs. The positive pressure keeps the airway open during sleep. Help with weight loss is important, and all patients with OSA are encouraged avoid alcohol several hours before sleep.

CHAPTER SUMMARY

- Being sick is a social definition.
- The illness definition suggests that symptoms are the key to defining who is sick. Problems with this definition include the frequency of symptoms in healthy individuals and the importance that a person attaches to the meaning of a particular symptom.
- The disease definition emphasises diagnosis by a health professional as the key element in deciding who is sick. Problems with this definition include differences in how diagnoses are made from time to time and from place to place, and the need for professionals to respond to the information provided by patients.
- Health cannot simply be defined as the absence of disease, but must take into account the social environment and sense of well-being of the individual.

- Health is measured using the amount of sickness (morbidity) and the number of deaths (mortality). The total number of cases (prevalence) and new cases (incidence) are important in judging the health of a community.
- The medical and biopsychosocial models provide different ways of thinking about the causes and management of illness, and how health can be maintained.

SELF TEST

1 Which of the following best fits the concept of a disease but not that of an illness?
   a Mary has a painful splinter under her fingernail.
   b Carlos has tested positive for hepatitis B, but does not know it yet.
   c Grigor's arthritis is so bad that the doctor recommends he have his hip joint replaced.
   d Meg has a serious reaction to a bee sting and needs to be hospitalised.

2 One definition discussed in the chapter is that the sick are those who have signs and symptoms. Which of the following is not a criticism of that definition?
   a It is not normally the symptom but its meaning that matters to the individual.
   b For a given individual and symptom, the meaning may vary with mood, knowledge and other factors.
   c The diagnosis and treatment of medical conditions varies from time to time and place to place.
   d Most symptoms are trivial and easily forgotten.

3 Which of the following statements is true?
   a Definitions of disease are fixed and based on biomedical science.
   b Illnesses are patterns of symptoms and signs identified by doctors.
   c Patients can recover from diseases but not from illnesses.
   d Definitions of illness and disease may differ between cultures.

4 A negative definition of health is based on:
   a pathological changes diagnosed by a health professional
   b the person's belief that something is not right
   c absence of disease or illness
   d a state of complete mental and physical well-being.

5 Morbidity:
   a can be used as a measure of the health of a community
   b refers to the number of deaths in a given year
   c can be used as a measure of illness in a person
   d indicates to a patient whether their treatment is the correct one.

FURTHER READING

Agus, D. (2012) *The End of Illness*. New York: Free Press.

National Sleep Foundation (2006) Prevalence of symptoms and risk of sleep apnoea in the US population: results from the National Sleep Foundation 'Sleep in America 2005' poll. *Chest*, 130(3): 780–6. www.sleepfoundation.org.

Sleep Alliance (UK) *The Sleep SOS Report. The impact of sleep on society*. Sleep Alliance (UK). www.orsa.org.uk.

World Health Organization (1986) *The Ottawa Charter for Health Promotion*. Copenhagen: WHO, Health Canada, CPHA.

USEFUL WEBSITES

Australian Sleep Association (ASA):
www.sleep.org.au

Evaluating breast lumps:
www.imaginis.com/cervical-cancer-symptoms-diagnosis/evaluating-a-breast-lump-1

Sleep education for nurses, therapists and doctors, plus the Epworth Sleepiness Scale:
www.faultywinks.com

CHILDHOOD AND ADOLESCENT DEVELOPMENT

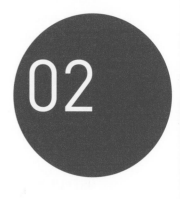

CHAPTER OBJECTIVES

By the end of your study of this chapter, you should be able to:

- understand the importance of an individual's development across the lifespan for their behaviour, cognitions and emotions, and how this impacts on health behaviour
- know how concepts from the study of development can influence understanding of health and illness, reactions to illness, and treatment by others
- describe and compare different life stages during childhood and adolescence within major developmental theories.

KEYWORDS

accommodation
assimilation
biopsychosocial model
chronological age
emotional intelligence
myelination
personal fable
physical age
prepubertal growth spurt
puberty
reaction range
reflex
rooting reflex
social age

INTRODUCTION

A developmental approach to the individual fits very well with the **biopsychosocial model** of health (as discussed in Chapter 1). Adopting a medical model often leads to overlooking important influences of age on health and illness. Our understanding of what is 'acceptable health' differs according to age. Old people often report that their symptoms of pain are overlooked by health professionals because old people always have aches and pains. Conversely, children may have their fears ignored because health professionals think that kids are always frightened about something. Even adults may be treated as if they were completely healthy up to the very moment when they became ill, simply because most adults are healthy most of the time. An understanding of some of the differences between different age groups can be very useful in understanding the experience of illness and health, and how to help people of various ages to cope with illness and its management.

Biopsychosocial model: a model of health that considers the individual as a whole person in a social setting, who may or may not be ill at any given moment.

DETERMINANTS OF HEALTH AND ILLNESS

During a person's lifetime, the basic genetic building blocks of the individual (their nature) are exposed to the influence of biological, psychological and social experiences (nurture). There has been a great deal of debate over whether nature or nurture is more important. The answer depends on what aspect of the person you are looking at, and which person.

The most important concept in understanding the interactions between nature and nurture is the concept of **reaction range**. As illustrated in Figure 2.1, the reaction range describes the total range of outcomes that are possible for a particular individual as a result of their genetic potential. Some things about us are relatively fixed by our genes, and there is little we can do about them under normal circumstances. Our height will be similar to that of our parents, as will our weight and body shape, our facial features and our eye colour. These physical things tend to be well accepted. Less recognised is the fact that psychological features such as temperament, intelligence and predisposition to develop certain psychiatric illnesses also have a substantial genetic component.

Reaction range: the total range of outcomes that are possible for a particular individual as a result of their genetic potential.

Figure 2.1   Reaction range

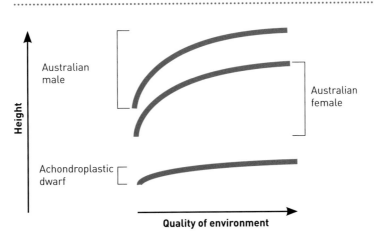

In a severely deficient environment, including starvation, war or abuse, development will tend to be at the bottom end of the reaction range. As can be seen from Figure 2.1, even a moderately supportive environment tends to produce close to optimal development. In spite of speculative theories about turning children into geniuses by playing music to them while they are in the womb, or teaching them maths by playing tapes to them before they can talk, the gains that can be achieved by a very enriched environment over a satisfactory one will always be marginal. The major factor that seems to distinguish geniuses is hard work and obsessive fascination with the area of their genius—factors of motivation that can be nurtured rather than capabilities.

PAUSE & REFLECT

A doctor takes a holiday in Samoa. While there, he is impressed by the fact that children are, typically, taller than children of the same age in Australia and concludes that reaction ranges are different in the two countries.

1   Why would this observation lead him to that conclusion?
2   Does this mean that Samoan children will be more advanced in all areas of development than Australian children?
3   Do you have any areas of development in which your reaction range was probably different from the average?

Science allows us to modify the biological environment to make up for problems in some areas of genetics. We can now prevent some types of dwarfism by using injections to boost deficiencies in human growth hormone. It is possible to prevent some types of intellectual disability by modifying diet, or supplying missing hormones or minerals. We can easily change superficial features by use of chemicals (for example, hair dye) or surgery (for example, breast implants). However, many of the genetic limits are beyond our capacity to control, and some are likely to remain so for many years. The concept of reaction range emphasises the interactions between determinants of development, and this is typical of the view of development taken by experts today. Few people would argue for a pure nature or pure nurture perspective these days; those who do are often restricting their arguments to a limited area of the total developmental picture.

MEASUREMENT OF AGE

A very common error in dealing with children is to assume that they are just like adults, only smaller. There are quite dramatic differences between children and adults, and between children at different ages and stages of development. Many of these differences are linked to biological changes, particularly in the nervous system. As these are very likely to occur in a certain sequence, and to take a roughly similar amount of time to happen with each child, age is a fairly good measure of child development. Even so, there are still individual differences in the speed of change; as a general rule, the older a person is the less useful their age is as a guide to their development. As a result, several different concepts of age have been developed.

The first of these is the familiar one: how many years have passed since the person was born. This is called **chronological age**. Some characteristics of individuals change more rapidly or slowly than others, and a lot of development depends more on these rates of change than it does

Chronological age:
the number of years that have passed sequentially since a person was born.

on the passage of time. The concept of **physical age** refers to the state of the person's biological machine, and we often hear terms like 'small for his age' or 'looking very old' that describe differences between chronological and physical age.

Physical age: the state of a person's biological machine.

Some events tend to happen at certain points in life, and these can have a powerful effect on our development, but they are not really linked to age. These events include finishing school and getting a job, getting married and having children, and retiring. A person may experience such events at widely varied points in life, from much earlier than the average to much later. **Social age** refers to the points at which a person has achieved these milestones. A teenager who marries early, gets a job and takes on family responsibilities may seem to be socially like an adult, while most of their friends still look like adolescents. For many teenage girls, their physical age, as measured by appearance, is quite different from their chronological age and their social age.

Social age: the points at which an individual has reached milestones in their life.

PAUSE & REFLECT

Think about your friends and classmates. Can you identify someone who stands out as having a physical age that is different from their chronological one? Consider the situation of a 15-year-old boy who needs to shave very day and plays tennis in adult competitions. Can you identify someone whose social age is different from their chronological age, perhaps someone who became a parent at 15, or someone at age 40, who still lives at home with their parents?

STAGES OF DEVELOPMENT

Some popular theories of development have looked at the human being in terms of the apparent stages that we all seem to move through as we age. These theories are popular to a large degree because they are simple and they agree with the ways in which Western developed countries think about typical activities of living. They have some major problems, however. They imply that the stages of development are fixed and that they occur to the same extent and the same time in everybody. These theories also suggest that the shift from one stage to another happens all at once, as if a switch was being turned on, whereas change is often gradual, partial, incomplete and even reversed. Theories of development also can be interpreted to suggest that what is typical is 'normal'; that is, the only healthy or desirable state for someone to be in at a given age. Despite this, such theories are so useful that to try to study development without them can be difficult and confusing. While much of the discussion that follows about age groups is based on a few stage theories, we suggest that you should always be critical about the way in which conclusions are drawn from them.

ALEX COLINI AND TYPE 1 DIABETES

CASE STUDY

The aim of this case is to look at differences in the individual's experience of the same illness at different ages.

Alex Colini is a 6-year-old boy. One night he complains of acute abdominal pain and vomiting. His mother takes him to a 24-hour general practice clinic. Alex's mother is aware that he is being bullied at school by some older boys. His mother believes that his recent onset of bed wetting is a result of this stress and does not mention this symptom to the GP.

The GP initially thinks that the pain may be appendicitis but first decides to rule out a urinary tract infection. A urine dipstick test is positive for glucose and ketones. She refers the child to a paediatrician for immediate management of his condition. Alex is subsequently diagnosed with type 1 (insulin dependent) diabetes, which means he needs to have daily insulin injections and to eat a special diet. Exercise can affect his diabetes. If his blood sugar levels drop too far, he may go into a coma and he could die.

1   What would you expect Alex to be able to do to manage his diabetes?
2   How much would you expect him to understand about the illness?

PAUSE & REFLECT

An international report predicted that the number of cases of type 1 diabetes among children in Europe under the age of 15 will increase 70 per cent from 94,000 cases in 2005 to 160,000 in 2020. The authors of the report say that genetic factors alone cannot explain the increasing numbers (Patterson et al. 2009). What might be some of the other contributing factors?

CHILDHOOD

PHYSICAL DEVELOPMENT

Prepubertal growth spurt: a period of dramatic physical growth that occurs just before puberty.

The most obvious component of development over the first fifteen or so years of life is physical. A baby usually doubles its birth weight in five months and triples it in the first year of life. Over that same year, height increases by 50 per cent. During middle childhood, the child adds about 5–7 centimetres and 2–3 kilograms per year, up until the **prepubertal growth spurt** when height and weight increase dramatically.

Myelination: the development of a fatty insulation on nerve cells that helps them work faster.

Some of the early physical changes are not just steady increases in size; they also create dramatic change in the behaviour of the baby. For example, **myelination**, the development of a fatty insulation on nerve cells that helps them work faster, is incomplete in the newborn. Although it does not actually reach its maximum levels until around age 15 or even later, most of the growth in myelination takes place in the first few years. One result of this is that the nervous system of the newborn is very primitive compared with that of the child it will become. The newborn is not capable of much control over movement, lacks the ability to perceive or interpret the world in any complex way, and is highly vulnerable to environmental change.

Reflex: an unlearned response to stimulus.

Rooting reflex: an automatic pattern of behaviour in newborn babies, where stimulation of the lips and tongue lead the newborn to turn towards the stimulus and initiate sucking activity.

The newborn comes equipped with some automatic behaviour patterns, called **reflexes**, that are essential to survival. These reflexes are unlearnt responses by the body to specific stimuli and do not require the intervention of higher brain functioning. Some, such as the breathing reflex, stay with us throughout our lives. Others are only useful in the earliest stages of life and, were we to retain them, could actually interfere with later ways of doing things. Such reflexes include the **rooting reflex**, where stimulation of the lips and tongue lead the newborn to turn towards the stimulus and initiate suckling activity, and the swimming reflex. During the first year these reflexes are gradually replaced by learnt behaviour that usually results in voluntary control becoming dominant over the reflexes. Without voluntary control over reflex actions, we could never be toilet trained or let go of objects we have grasped.

Development continues in all areas at the same time, of course, but it is possible to identify some central themes during the early years. In general, the first year of life involves growing larger and stronger, and bringing perception under control. The second year of life involves gaining mastery over the motor functions of the body—walking and jumping, holding and dropping, throwing and catching, and the early stages of toilet training. The third year of life brings language. Though steady physical development continues until just before puberty, the big areas of change become social and cognitive.

Physical development tends to follow three basic principles (Sigelman & Rider 2006). The first is that babies seem to be very top heavy: the head of a newborn represents about 25 per cent of its weight. Subsequent growth proceeds from the head towards the extremities, so it is said that physical development follows a *cephalocaudal* (from head to tail) pattern. It is also noticeable the arms and legs tend to lag behind the body in growth. So the second principle is that growth is *proximodistal* (from near to far) because the central parts approach their adult size and function faster than the extremities. The third principle, the *orthogenetic* principle, refers to the observation that the organism begins as undifferentiated, but gradually changes in the direction of more differentiation and better integration of function. Most of you would know that stem cells can develop into a large variety of other cells, leading to new treatments for everything from heart disease (where they are trained to become heart muscle) to Parkinson's disease (where they are trained to become brain cells). This is a demonstration of the orthogenetic principle.

SOCIAL DEVELOPMENT

The most visible part of social development in the early years of life is the attachment that quickly develops between baby and parents (or other regular caregivers). This attachment helps to ensure the survival of the baby by keeping it close to the caregiver and keeping the caregiver close and attentive to the baby (Ainsworth 1993). Attachment has two components for the baby: first, it attempts on several levels to maintain contact with or nearness to the caregiver; second, it expresses anxiety when separated from the caregiver. Even in the very early days of life, babies maintain eye contact with their caregivers, recognise their individual smells, and cling to them when distressed. As the first year progresses, babies begin to smile, to tug and to give certain cries or other sounds to attract attention. Some patterns of attachment are clearly desirable for the baby—dependability, consistency and responsive caregiving; but others are clearly bad—neglect, unreliability and abusive caregiving. Variations in the care received can produce variations in attachment, with some babies being securely attached (the caregiver serves as a secure basis for exploring the world) and some being insecurely attached (fearful of loss of contact and of strangers, and anxious about the world). Some may even become avoidantly attached, preferring to avoid the caregiver and rejecting contact with others.

Erikson (1950) proposed a stage theory of psychosocial development that may help to draw together some of the strands of early physical and social development (see Table 2.1). Erikson saw each stage as presenting the individual with a social task that needed to be achieved if development was to continue in an orderly fashion. For example, the task that the baby needs to achieve in the first year is to develop basic trust; if this is not accomplished, the child has a tendency to distrust the world and may find it a frightening and incomprehensible place. If trust is developed, at least to some extent, the child is able then to move on in the second year to attempt to gain mastery over bodily functions and the self, producing a feeling of autonomy. (Failure at this stage will produce self-doubt.) A sense of autonomy allows the child to move on to developing initiative, and so on, through the lifespan.

Table 2.1   Erikson's stages of childhood and adolescent development

Birth–1 year Trust versus mistrust	Babies learn either to trust that others will care for their basic needs (including nourishment, warmth and physical contact) or to lack confidence in the care of others.
1–3 years Autonomy versus shame and doubt	Children learn either to be self-sufficient in many activities (including toileting, feeding, walking, exploring and talking) or to doubt their own abilities.
3–6 years Initiative versus guilt	Children want to undertake many adult-like activities, sometimes overstepping the limits set by parents and feeling guilty.
7–11 years Industry versus inferiority	Children busily learn to be competent and productive in mastering new skills, or feel inferior and unable to do anything well.
Adolescence Identity versus role confusion	Adolescents try to figure out who they are. They establish sexual, political and career identities or are confused about what roles to play.

From Berger (1998).

COGNITIVE DEVELOPMENT

Anyone who has much to do with children quickly learns that they do not think like adults. People are often less aware that the thinking of children gradually changes over a number of years to become more and more like that of adults. Language, and the way in which children use language to organise the world they live in, is critical to these changes in thinking. Psychologist Jean Piaget (1985) provided a stage theory of cognitive development (see Table 2.2) that can help to understand changes in thinking that take place during childhood. By comparing the ages in Table 2.1 and Table 2.2, you should be able to see how these stages line up with Erikson's, which should help you to understand how development in one area parallels development in others.

Table 2.2   Piaget's stages of childhood and adolescent development

Birth–2 years Sensorimotor	The infant uses senses and motor abilities to understand the world. There is no conceptual or reflective thought: an object is known in terms of what the child can do with it.
2–6 years Preoperational	The child uses symbolic thinking, including language, to understand the world. Sometimes the child's thinking is egocentric, causing the child to understand the world only from one perspective: his or her own.
7–11 years Concrete operations	The child understands and applies logical operations, or principles, to help to interpret experiences objectively and rationally rather than intuitively.
12+ years Formal operations	The adolescent or adult is able to think about abstractions and hypothetical concepts, and is able to speculate in thought about the possible as well as about the real.

From Berger (1998).

Assimilation: the use of a reflex or an existing habit to allow the individual to deal with a new experience.

Accommodation: the modification of existing behaviours, or the development of entirely new behaviours, to allow an individual to deal with a new experience.

Basic to Piaget's theory of development is the idea that children organise the world by the use of two strategies. When they encounter an object or experience, they first try to deal with it by **assimilation**, which involves using a reflex or an existing habit to deal with it. Babies, for instance, usually put any new object that they encounter into their mouth. This is assimilation of new things into the existing behaviour. The other strategy, **accommodation**, generally comes into action if assimilation fails. The existing behaviours are modified to deal with the experience, or entirely new behaviours are developed to allow the baby to accommodate to the new experience. Piaget believed that play was accommodation, with the baby trying out a variety of new behaviours with objects or experiences and finding pleasure in this experimental activity.

OTHER VIEWPOINTS ON COGNITIVE DEVELOPMENT

Not everyone agrees with Piaget's conceptual approach. Sigelman and Rider (2006) identify five criticisms that have been made of his theory of cognitive development:

1   underestimating the capabilities of young minds to learn
2   failing to distinguish between what a child usually does (performance) and what it may be capable of doing (competence)
3   claiming that broad stages of development exist, when development may vary a great deal from one area of thinking to another
4   describing patterns of development rather than explaining what causes them to occur
5   paying too little attention to social influences on children's thinking, emphasising the child as an individual explorer of the world.

This last problem may be particularly important when we think about health and health behaviour. How much about health can a child learn by trial and error? Often, the effects are remote in time from the cause. A child who eats something that makes them immediately sick will learn to avoid that behaviour (this is known as conditioning). But the incubation time for infectious diseases may be days, so how is a child to learn that being coughed on by another child will make him/her sick next week? Many of the behaviours that lead to health (for example, eating fruit) or illness (for example, eating too much fried food) become habits before the child has the necessary control over the environment to do the exploring.

CROSS-REFERENCE
The concepts of conditioning, habit and learning are discussed in Chapter 6.

Alternative viewpoints have been offered for understanding the way children's cognitions develop. One is to focus on the observation that learning takes place within a social and cultural context. The child learns rules ('Coughs and sneezes spread diseases') and behaviours ('Cover your mouth when you cough') when engaged in interactions with adults and other children, sometimes through direct instruction and sometimes through observation.

Fifty years after his death in 1934, Russian psychologist Lev Vygotsky attracted the attention of Western psychologists and educators for his sociocultural theory of cognitive development (Daniels 2008). According to Vygotsky, there was a difference between what children were able to learn by independent exploration and what they could learn through guided participation in an activity with an adult or more capable peer. Development of cognitions was dependent on the interaction, and the guided participation that the child received during interactions. Speech between the child and the adult about the world, for example, eventually provides the basis for language within the child about the world, or the content of their thought processes (Daniels 2008). A child who grows up in an environment where there is instructive conversation is likely to have better developed verbal and thinking skills than a child who is neglected.

CROSS-REFERENCE
The role of language in memory is discussed in Chapter 6.

In looking at how children understand biological concepts such as life or the working of the body, Carey (1985) observed that there was a huge conceptual gain at about 9 or 10 years of age. In Carey's view, the crucial factor was not that the child had moved into a different type or stage of reasoning, but that there were changes in the amount and organisation of the knowledge that the child had to work with. This would particularly be the case if the child was highly motivated to learn.

CASE STUDY

ALEX (CONT.)

According to Erikson's theory, at the age of 6 Alex is probably in the stage of developing initiative. According to Piaget's theory, he is using preoperational thinking. He will almost certainly understand that his life is different from that of other children of his age, but he is unlikely to understand how great that difference is. Alex will need to have his injections administered by an adult—a parent or teacher—to ensure that the dosage is right for the conditions of food intake, that the time of day the injection is given is correct, that his exercise is completed or about to be done, and so on. If Alex finds out that an adult he knows has diabetes, he might think that is cool. His classmates are likely to be very interested in his injections, but not have the amount or organisation of information to be able to understand what is really different about him. Sometimes he is likely to find the attention fun, but he may become tired of the constraints on his activities. Alex might even wonder what he has done wrong to get diabetes (reasoning that bad consequences arise from bad actions).

1   How will Alex's understanding and behaviour change as he gets older?

2   How might Alex demonstrate his developing sense of initiative in managing his diabetes?

Many other processes, such as the development of moral reasoning and the development of concepts of health and healthy behaviour, follow cognitive development. In dealing with children in the clinical situation, physical, social and cognitive development must all be taken into account. There are many things that young children (as a general guideline, those under the age of about 7 years) simply cannot do, and others that they cannot understand in the same way that adults do. Trying to use adult modes of explanation simply will not work; behaviours that seem straightforward and sensible to you may seem threatening, stupid or unacceptable to a child. Even older children, who might understand the concepts, may not be able to understand the reasoning behind them. Although children can use adult concepts, they are likely to have a very limited understanding of the abstract meaning of those concepts, and may be very literal and concrete in their thinking.

PAUSE & REFLECT

Films and television shows occasionally present a story in which a baby or young child thinks, talks or acts like an adult. Such shows are always comedies. Why do you think people find children who do this funny? Think about it from the opposite perspective. If there was an adolescent whose mental development was normal, but whose physical development made them appear to be a child, would this be funny?

HEALTH IN CHILDHOOD

The health of children in developed countries is generally excellent. The number of deaths at birth and through the entire time period up to 14 years of age has been decreasing for a long time. The burden of disease and injury is also low. Australia comes roughly in the middle third of developed countries with regard to child health (AIHW 2011b). One significant reason for this middle ranking is the extremely poor health of one group: Indigenous Australians. The disadvantage in terms of survival is obvious from the beginning of life, with death rates for Aboriginal children aged 1–14 being three times that of the remainder of the population. The health disadvantage for Aboriginal children continues throughout childhood and adolescence, and contributes to the much higher rates of poor health for Indigenous adults.

CROSS-REFERENCE
Morbidity and mortality are defined in Chapter 1.

The main causes of illness in all children are infectious diseases (mostly those affecting the respiratory system) and injuries. Chronic illness is rare, and tends to be mild and relatively easily controlled problems such as asthma, hay fever and other allergies. Diabetes and cancer, although relatively rare, contribute substantially to the burden of illness because of the impact on the normal physical and social development in the early years.

ALEX (CONT.)   CASE STUDY

Now aged 10, Alex has been living with diabetes for four years. During this time he has received a lot of information about his condition, including not only what he needs to do to control the diabetes, but also how his internal body systems operate. By now he will probably have an idea of what his pancreas is, where it is located and how it is supposed to function. He may already have a clearer understanding of his condition than a typical adult would. The constraints placed on his behaviour are almost certainly an irritation to him.

Alex wants to do the same things as his friends, but it's not that easy. Exercise, for example, is an important part of his life. Exercise contributes to physical fitness, weight management and a sense of accomplishment, and offers opportunities for Alex to mix with his friends. However, for Alex, exercise involves much more than this, and can be a challenge. Alex is at risk for low blood sugar during and immediately after exercise, and again for seven to eleven hours afterwards. This is called the 'lag effect' of exercise and is due to different hormonal changes after exercise, as well as increased demand for glucose by the liver and muscles as they try to replenish the store of glucose that was depleted during the exercise. If there is insufficient glucose, Alex may feel sick, be unable to concentrate and even collapse.

As he moves towards adolescence, Alex may try harder to cover up his condition from other children, with the exception of those who are close enough to him to have learnt about diabetes from him or for his sake.

1   What would you expect Alex to be able to do to manage his diabetes as a 10-year-old boy?
2   As Alex moves toward adolescence, how would you expect his behaviour and thinking to change?

Let's look an example of how a child's behaviour and thinking change over time. The idea that a behaviour—such as taking off your clothes and letting another person touch your body—may be considered wrong in most settings but all right in others is difficult for most children to understand. This difficulty with abstract thinking can last until adolescence, and up to the stage of the development of formal operational thinking. Many others do not fully master abstract thinking at all, and so may never be able to make distinctions that may seem highly logical and obvious to most people.

ADOLESCENCE AND YOUNG ADULTHOOD
PHYSICAL DEVELOPMENT

Puberty:

a developmental stage defined by the appearance of secondary sexual characteristics, such as body hair and deepening of the voice in males, and menstruation and breast development in females.

The next major physical changes that do not involve a simple increase in size for the child are those associated with puberty. **Puberty** is defined by the appearance of secondary sexual characteristics, such as body hair and deepening of the voice in males, and menstruation and breast development in females. Physical puberty is seen as ending when the long bones of the body, especially arm and leg bones, have reached their maximum length and the individual reaches their full adult height. It is hard to use physical changes to define the developmental stage called adolescence, however, because some people (especially girls) may have reached adult size and development by 11 years of age, while others (especially boys) may not stop growing until they are aged 20 or more.

Despite the obvious physical changes associated with puberty that occur during adolescence, it is important to recognise that adolescence is a psychosocial stage as well, not just a physical one.

SOCIAL DEVELOPMENT

Adolescence represents the transitional time between childhood and adulthood. This means different things in different societies, during different historical periods, and to different individuals. The modern Western view that adolescence is always a time of stress and rebellion is an exaggeration. Although adolescence tends to be a time of developing personal values and independence, it does not always involve rejection of parental values or large-scale conflict with them. Nor does it necessarily involve wild experimentation with sex, drugs or music, or with politics, religion or personal hygiene for that matter. The fact that it frequently does is as much a matter of family and cultural context as anything else. Some cultures maintain that adolescence as we know it—a period of life change and upheaval during the teenage years—does not even exist. Some societies actively encourage sex play among prepubertal children; in others, children are never permitted to question their parents' values until after the parents have died.

In the developed world, many of the experiences of adolescents revolve around education; the move from secondary education to tertiary education—or to work—and are likely to result in major changes in the person's lifestyle.

COGNITIVE DEVELOPMENT

Looking back to the theories of Erikson and Piaget, some things about adolescence become clear. Their theories involve new ways of dealing with the environment. The development of formal operations can lead to conflicts between the individual's abstract understanding of what matters in life and other people's understandings.

Adolescence involves, for most people, a need to be independent and to move into different social relationships with other people. Friendships and emotional relationships become particularly important, and can cause problems with parents who have trouble accepting their reduced influence in the life of their child. As part of learning how to deal with the world, adolescents sometimes do things that look dangerous or stupid to outsiders, but most adolescents have as highly developed a sense of self-preservation as anyone else, and so keep their experimentation to a minimum. It is important to keep in mind that not everyone develops formal operational thinking, and many function on the basis of concrete operational thinking for all of life.

Throughout childhood and adolescence, cognitive development also involves the management of feelings and formation of relationships with others. **Emotional intelligence** (EI) has been defined as an individual's ability to perceive, use, understand and regulate emotion (Mayer & Salovey 1997). EI is a measure of a person's overall emotional capability and contributes to optimal emotional health and social functioning. Children who are able to accurately detect, understand and appropriately respond to their feelings and the emotions of others are likely to have more friends and adapt better in demanding social and emotional situations (Denham 2007). In addition, managing one's own emotions effectively enables the child to express emotions and act in ways that are socially appropriate. The extent to which a person develops emotional intelligence varies. A study with older adolescents found that those with low EI were more likely to experience loneliness, depression and aggression than their peers (Chapman & Hayslip 2005).

> **Emotional intelligence:** the ability to perceive, use, understand and regulate emotion.

PAUSE & REFLECT

Why do adolescents find it difficult to resist peer pressure, particularly with regard to unhealthy behaviours such as binge drinking? Do you think university students are different from others of the same age in terms of resisting peer pressure?

In the health care situation, adolescents (and young adults) are usually the easiest patients or clients to deal with. They tend to be less intimidated by technology, and are more confident of their physical strength, balance and knowledge than younger or older people. This is most likely to be true once the physical changes of puberty have been accepted by the individual and they have begun to develop an independent identity. Until these changes have occurred, young adolescents may be painfully shy and uncertain. They may be embarrassed by their bodies, the changes in their bodies, or their bodily functions. They may also be prone to seeing everything through their own **personal fable**—a belief that the world revolves around them—and tend to take everything very personally.

> **Personal fable:** the belief a person has that the world revolves around them.

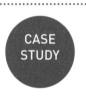

ALEX (CONT.)   CASE STUDY

Alex is now 16 years old. He has been living with the reality that he has diabetes for ten years. Over that time, there has been no significant change in his condition, although he has now had experience of what happens and how it feels if he fails to have his insulin on time.

Alex probably knows a great deal about diabetes by this stage (his adolescence). As part of developing his identity, he will have had to try to incorporate his diabetes into it. He has a formal operational understanding of it—its causes, mechanisms of action and what insulin actually does to his body when injected. He may bitterly resent the fact that he has diabetes and others do not, but he will understand that he is not to blame for having it.

He said, 'Sometimes I don't have time to test [blood glucose] between classes. It's embarrassing and I don't like to make an issue of it. I know I shouldn't, but I've got into a routine of not testing when I'm at school. I feel okay most of the time, but I test when my bloods are high [glucose level] and I feel sick, and can't concentrate.

He sometimes daydreams about a cure being found, which would mean that he would no longer be sick or different from his friends. Alex understands the problems that alcohol causes for people with diabetes. While he tries to avoid typical teenage drinking, he has also tried drinking in spite of the fact that it puts him at risk of a health crisis.

1 What would you expect Alex to be able to do to manage his diabetes?
2 How much would you expect him to understand about the illness?
3 How would Alex's understanding of diabetes change as he becomes an adult?

HEALTH IN ADOLESCENCE

In the years 15–24, the vast majority (70 per cent) of young people in Australia rate their health as good to excellent, and the statistics on the burden of disease and injury bear this out (AIHW 2010). The principal source of burden of disease in this age range is mental rather than physical health. Almost half of the estimated burden of disease comes from mental health problems such as anxiety and depression, with much smaller contributions from other problems such as drug abuse, schizophrenia, eating disorders and personality disorders (AIHW 2010). Mortality due to disease in this age group is rare, with injuries (accidental or self-inflicted) accounting for two-thirds of all deaths. Overall, this is the healthiest time of the life cycle, with the immune system working effectively and lifestyle disorders not yet playing a significant role in health and well-being.

CASE STUDY

LIONEL McDONALD AND INDIGENOUS YOUTH SUICIDE

The aim of this case is to look at possibly psychosocial stressors experienced during adolescence, particularly for those living in marginalised communities.

Lionel McDonald is a 16-year-old Indigenous boy living in the community of Cherbourg, Queensland. He is going through a tough time. His father was an alcoholic and unemployed. When intoxicated, he was physically and emotionally violent towards Lionel, his mother and his younger siblings. Lionel was glad when his father left five years ago, but he knew it was hard for his mother to raise the family of four children. His uncle's family lives in the community and gives practical and financial support to Lionel's family. Lionel recently went through a stressful time. He didn't know who he was or where he wanted to be. He said:

I was trying to finish high school. Although my teacher said that if I worked hard I was smart enough to go to technical college (TAFE), I didn't know what that would be like. I knew it would mean moving away from home into the city. I was in limbo. I didn't know how to build my life for myself. Doing HSC was hard. I constantly felt the pressure of studying and tests. I never let on that I was feeling so pressured. My mum tried to do the 'It doesn't matter how you go …' thing … but I knew she would be disappointed if I didn't do well. My brother and sisters tried to give me space and some peace and quiet, but it wasn't good enough, being younger, they just couldn't understand.

I tended to bottle my problems up. I held everything in, and never told anyone what was zipping through my mind. Soon enough, I became depressed and on edge all the time. At the start of the year, a very good friend of mine attempted suicide. He tried to hang himself, but his brother found him just in time and I walked in soon after. He was sent to a hospital in Brisbane. This was perhaps the lowest point in my life yet. I was very shocked and didn't have a clue how to handle how I was feeling. I didn't know how he was for a bit over a fortnight.

Then I started having nightmares about my friend. These weren't your regular nightmares; these were powerful sharp images of my friend hanging there that would haunt me most nights, and I would wake up in a sweat. The nightmares started to make me very tired during the day, and I couldn't study or concentrate on anything. The only way I could see to stop the nightmares was to not sleep. I was so screwed up. My concentration, study habits and health went downhill fast. I didn't want people to know about the nightmares because I felt there was something wrong with me. No one knew how much I was missing my friend, or how worried and scared I was that he was in hospital and sick. But finally I cracked ....

1   Lionel had a number of experiences during childhood that may have challenged his development. Can you identify possible psychosocial and cultural risk factors for Lionel? Relate these challenges to Piaget's stages of development.

2   As a teenager, Lionel reached the developmental stage of identity formation (according to Erikson 1986). What might be some of the challenges being faced by Lionel at this time? Can you explain why he is feeling suicidal?

Points to consider

Aboriginal and Torres Strait Islander people are exposed to four times more stressful life events than other Australians (AIHW 2009). As a young child Lionel was exposed to alcohol abuse, violence and socioeconomic disadvantage. According to Piaget, children aged 6–12 years need to gain a sense of competence. Children will consistently evaluate their social, physical and intellectual skills and compare them to their peers. If they view these positively then achievement will take place. However, negative views and self-criticism will produce feelings of inferiority. Although Lionel was coping at school, at home he was subjected to humiliation and rejection by his father. Fortunately, Lionel's uncle taught him how to discipline himself to sit down and focus on his schoolwork. Failure to develop these skills may lead to feelings of hopelessness.

Suicide is a complex problem. Social and cultural beliefs help shape identity. One factor underlying suicide concerns the failure to construct a healthy identity. According to Erikson (1968), in instances of delayed and prolonged adolescence, complaints of 'I give up' and 'I quit' are more than signs of mild depression—they are expressions of despair. Erikson acknowledged that suicide itself is an identity choice for some adolescents. For some Indigenous youth, their sense of identity is fragmented due a range of factors such as violence; drug or alcohol problems; sexual, physical or mental abuse; unemployment; and cultural dislocation (Silburn et al. 2010). For Indigenous youth around the age of 15 years, the rate of suicide is almost ten times higher than of non-Indigenous youth. More than 90 per cent of Indigenous suicides in the period up to 2007 occurred by hanging (De Leo et al. 2011).

CHAPTER SUMMARY

- Behaviour, cognitions and emotions differ at different stages in the lifespan.
- Determinants of development include the individual's genetic endowment and the biological, psychological and social experiences that they are exposed to.
- Reaction range describes the total range of outcomes that are possible for a particular individual as a result of their genetic potential.
- Age can be measured in terms of time from birth (chronological age), characteristics of the body (physical age) or events in the life of the individual (social age).
- During childhood, physical development—which includes growth in size and maturation of systems in the body—is rapid.
- Social development is influenced by the attachment of the child to caregivers.
- Erikson proposed that psychosocial development consisted of a series of tasks that must be resolved if the child is to develop in a healthy manner. Piaget looked at the gradual development of thinking.
- During adolescence, identity is formed and the individual begins to develop intimate relationships with others.

SELF TEST

1 The principal reason why newborn babies are regarded as 'relatively primitive organisms' compared with older children and adults is:
   a They are not able to talk.
   b Myelination of nerve fibres is incomplete.
   c Their brains are only one-tenth of adult size.
   d They have no self-control.

2 According to Erikson's theory of psychosocial stages, a child aged about 7 years will either be learning to be confident and productive and mastering new skills, or:
   a learning to be self-sufficient in many activities
   b becoming confused about their identity and what roles to play
   c coming to feel inferior and unable to do anything well
   d becoming isolated from others through fear of rejection.

3 Thani is a 3-year-old who has secure attachment to her mother and father. She will make attempts at several levels to stay close to them, and:
   a get angry if they don't pay attention to her
   b have trouble adapting to school when she is aged 5
   c show anxiety if she is separated from them
   d be a difficult child for her parents to deal with.

4 A major criticism of theories that describe separate stages of development, such as Piaget's theory, is that:
   a Development is characterised by major changes followed by periods of stability.
   b They do not consider changes in thinking, only describing physical change.
   c They do not seem to agree with most people's ideas about intelligence.
   d Not everyone goes through the same stages of development in the same order.

5 You see a patient who not only understands the procedures that you are performing, but also why they are being done. You have a discussion about the ethics of the procedures with them. This patient is demonstrating:
   a formal operations
   b concrete operations
   c pre-operational thought
   d superstitious thought.

FURTHER READING

AIHW (2011). *Headline indicators for children's health, development and wellbeing*, 2011. Cat. No. PHE 144. Canberra: Australian Institute of Health & Welfare.

Daniels, H. (2008) *Vygotsky and Research*. London: Routledge.

Lantieri, L. (2008) *Building emotional intelligence: techniques to cultivate inner strength in children*. Boston: Sounds True.

Purdie, N., Dudgeon, P. & Walker, R. (eds). *Working together: Aboriginal and Torres Strait Islander Mental Health & Wellbeing Principles and Practice*. Canberra: Australian Government Department of Health & Ageing.

USEFUL WEBSITES

Centre for Adolescent Health:
www.rch.org.au/cah/research.cfm?doc_id=11036

Diabetes animation (YouTube):
www.youtube.com/watch?v=NnIWDxuZKUo&feature=related

Juvenile Diabetes Research Foundation:
www.jdrf.org.au/living-with-type-1-diabetes

LIFE: Living Is For Everyone:
www.livingisforeveryone.com.au/Indigenous.html

ADULT DEVELOPMENT
AND AGEING

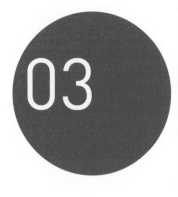

CHAPTER OBJECTIVES

By the end of your study of this chapter, you should be able to:

- understand the importance of the individual's position in the lifespan for their behaviour, cognitions and emotions, and how this impacts on health behaviour
- know how concepts from the study of development can influence understanding of health and illness, reactions to illness, and treatment by others
- describe and compare different life stages during adulthood within major developmental theories
- understand end-of-life issues, including the process of grieving and its impact on the well-being of the individual.

KEYWORDS

advanced healthcare directive (living will)
Alzheimer's dementia
anticipatory grieving
crystallised intelligence
disengagement theory
fluid intelligence
morbid grief
multi-infarct dementia (MID)
practical intelligence

ADULTHOOD

The point at which an adolescent becomes an adult is not really very clear. Some societies or cultures use markers such as high school or university graduation, confirmation, bar mitzvah, marriage or leaving the parental home to define the beginning of adulthood. These events may take place at almost any time between the onset of puberty and the early twenties. In reality, the change is most likely to be gradual and piecemeal. The usual experience reported by most people is that they were not aware of becoming an adult, but simply started thinking of themselves as one somewhere along the line. Usually, this will vary from one part of the person's life to another; that is, they may regard themselves as an adult with regard to independence but not with regard to family responsibility or work.

Erikson's stage theory of psychosocial development continues throughout the lifespan. As in childhood and adolescence, adulthood and old age present the person with social tasks that needed to be achieved if development is to continue in an orderly fashion. The tasks at these times of life involve forming intimate relationships, contributing to the next generation and being able to look back on life with a sense of meaningful satisfaction.

CROSS-REFERENCE
Erikson's stage theory of psychosocial development is discussed in Chapter 2.

Table 3.1   Erikson's stages of adult development

Intimacy versus isolation	Young adults seek companionship and love with another person, or become isolated from others by fearing rejection or disappointment.
Generativity versus stagnation	Middle-aged adults contribute to the next generation by performing meaningful work, creative activities and/or raising a family, or become stagnant and inactive.
Integrity versus despair	Older adults try to make sense out of their lives, either seeing life as a meaningful whole or despairing about goals they never reached and questions they never answered.

From Berger (1998).

The start of adulthood can be delayed by some experiences, and university education is one of the most common in developed countries. It results in a longer period of dependence on others for training and support, and often produces a delayed sense of development. People going on to tertiary education usually postpone other adult experiences, such as marriage and full-time work, until they have at least developed a sense of a stable future path. Those who do move into more adult experiences while still in full-time education often report feeling out of things, or not being like all the other students.

PAUSE 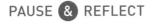 REFLECT

Has being a university student stopped you from being an adult? What are some of the areas of your own life where you think you are an adult? Are there other aspects of your life where you still feel like a child?

ALEX COLINI AND TYPE 1 DIABETES

CASE STUDY

This is the continuation of Alex's case, outlined in Chapter 2. The aim of this case is to continue to look at the differences in a person's experience of the same illness at different ages.

Alex is now 36 years old. He is married and has two small children, aged 4 and 6 years, and works in a men's clothing store as a sales clerk. After high school he continued to play football with his local club and attended training twice a week. Once he married he didn't have time for sport and is finding it harder to maintain his weight. There are always family occasions to attend and he has always loved his mother's cooking, so he tends to over-indulge at these times as well as drink a bit too much. There is still no significant change in his condition, but the constant daily routine of monitoring his blood glucose levels and all the other associated care (such as regular doctor's appointments, podiatrist and optometrist appointments, and making sure he always has enough insulin on hand) gets him down sometimes.

Alex's wife, Lyn, is supportive and has tried to learn as much as she can about type 1 diabetes. Lyn is aware that Alex is at greater risk for other life-threatening conditions such as renal and cardiac diseases. She tries to prepare healthy meals and encourage Alex to watch his diet. Lyn also believes that the children may have a predisposition to diabetes and so watches their health as well.

1 What would you expect Alex to be doing at this stage to manage his diabetes?
2 How can a supportive family environment help Alex to cope with the condition now and in the future?

PHYSICAL DEVELOPMENT

Few of the physical changes of adulthood are obvious, and hardly any of them are apparent in early adulthood. Exceptions, such as premature baldness or grey hair, are generally considered to be premature. However, this overlooks the fact that baldness and greying have a large genetic component: although they may occur earlier for some than for others, there is nothing abnormal or premature about them at all.

Most of the overt physical changes that occur are gradual, such as loss of skin elasticity leading to wrinkles, the tendency to increase body weight and the loss of pigment in the hair. Most of the physical changes are internal, and not even the individual is aware of their occurrence. They include processes that may eventually result in significant health problems, such as atherosclerosis (the build-up of fatty deposits in the arteries) and a progressive decline in bone density (osteoporosis). Most adults are not aware of these changes until they begin to significantly affect their ability to do things. The most common complaint that people have about getting older is that they do not like looking older.

SOCIAL DEVELOPMENT

The key themes of adulthood tend to have to do with responsibility: the adult gradually becomes enmeshed in a network of obligations to other people that can be summarised under the general headings of family, work and society.

FAMILY

The majority of adults will marry (that is, form a legal relationship between a man and a woman) at some time in their lives. Although the proportion of the population who marry has been dropping for about four decades, there has been a trend towards marriage since 2001 (ABS 2011). At its peak in the 1970s, 86 per cent of women and 79 per cent of men married at least once during their lives (De Vaus, Qu & Weston 2003). In 2010, there were 121,176 marriages, representing an increase of 1058 (0.9%) marriages registered in Australia in 2009. This is the highest number of marriages registered in a single year and continues the relatively steady increase in the number of marriages since 2001. Although the number of marriages is now the highest on record, the population has also increased over time. The rate of marriage has actually decreased to 5.4 marriages per 1000 in 2010, compared with 6.9 marriages per 1000 in 1990 (ABS 2011). Even people whose predominant sexual orientation is homosexual have a fairly high probability of heterosexual marriage, largely because of parental pressure, societal expectations or a desire to have children.

Around one in every three first marriages in developed countries such as the USA, New Zealand and Australia will end in divorce, and the proportion is higher for subsequent marriages. However, the number of divorces granted in Australia has been decreasing each year since reaching a peak in 2001. As the number of divorces granted decreases and the population increases in Australia, the crude divorce rate has declined steadily since 2001 to around 2.3 divorces per 1000 (ABS 2011). Furthermore, a number of trends are decreasing the proportion of marriages that look like the traditional image of marriage. These include:

- fewer people getting married
- later marriages
- increasing divorce rates
- increasing numbers of childless marriages
- more remarriages.

Nevertheless, the most common family type is still two adults living with two children, closely followed by two adults living alone (ABS 2010b). Couple-only families are projected to increase the most rapidly of all types of families over the next 25 years. If recent trends continue, couple-only families will overtake the number of couple families with children in either 2013 or 2014. This is mainly related to the ageing of the population, with baby boomers becoming 'empty nesters' (ABS 2010b).

WORK

During adulthood, work serves a variety of functions. It occupies most of one's waking hours, provides the income that determines lifestyle, and provides identity. All of these functions are important, but for men in our society the last is probably the most important. The same tends also to be true for women who work through their childbearing years, and particularly for professional women.

Women living more traditional lives—that is, spending a significant part of their childbearing years working in the home—tend to take their identity from their family and from their husband's occupation. They also tend to see their own work outside the home as a source of additional income and social contact, rather than a source of personal identity. However, as more and more women are obtaining higher degrees and moving into professions, a woman's identity is increasingly being based on herself as an individual and less on her role within a marriage. In the developed world, the choice of a career is influenced to a great extent by education rather than family factors, and social class is more likely to be earned than inherited.

SOCIETY

There are various responsibilities people have to their society. Some are legal requirements. Australian adults must, for example, register with the electoral office and are required by law to vote. Many other responsibilities come with chosen life activities. If you wish to drive a car, you must have a licence, car registration and insurance. If you have children, they must be educated, housed, inoculated and supported. If you buy a property, you must pay rates. If you work for a living, you must pay taxes. The more involved the individual becomes with other people, the more they become involved with these kinds of social obligations. As with physical ageing, the development of social involvement is often so gradual that a person only realises how involved they were when they look back on their lives, or if they are no longer able to carry out their obligations.

COGNITIVE DEVELOPMENT

CROSS-REFERENCE
The role of cognition in health is explored in detail in Chapter 7.

Thinking also tends to show mostly slow and gradual change during adulthood. Rapid change in cognitive functioning is likely to be the result of physical change, and health professionals now use cognitive change as an important sign of the presence of disease. Many illnesses, such as heart disease, cancer, respiratory disease and AIDS, produce changes in behaviour or in cognition. In the absence of illness, the changes that take place during adulthood are minor.

CASE STUDY

ALEX (CONT.)

As an adult, Alex will probably have the management of his diabetes down to a fine art. It will not require much thinking for him to know what he needs to do, when he needs to seek help or how to recognise and prevent problems before they occur. He is likely to be very skilled at calculating doses and injecting himself. His eating habits will be well established, and most of the time he won't even have to think about being a person with diabetes—it will be fully incorporated into his sense of who he is. He is likely to have accepted the limitations placed on his activities and no longer be resentful of them. His wife will also understand his condition, and may actually worry about it more than Alex does.

Lyn worries that Alex sometimes neglects his scheduled appointments. Recently, his vision has been blurred at times and yet he refused to make an appointment to see the optometrist. Lyn thinks that Alex does not want to face the long-term realities of his condition and they had an argument about it. Alex's mother told Lyn that he went through a bout of depression when he left school and started work. Lyn is worried that Alex's irritable mood may be masking more serious worries.

1   What factors may be contributing to Alex's sense of depression?
2   In what way would this picture be different if Alex had only recently been diagnosed with diabetes?

Fluid intelligence:
using flexible reasoning to draw inferences, solve problems and understand the relationships between concepts.

One gradual change in cognitive functioning throughout the lifespan relates to intelligence. Researchers noted changes away from fluid intelligence towards more crystallised intelligence (Cattell 1971). **Fluid intelligence** refers to the use of flexible reasoning to draw inferences, solve problems and understand the relationships between concepts. Theorists have suggested that mathematical geniuses tend to make their major contributions early in adulthood because of their fluid intelligence. By contrast, **crystallised intelligence** refers to the accumulation of knowledge that comes with experience and education. Because the world of ideas is more complex than the world of mathematics, more experience appears to be required to make discoveries in philosophy or psychology, and geniuses in these areas tend to make their major contributions much later in life.

Another kind of intelligence also tends to become more important during the adult years, and that is **practical intelligence** (Sternberg et al. 1995). This is the kind of common-sense thinking that allows a person to successfully negotiate their daily activities. It has been noted, for example, that some people who are unable to read are still able to lead successful lives because they have organised themselves so that reading is not necessary. Individuals with an intellectual disability can develop the practical skills necessary to cope with their lives in a highly successful fashion, in spite of gaps in both fluid and crystallised intelligence.

Crystallised intelligence: the accumulation of knowledge that comes with experience and education.

Practical intelligence: common-sense thinking that enables a person to successfully negotiate their daily activities.

HEALTH IN ADULTHOOD

It is in middle adulthood that the effects of lifestyle first begin to have a significant impact on physical health. Diet, smoking, exercise (or lack of it), drinking, risk-taking, stress and repetitive activity begin to cause permanent changes in the body and its functions. The onset of problems varies greatly, and most people only become ill during their later years. Change in behaviours during the young adult period is often able to postpone the onset of these problems, and even prevent their occurrence. The lack of symptoms can make it difficult to persuade young adults that these changes are necessary. In addition, early adulthood is a busy time for the establishment of family, work and societal connections, so people often place a low priority on healthy habits due to a lack of time or energy. It is common for this low priority to continue as it becomes habitual.

AGEING

There are four main reasons why some people live to be very old while others do not: good genes, good overall health throughout life, good psychological resilience and a lot of good luck. This statement matches the views of scientists about the determinants of development overall.

MARCUS COLINI AND TYPE 2 DIABETES

CASE STUDY

The aim of this case is to look at a one person's experience of illness during old age.

Alex's father, Marcus, is 68 years old. Although he was athletic as a young man, he gained a lot of weight in his late forties and has been obese (with a body mass index of 32) for the last twenty years. But he remains active and has lots of interests as well as a wide circle of friends. Two months ago, Marcus started to notice some changes. He was losing weight without trying—which he was really pleased about—but he was urinating often, was always tired, had problems thinking clearly and his vision was blurry. He enjoys doing woodwork in his shed at home, but lately felt clumsy and his hands tingled. He actually cut his hand on one of his tools, and the wound would not heal. His wife Maria, urged him to see a doctor. A blood test revealed a glycated haemoglobin level of 8.1 per cent, indicating type 2 (non-insulin dependent) diabetes.

1   What would you expect Marcus to be able to do to manage his diabetes?
2   How much would you expect him to understand about the illness?

The links between physical, social and cognitive development become more significant as people age. In general, as long as physical health holds up, there is little reason for an individual's life to change as they age. It is now recognised that a person's intelligence does not decrease with age but as a result of illness. The more similar the ageing individual's lifestyle is to that of their middle years, the more active and contented they will be, regardless of their chronological age. There is no separate section about 'Health and Ageing' in this text because it is actually difficult to separate the concepts of ageing and disease.

This recognition that ageing is linked directly to the breakdown of the biological machinery has led to a number of theories of ageing, including the following: wear and tear theory, free radical theory, errors in copying theory and obsolescence theories.

WEAR AND TEAR THEORY

In one model of the wear and tear theory, the human body wears out merely by being lived in and exposed to environmental stressors. The body is seen as a biological machine that wears out with time and use. Even young people experience health problems of wear and tear. When professional athletes retire, usually in their thirties, the commonly cited reason is that the body just can't take the stresses of training and competition any more. Even if there are no specific sites of damage, such as scar tissue from repeated injury, it takes longer to recover from each contest. Popular treatments for the effects of ageing through wear and tear include cosmetics that are advertised to replace or restore tissue, such as collagen. Another model is based on the idea that the body wears out as a result of the effects of the gradual accumulation of waste products. These include substances such as heavy metals and chemical compounds that the body can't dispose of through normal processes.

FREE RADICAL THEORY

This theory posits that atoms with unpaired electrons react violently with molecules in body cells, tearing them apart and making the cells work less efficiently. This theory has received a lot of media attention, with the focus on the idea that free radicals cause their negative effects through oxidation. Many naturally occurring products are advertised as containing antioxidants, including tea, red wine, dark chocolate, fruit and vegetables, the implication being that these products will prevent disease or slow ageing. Additional treatments, such as dietary supplements, are being manufactured to contain antioxidants, specifically with the intention of slowing or reversing the effects of ageing.

ERRORS IN COPYING THEORY

One of the basic processes of life is that the cells that make up the body regularly copy themselves to replace the loss of the original cells. This theory suggests that sometimes these copies are not exact: they have errors that can be anything from totally unimportant to something so dramatic that the copy cannot survive. Many of the errors are small enough to allow the copy to survive, even if it is flawed in some way. Early in life, most copies are quite accurate. Errors in copying cells gradually increase as a person ages, leading to further errors in subsequent copies, and poorer repair by other cells. Part of the effect of errors in copying is purely mathematical; that is, the longer a person lives, the more likely it is that a copy of a cell will be faulty. Another element of the errors in copying theory is related to the wear and tear theory: it suggests that exposure to environmental influences will increase the likelihood of faulty copies (known as somatic mutation theory). The range of environmental influences is large, from sunlight and industrial pollution to ordinary food or cooking processes, and includes the heavy metals and chemicals already mentioned among accumulated wastes. Cancers represent a special case of errors in copying, where the faulty cells reproduce themselves vigorously at the expense of accurately reproducing cells.

OBSOLESCENCE THEORIES

Several theories claim that the body has an internal program, determined by genes or cells, that sets a limit to how long it can work efficiently. The simplest version of this theory is that the body has an internal clock built into the nervous, endocrine or immune (known as auto-immune theory) system that simply runs down. A recent variation of this theory, related also to errors in copying, concerns telomeres. Telomeres are repetitive segments on the ends of strands of DNA that serve to protect the important information coded in the strand from being lost. The theory states that each time the cell replicates itself, some of the telomere material is lost. Eventually, enough is lost that the core information is affected. There is growing evidence that telomere length is associated with human ageing (Aviv 2004). Other research has found that stress accelerates the loss of teleomere length (Espel et al. 2004).

Because the supposed changes of ageing are really changes resulting from illness, there are no essential differences between the functioning of elderly people and other adults. However, social changes brought about by particular societies, such as compulsory retirement and the payment of a pension to retired people, have a considerable effect. Some theorists have suggested that elderly people and society disengage from one another, and that this is appropriate (Cumming & Henry 1961). A more recent form of this **disengagement theory** suggests that ageing individuals tend to modify the amount of interaction they have with the society around them to suit their capabilities. This suggests that those who are physically fit, mentally alert and financially secure tend to maintain a high level of social engagement into their eighties or even later. Some individuals—Pablo Picasso, George Burns and Mother Theresa are examples—remained highly active and effective past the limits of normal life expectancy.

As age increases, the probability that disease will cause significant loss of function increases, and most people over 75 years of age experience major disabilities in the areas of sight, hearing and mobility, which tend to result from the continuation of the physical changes that began in young adulthood—atherosclerosis, loss of bone density and the development of cancers. Among the very old, fragility is a significant problem.

By far the most common mental health disorder among the aged is depression—exactly as for middle age—but various kinds of dementia are increasingly being observed. Dementia used to be called senility. The mistaken assumption was made that senility was a general characteristic of ageing, but it is now recognised that dementia results from illnesses of

Disengagement theory: the idea that aging individuals tend to modify the amount of interaction they have with the society around them to suit their capabilities.

CROSS-REFERENCE
The effects of dementia on memory are discussed in Chapter 6.

Alzheimer's dementia:
a significant loss of
thinking, memory
or problem-solving
ability resulting from
abnormalities of cells in
the cerebral cortex.

Multi-infarct dementia:
a significant loss of
thinking, memory
or problem-solving
ability resulting from
small blockages of the
blood supply that kill
off localised groups of
cortical cells.

various kinds, and can occur well before old age. Dementia is not an inevitable part of ageing, but is a growing problem (Brodaty & Cumming 2010). In line with the ageing population, the prevalence of dementia in Australia is expected to increase fourfold from 245,000 in 2009 to around 1.13 million by 2050 (Access Economics 2009). Dementia is the third leading cause of death in Australia (ABS 2010a) and is prevalent across ethnic groups. Furthermore, one small study found that dementia prevalence among Aboriginal Australians in a remote area of Western Australia was substantially higher (12.4 per cent) than that found in non-Aboriginal Australians (2.4 per cent) (Smith et al. 2008).

The two most common causes of dementia in ageing are **Alzheimer's dementia** (about 70 per cent of all dementias) and **multi-infarct dementia** (MID; 15 per cent). Alzheimer's results from abnormalities of cells in the cerebral cortex. MID results from small blockages of the blood supply that kill off localised groups of cortical cells. In both cases, the first symptoms usually noted are problems with short-term memory, such as an inability to remember names or where things have been put. This is followed by more general memory problems (such as loss of recent events) and increasing confusion. Personality may seem to change, as sufferers become irritable about their losses and anxious about their ability to cope. Finally, the losses become serious, with sufferers forgetting things such as eating and dressing properly, and even who they are or where they live.

In health care settings, elderly patients may be slow to understand or respond to instructions not because of loss of mental abilities but because they are assessing the instructions against their capabilities. The frail aged, and those who suffer from dementia, may be fearful in health care settings. These fears may result from uncertainty about the equipment, about the stresses that will be placed on them, or about the loss of personal dignity involved in the procedure. It is important that health professionals keep quality of care and not speed of treatment in mind when working with all patients, but this is particularly true with the elderly.

MARCUS (CONT.)

CASE STUDY

The diagnosis of Type 2 diabetes was a shock for Marcus. Even though his son, Alex, developed diabetes as a young child, Marcus thought it would not happen to him. Maria, on the other hand, thought that it was inevitable. Maria knew the risks as his mother and an uncle had diabetes. She said, 'I was expecting it because Marcus had gained a lot of weight, and so many people in his family had it. He loves my cooking and we have such a good time with our friends and family. I suppose it's all my fault that this has happened to him.'

Maria was also worried because she had watched Marcus's family members develop severe complications, including gangrene, foot problems and heart disease. She said, 'I knew diabetes was serious. His uncle died at age 57 after having a leg amputated and a heart attack. So when Alex was diagnosed as a young boy, I was scared and I am still scared.'

Not only was life now different for Marcus and Maria, but she feared that diabetes would limit the length and quality of remaining life they would share. There were already incidents of arguing and nagging about changes to their daily lives and ongoing management of the condition. Maria was concerned that Marcus was not managing the disease as well as he should be. Maria said, 'Marcus saw me care for Alex as a young boy and expects me to do the same for him. He says, "You have to do this for me, and you have to do this for me," and I say, "No! You can read and you have two hands, and if you don't like what I am doing, then you can go in the kitchen and do it."

1 Why is Marcus experiencing difficulty in managing his condition?
2 How could Maria and Alex support Marcus at this time?
3 What are some possible psychosocial consequences that Marcus may need to face in managing his condition successfully?

Points to consider

Marcus may have more trouble dealing with his diabetes than Alex does with his. Mostly, this will be due to the fact that it represents change for him. His lifestyle has led to his weight problem, which has in turn led to his condition. The management that is needed also requires changing long-established patterns of behaviour. Marcus may have to give up preferred foods and quit or greatly reduce his alcohol intake. He may have to increase exercise and modify a number of other behaviours. And, he will have to face the knowledge that increased risk of other serious health problems, from heart disease to blindness, accompanies his condition.

DEATH AND GRIEVING

In most people, the final stages of life involve simple physical deterioration without major mental suffering. People who have worked with the elderly generally find that they are not afraid of dying. Instead, they see death as familiar. Patients who are in pain, or who are lonely after losing a life partner, often see death as a welcome release from their situation.

The elderly in health care settings are often more concerned with the quality of their remaining life than the quantity. They may refuse treatments that offer them a short extension of life on the grounds that the loss of dignity, awareness or personal control is not worth the small gain in time. Treatment of dying patients has been regularly criticised, even within the health professions. Several commonly mentioned problems are that:

1 Patients are often not told that they are dying, and often find out by accident from people around them, or have to wait until family members tell them.
2 Patients often die in too much pain.
3 Patients often have little or no contact with their doctors once it is decided that medicine cannot offer a lengthening of survival time, so that care of the dying is not optimally managed.

In order to exert more control over the process of dying, many people now sign an **advanced health care directive (living will)**. Although there are a number of slightly different versions, the common elements of a living will are statements that the patient wishes to receive adequate pain relief to avoid suffering, even if that hastens death, and that the patient wishes to be allowed to die and to not be kept alive by artificial means or heroic measures. Many doctors and hospitals abide by living wills, but some choose to disregard them.

Advanced health care directive (living will): a statement—not legally binding on health professionals—signed by a patient about the treatment they would like to receive when they are dying.

KÜBLER-ROSS'S FIVE STAGES OF DYING

It has long been recognised that dying is a process rather than a point in time. One of the first authors to offer a theory of dying was psychiatrist Elisabeth Kübler-Ross (1969). After lengthy experience working with dying patients, Kübler-Ross proposed a five-stage process:

1 Denial—In this stage, the person's reaction is described as 'Not me!' The person simply does not take in the information. They may continue with life activities as if they had been told nothing. This can be frustrating for health professionals, and often for families, but has a protective effect for the individual. Even though their denial may appear irrational, it can provide them with time to take actions that will enable them a better adjustment later.

2 Anger—In this stage, the person has accepted the truth of their situation but experiences anger over the unfairness of it. The typical reaction is 'Why me?' Their anger may have any of a number of targets: themselves, others who may have exposed them to risk, parents for passing on a genetic vulnerability, health professionals or their god.

3 Bargaining—Having now recognised that the end cannot be changed, the person begins to try to bargain about the details. The typical reaction is 'Not now'. They may try to bargain a reprieve from the doctor if they promise to change their behaviour. They may make promises to their god in exchange for a little more time or a miracle.

4 Depression—In this stage the person recognises the reality of the end of their life and experiences the sadness of it. They may withdraw into a true clinical depression, but are more likely to experience an appropriate and transient sadness. It is likely that they will begin to make plans for their death, to change their life activities and to disengage from many people and events.

5 Acceptance—By this, Kübler-Ross meant far more than simply admitting that death is inevitable. She describes a complex pattern of withdrawal from life. The dying person begins to say goodbye to things and people, and progressively cuts off contact with others until they reach a point where they prefer to be with only a few close people, usually family. They also withdraw from activity, spending more and more time in sleep. They may experience a loss of sensation, with even severe pain fading away. At the very last stages, they often want to be alone with a single spouse or child, and they may prefer to avoid talking in favour of simply holding hands or being in the same room. In Kübler-Ross's view, this was a positive stage in that it allowed the individual to die in comfort and with dignity.

GRIEVING

Some have been critical of Kübler-Ross's theory. It has been criticised for suggesting that all the stages occur for every person, that they occur in a fixed order, that once past a stage the individual does not return to it, and for a number of other perceived flaws (Kastenbaum 1992).

Figure 3.1 depicts a more general grieving model, which is adapted from LoCicero (1991). The advantages of this model are that it can be used to describe the experience of those who survive a life-threatening illness as well as those who die, and that it also can describe the experience of those close to a dying person. It also deals with the criticism that theories of dying are too negative, and that by encouraging acceptance they may be reducing survival.

Figure 3.1   The grieving cycle

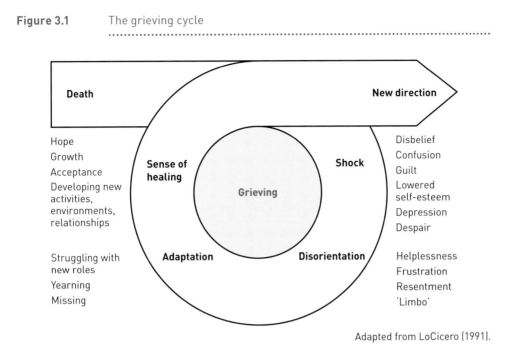

Adapted from LoCicero (1991).

Grieving actually takes place at any time a person experiences a significant loss. This could include loss of another through death, divorce or moving away; loss of function through amputation, stroke or ageing; loss of activities due to disability or other barriers; and loss of self through any of the above, plus dementia or impending death. Because those who are grieving seem so miserable, it is natural that we have an urge to prevent or stop the process. However, the work of grieving needs to be done before recovery can be complete.

It is possible for grieving to take place before the loss has occurred. This **anticipatory grieving** (Brown & Stoudemire 1983) is common in any case where the impending loss is known ahead of time. If the time scale of the loss is long enough, grieving may well be complete almost as soon as the loss is experienced. Sometimes outsiders are amazed by how little grief seems to be experienced by the surviving partner of an elderly couple. This does not mean a lack of feeling for the lost partner, but simply that there has already been sufficient time for grieving to take place. The surviving partner may feel that everything that needed to be said was said, and that with their partner's suffering over, there is no grieving left to do.

Anticipatory grieving: grieving that takes place before an expected loss has actually occurred.

Grieving can also cause problems if it continues for too long without change or a sense of being adapted, if it is too intense or if it is inappropriate to the loss. This is known as 'morbid grief' or complicated grief and is usually a sign of other psychological problems. Grief can produce problems if it is blocked, prevented, postponed or denied.

Morbid grief: grieving that is too intense, or inappropriate to the loss.

Grieving can also produce problems if the people involved get out of sync with one another; that is, if they are at different stages of grieving at the same time. Imagine, for example, the case in which doctors inform an elderly male parent that he has only six months to live. He and his surviving partner, if there is one, will begin the process of grieving. Their middle-aged child who lives at some distance from them may only arrive on the scene for the final stages of grieving. They may be angry, bargaining or depressed at a time when the parents have achieved adaptation and acceptance. The adult child may feel rejected, or feel that the parents are indifferent to the seriousness of the situation. If the adult child then tries (appropriately to their own stage of grieving) to get doctors to take heroic measures to save the dying parent, this may cause more friction between child and parents.

In the same way, an individual with Alzheimer's dementia may lose so much of their memories, thoughts and personal characteristics as a result of their disease that their partner regards them as already lost long before they are dead. In this case, the partner may have completed grieving for the person, and continue taking care of the body—which, as the partner sees it, is all that remains. When death finally occurs, the major feeling may be relief.

CASE STUDY

DOROTHY, DEMENTIA AND MENTAL HEALTH

The aim of this case is to look at an individual's experience of illness during old age that involves different elements.

Dorothy is 82 years old, and until recently has been in good health. She lives independently in a ground-floor unit in a suburb in Adelaide. She has a good relationship with her three children and their families. Dorothy is particularly fond of her grand-daughter Kylie who recently graduated with her pharmacy degree. Dorothy had a fall two months ago and was hospitalised with a fractured femur. She had a hip replacement and her recovery was non-eventful, but Dorothy is concerned that she doesn't feel like her usual self. Her family are also worried that she may be showing signs of Alzheimer's disease. Her daughter June decided to meet with Dorothy's GP to talk about her mother. The GP agreed to arrange a home visit for a detailed assessment. Dorothy was diagnosed with mild Alzheimer's.

Dorothy acknowledges that her memory isn't as good as it had been. Since her fall she's had difficulty remembering things that happened earlier in the week. Sometimes in conversation she can't find the right word to describe something or to say what she wanted. Only last week she walked to the local shopping centre, but when she got there she couldn't remember what she needed to do. She also seemed to be forgetting where she put her handbag.

June told the GP that she thought Dorothy's personality had changed. She used to be bubbly and lively, but now had become subdued and withdrawn. This was particularly the case when the family gathered to celebrate Kylie's graduation. June believes that Dorothy gets irritated by little things. She seems to have difficulty concentrating and doesn't seem motivated to complete tasks around the house. The GP was interested in the family's perceptions of changes in Dorothy's mood. He wondered if perhaps she was suffering from depression.

A domiciliary care nurse has been visiting Dorothy twice a week. She noted that Dorothy did seem depressed and spoke to her at length about what had been happening in her life. Dorothy's recently fractured femur had been causing her considerable pain. It was difficult for Dorothy to get around the house and to go out and meet her friends. She was feeling lonely and her circle of friends was dwindling. The fall also prompted feelings of death. She feels anxious most of the time. She is particularly worried that she might fall again and no one would find her.

1 What are some of the cognitive changes that may indicate the development of mild Alzheimer's?
2 What are some of the risk factors that contribute to depression in the elderly?
3 Is it possible that Dorothy's depressed mood could also related to a sense of loss?

Points to consider

Loss is painful, and Dorothy could be grieving her loss of independence, mobility and health. Distinguishing between grief and clinical depression can be difficult as both conditions share many symptoms. However, grief involves a wide variety of emotions and a mix of good and bad days. There can be moments of pleasure or happiness. With depression, on the other hand, the feelings of emptiness and despair are constant. It is likely that Dorothy was experiencing both grief and depression. This is understandable given her chronic pain and physical disability as a result of the fall.

It is important to be aware that medical problems can cause depression in the elderly, either directly or as a psychological reaction to the illness. Any medical condition in the elderly, particularly if it is painful and disabling, can lead to depression or make depression symptoms worse and should be investigated.

CHAPTER SUMMARY

- The important themes of adulthood revolve around responsibility towards family, work and society.
- Health impacts of lifestyle begin to appear and the development of the individual becomes more variable.
- During middle years, health becomes a more important determinant of lifestyle than does age.
- Ageing brings life changes as a result of societal expectations.
- Deterioration during old age is related to the health of the individual.
- Healthy older people live a life that is very similar to that of the middle aged.
- Death and dying are important issues at the end of life.

SELF TEST

1 Your new neighbour has two children under the age of 2, and has just completed teacher training. Your judgment that he is a young adult is based on his:
   a chronological age
   b mental age
   c terminal age
   d social age.
2 During middle adulthood:
   a the habits we have had during earlier years begin to affect our health
   b Australian men tend to marry for the first time
   c work is relatively unimportant to us
   d we change from using mostly our crystallised intelligence to our fluid intelligence.

3   Dr Elgar believes that nothing can increase the average lifespan of healthy people
    much past the age of 85. The theory of ageing that is most consistent with Dr Elgar's
    belief is:
    a   obsolescence theory
    b   wear and tear theory
    c   free radical theory
    d   errors in copying theory.

4   Grieving is least likely to cause problems for a bereaved individual if it is:
    a   blocked
    b   prolonged
    c   encouraged
    d   intense.

5   Mr Ch'ng is suffering from dementia. Of the following symptoms, it is least likely that
    he will show:
    a   short-term memory loss
    b   reduced anxiety levels
    c   confusion
    d   changes in personality.

FURTHER READING

AIHW (2007) *Dementia in Australia: National data analysis and development.* AIHW cat. no.
    AGE 53. Canberra: Australian Institute of Health and Welfare.

Ames, D., O'Brien J. & Burns, A. (eds) (2010) *Dementia*, 4th edn. London: Hodder Arnold.

Craft-Rosenberg, M. & Pehler, S. (eds) (2011) Death and the grieving process in families. In
    Encyclopedia of family health. Thousand Oaks, CA: Sage Publications.

Goymer, P. (2007). New syndrome reconciles theories of ageing. *Nature Reviews Genetics*,
    8(2), p. 90.

Martin, T.L. & Doka, K.J. (2010) *Grieving beyond gender: Understanding the ways men and
    women mourn* (rev. edn). Hoboken: Taylor & Francis.

USEFUL WEBSITES

Alzheimer's Australia:
www.alzheimers.org.au

Black Dog Institute (support groups):
www.blackdoginstitute.org.au/public/gettinghelp/supportgroups.cfm

Health Insite (personal stories about depression):
www.healthinsite.gov.au/topics/Personal_Stories_about_Depression

04 REACTIONS TO ILLNESS

CHAPTER OBJECTIVES

By the end of your study of this chapter, you should be able to:

- understand the common ways in which individuals react to illness, and the process of illness behaviour, by which a well person becomes a patient
- know the rights and obligations of the sick role and how they influence the way others treat sick people
- understand how illness behaviour may be considered abnormal
- understand how characteristics of the individual may increase vulnerability or resistance to illness and disease
- know the factors that influence vulnerability and capability in an individual
- describe and contrast stable characteristics of the individual and situational strategies as they affect health
- apply the principles of perception to explain varying reactions to illness.

KEYWORDS

abnormal illness behaviour
arousal
capability
conservation withdrawal
foetal alcohol syndrome (FAS)
gestalt
hardiness
illness behaviour
illness perceptions
in utero
learning
neuroticism (N type)
optimism

perception
perceptual constancy
perceptual set
perinatal
phi phenomenon
self-esteem
sensation
sick role
stereotyping
temporal extension
type A (coronary prone) behaviour
  pattern
vulnerability

INTRODUCTION

Reactions to illness vary considerably. For the majority of people, minor aches, pains and other illness symptoms are an inescapable, and even expected, aspect of daily living. There are a large number of possible responses to a given symptom, ranging from ignoring the symptom to immediately seeking professional emergency medical care. In between these extremes are self-care responses ranging from relatively passive (getting more rest) to active behaviour (taking over-the-counter medications). This chapter explores the range of factors that influence individuals' reactions to illness. These reactions can be influenced by the illness itself, the situation and the person. Following your reading of Chapter 2 and 3, you can appreciate that individual responses to illness will differ according to the person's stage of development. There has been increasing interest in the factors that appear to be involved in the individual's decision to seek medical care, including the severity of the symptom, cultural and family background, social networks, psychological distress, illness beliefs, locus of control, learning history and personality factors. Although some of these factors remain constant, others (perhaps the majority) are subject to change. The variability of the different factors make it difficult to build a consistent picture of who is likely to use medical care a lot—perhaps unnecessarily—and even more difficult to identify those people who are seldom seen by health professionals, even though their condition warrants care and attention.

The typical reactions to illness are very similar to the typical reactions to any other stressful event in life—whether it is a loss or a pleasant experience. These typical reactions can be examined under four headings.

1 *Physical responses* (that is, changes in bodily states and processes). Physical responses include loss of or change in appetite, sleep problems and tiredness. These may result directly from the illness—as when body temperature rises, or tissues become irritated—or indirectly as a result of the other kinds of responses (discussed below).

2 *Emotional responses.* Emotional responses could include sadness, anxiety, anger or irritability. In some cases, when the individual sees that blame can be assigned for their illness, specific emotional reactions are common. If the blame for an individual's situation rests with themselves—say, a smoker who develops lung cancer—that person may experience feelings of guilt. Where the blame can be seen to rest with another—say, lung cancer resulting from exposure to pollutants—anger is common. Again, these emotional reactions may result directly from illness processes or indirectly.

3 *Cognitive responses* (that is, responses having to do with thinking, judging etc.). Cognitive responses include preoccupation with symptoms, changes to self-image, memories and dreaming. These kinds of reactions are often overlooked because the physical and emotional ones are more obvious. However, loss of **self-esteem** is common in many health conditions, and may interfere with many aspects of the individual's life. Men with problems getting or maintaining an erection as a result of medical conditions associated with ageing, for example, may feel that they have become less manly, that they will be a target of jokes, or that they will have difficulty maintaining their relationship with their partner. Like physical and emotional reactions, cognitive reactions may have direct or indirect causes. A direct cause that could change thoughts could include confusion as a result of physical changes to the brain during a high fever. An indirect cause that could alter thoughts could include preoccupation about the condition and subsequent anxiety.

Self-esteem: the perception on the part of an individual that they are a good and worthy person.

4   *Behavioural responses.* Behavioural responses to illness could include changes in habits, restlessness, withdrawal from people, help seeking and information seeking. Many such changes are seen as normal in the initial stages of an illness, but regarded as abnormal if they continue. Behavioural responses could range from something as simple as beginning to take vitamins to a complete lifestyle modification. A substantial part of the behavioural reaction consists of an attempt to cope with the stress of a situation; this is discussed in later chapters. As you can imagine, the more serious the illness, the more likely we are to expect and accept these reactions from individuals. In a similar way, the more serious the illness, the longer we will see these reactions as being normal and appropriate. If an illness is chronic—that is, occurring regularly or repeatedly over a period of time—or even permanent, we will expect and accept some persistence of the reactions. An individual who is confined to a wheelchair as a result of injury, for example, may be forever exempted from a range of activities.

PAUSE & REFLECT

Think back to the last time you were ill. What kind of physical, emotional, cognitive, and behavioural reactions did you experience?

EDITH KARMI, ASTHMA AND HEART DISEASE

CASE STUDY

The aim of this case is to consider how people react to the experience of being ill and to examine the factors that influence these reactions.

Edith Karmi is 76 years of age and lives in her own home in inner Melbourne. Her husband of 53 years died eight months ago after a long illness due to cancer. She misses him every day. They had three children, and her married son lives in the next suburb. Since his father's death, Peter calls in regularly to visit his mother to provide company and make sure that she is all right. One very cold July morning Edith walked outside to collect her newspaper and suddenly began to gasp for breath. She felt that it was impossible to pull enough air into her lungs.

Edith is annoyed with herself for not taking her usual dose of respiratory medication before going out on such a cold, dry day. Nor did she take any additional precaution such as wearing a scarf over her face to help warm the air before each breath. Edith knows that she suffers from asthma. She was first diagnosed with asthma a child and, as a result, usually carries a puffer with her to deal with sudden asthma attacks. Over the years, Edith has gained quite lot of information about asthma from health professionals and from her own reading. She always tries to keep up with news about the latest treatments and theories about asthma. Edith, who also suffers from heart disease, has been warned by her doctor that a severe asthma attack may trigger a heart attack. Edith was able to make her way back inside the house and take a dose from her puffer.

1   How might the information from Edith's doctor change your ideas about Edith's reactions to her sudden breathlessness?

2   What might lead Edith to decide to go to her doctor about this particular attack of breathlessness? What kind of decisions could she make?

Points to consider

Because there is a certain amount of risk that comes with any serious asthma attack, as well as with Edith's heart disease, we would expect Edith's reaction to be considerably greater than her reaction to feeling nauseated or to a having a sprained ankle. If her breathlessness were to continue for an extended period of time, or if the puffer didn't control the attack, her reactions would probably include fear, anxiety, restlessness and thoughts about death, all of which would be worse because her heart disease increases the risks.

ILLNESS BEHAVIOUR

Illness behaviour:
the process by which an individual goes from being a well person to an ill patient.

Illness behaviour is the process by which an individual goes from being a well person to being an ill patient. The focus is on the nature of the individual's response to their experience of being ill. This response can also be thought of as a coping response to the stress of being ill, according to Mechanic (1968). It involves a series of decisions something like the following, although each situation may be different.

ARE MY SYMPTOMS NORMAL?

Some symptoms may be perceived to be common or of no great significance when they occur and are likely to be considered normal. It has been estimated, for example, that only one out of every 200 headaches is ever actually reported to a doctor. A chronic symptom, such as back pain, may also be accepted, whereas the same symptom as a one-off (acute) symptom of pain would send most people screaming for help. Non-professional people, such as family and friends, may be consulted to see if they think that the symptom is real ('Is it just me, or is it hot in here?') or serious ('Do you ever have headaches on one side of your head?').

WHAT CHOICES ARE AVAILABLE FOR DEALING WITH THE SYMPTOM?

The most common response is probably to ignore the symptom until it goes away, but—as you can imagine—there are no statistics on how many people do this. Self-treatment is very common, particularly for expected and recurrent symptoms. Most of us take pain relievers (analgesics such as aspirin and paracetamol) as needed without regarding ourselves as sick. Many of us take preventative measures (such as regular asthma or blood pressure medication) without experiencing symptoms or feeling ill. The next step beyond self-treatment is to consult non-professionals for advice: friends and family. If these people advise seeking professional help—'You look pale. You should see a doctor'—then the individual is more likely to take that next step.

SHOULD I SEE A PROFESSIONAL NOW?

It is important to remember that 'professional' does not necessarily mean a doctor, particularly in some cultural groups. Some people will prefer to see a massage therapist, a herbalist or a faith healer. Regardless of the professional involved, the general process of becoming a patient follows the same path. The question of when to consult must be settled.

Five common triggers for the decision to seek professional help have been identified.

1   *Perceived interference of symptom with vocational or physical activities.* The person feels that they cannot work or do other things that they need to do because of the symptoms they are experiencing.

2   *Perceived interference with social activities or personal relationships.* The person may be well enough to do the things they have to do, such as going to work, but feel too tired or ill to do things that they would like to do, or others would like them to do.

3   *Occurrence of a personal crisis (for example, the loss of a job or a bereavement) that disturbs usual coping.* A symptom that we could tolerate if everything else is normal may not be tolerable if we also have to deal with the stress of an unusual or unexpected event.

4   *The symptom has gone on long enough or past a self-imposed deadline.* Often, the length of this deadline is affected by the severity of the symptom. We will tolerate low levels of symptoms or symptoms that do not appear to mean anything major much longer than we will tolerate severe or worrying symptoms.

5   *Pressure from others to seek help (sanctioning).* Family and friends, who are often the trigger for people consulting professionals, may be more concerned about interference with activities or the duration or meaning of a symptom than the individual who actually has the symptom.

WHAT CAN THE PROFESSIONAL PROVIDE?

Usually, health professionals can help by making the symptom go away by means of treatment, reducing the anxiety about the symptom by explanation and reassurance, or simple validation of the presence of a real disease as indicated by the symptoms. Prior experience with professionals is very important in deciding what they can provide and if this service is useful to the person. If the individual has been disappointed with the outcomes or side effects of treatment, or even the kind of treatment they have received, they may look for a different kind of professional, such as a naturopath, osteopath or a religious healer, rather than go to a medical practitioner.

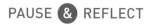

PAUSE & REFLECT

What things might lead someone to choose to consult a herbalist or a religious healer rather than a health professional?

EDITH (CONT.)   CASE STUDY

Edith's puffer controlled her breathlessness, so she decided not to visit the doctor for diagnosis, although she considered going for reassurance, and to keep her family from worrying and nagging her (even though she was not worried).

  Later that morning Edith began to have crushing chest pain. She made her way to the bathroom for a tablet to ease the pain. She sat quietly for 30 minutes praying for the drug to take effect. As the pain continued she recognised the need for help and was becoming frightened. Her first thought was to phone Peter, but then remembered that he was at work. She phoned 000 and was able to give her address before slumping to the floor. Because of the inner-city location of Edith's house, the ambulance arrived within 10 minutes. The officers were able enter the house, administer immediate care and transfer Edith to hospital for an emergency admission.

1   Because Edith has been diagnosed with both asthma and heart disease, how is her situation different from that of someone who does not have these diagnoses?

2   Is her treatment by others different? Is her place in the family or society different?

Points to consider

Edith's role suddenly changes at this stage. Her doctor or family will formally change her status to 'patient' because of the involvement of the ambulance in taking her to hospital. Her admission will involve Edith missing out on her usual appointments or social events, consulting other professionals, worrying about how to pay for her health care, and other such matters. It is very unlikely that there will be any problems with her being granted the rights of the sick role—from family, friends, hospital, employer or health insurer—even if the chest pain turns out not to have been a heart attack. In Edith's case, her entitlement to the sick role is very clear.

THE SICK ROLE

Sick role: a social agreement involving a balance of rights and obligations granted to an individual who is regarded by others as sick.

In looking at what it means for the individual to be sick, sociologist Talcott Parsons (1951) described the **sick role** as a social agreement involving a balance of rights and obligations. The rights are to be:

- excused from normal roles and responsibilities
- regarded as not personally responsible for being sick (which means that the individual has a real problem and cannot be expected to get better simply by will power or by deciding to do so).

The obligations are to:

- want to get better
- cooperate with technically competent help.

Parsons believed that the sick role was present in every culture and always included these rights and obligations. Obviously, different beliefs about the causes of symptoms (for example, germs or witchcraft) will affect what is meant by terms such as 'not personally responsible' and 'technically competent help'.

In most societies, the decision about who deserves the sick role is quite heavily loaded with moral judgments. We ask whether smokers (who are perceived to be personally responsible for their symptoms) should be granted the same rights as those who do not smoke. A number of health insurers have decided that they should not and that smokers should have to pay a larger share of their own health care costs. However, the more we know about the effects of behaviour and lifestyle on health and illness, the less clear some of these distinctions become. Automobile accidents can happen to anyone, but are far more likely to happen to at-risk drivers, including drink drivers, the impaired elderly, young males and just plain bad drivers. Should we then blame people in these categories in the same way that we blame smokers? The debates over treatment of HIV/AIDS, genital herpes and alcoholism often revolve around guilt and innocence, yet debates about treatment of obesity-related disorders such as heart disease seldom do.

As public awareness of the risks associated with obesity changes, so too are attitudes changing. We tend to agree that genetic predisposition is not something that the individual can be blamed for, but what about failing to take appropriate action to reduce the genetic risk? These arguments have a great deal to do with our responsibility-oriented culture. In many other cultures, these issues are never considered at all.

CROSS-REFERENCE
Risky behaviour is discussed in Chapter 7.

ABNORMAL ILLNESS BEHAVIOUR

Sooner or later, a point will be reached when continuing reaction towards illness on the individual's part will be judged to be an overreaction, or abnormal. This point will vary depending on who is doing the judging, and on things such as the nature of the illness, the age and sex of the sick person, and the nature of their responsibilities.

Pilovsky (1978) identified a pattern of behaviour that he called **abnormal illness behaviour**. (Note that it is very important to distinguish between this concept and the broader concept of 'abnormal behaviour', discussed below.) Pilovsky defined abnormal illness behaviour as 'the persistence of inappropriate or maladaptive modes of perceiving, evaluating or acting in relation to health' after the person has received an appropriate explanation of the nature and management of the illness from a professional. This could be shown in a variety of ways, most of which can be seen as either requesting the rights of the sick role when they are not actually needed, or avoiding the obligations when they do not need to be avoided. In what is clearly a most extreme example of abnormal illness behaviour, a woman in England who was ill with a bad cold was told by her doctor to 'go to bed and stay there until I tell you to get up'. Unfortunately, the doctor never returned, and even though the woman quickly recovered from the cold, she stayed in bed for over 40 years—becoming an invalid from inactivity and placing heavy demands on her family. When finally visited by a new doctor, it took months to get her to leave her bed and take up something like normal activities.

Abnormal illness behaviour: the persistence of inappropriate or maladaptive modes of perceiving, evaluating or acting in relation to health after the person has received an appropriate explanation of the nature and management of the illness from a professional.

What must not be assumed is that the patient is necessarily aware of how they are behaving and how it is perceived by others. Abnormal illness behaviour is frequently not conscious, which is why we used the word 'needed' with regard to the rights of the sick role in the paragraph above, rather than using a word such as 'deserved' or 'merited' that would have suggested that the sick role must be earned. The diagnosis of abnormal illness behaviour is always going to represent to some extent a value judgment on the part of the professional or the patient's family, friends or associates. Clearly, individual or cultural differences can have an enormous effect on what is judged to be inappropriate and maladaptive. A good example of abnormal illness behaviour—which might help you to understand some of the subtleties involved—is the persistent (chronic) pain syndrome, which is described in Chapter 11.

Illness may also serve as a trigger for a wide range of psychological problems, such as depression, anxiety disorders, adjustment disorders, substance abuse, so-called psychosomatic illnesses, family, social or occupational problems, and even psychosis (severe mental illness). Earlier, it was mentioned that a life event or crisis may serve as a trigger for consulting a health professional. If the individual is already predisposed to the development of a psychological illness, it is not uncommon for a physical illness to trigger that psychological disorder or make it worse.

FACTORS AFFECTING REACTIONS TO ILLNESS

The illness, the situation and the person are all factors that can affect reactions to illness.

THE ILLNESS

The nature of an illness can affect how people react to it. Severe or horrific illnesses are likely to cause greater reactions. Cancers—even those that are slow-developing, easily treated or present a low risk of disability or death—often produce very strong reactions due to the images produced by the word. So-called flesh-eating viruses combine very rapid onset, horrific damage and low probability of cure to produce a very fearful impact. Conditions that are known to produce long-term effects (for example, diabetes and epilepsy) or to affect many areas of life (such as spinal injury and Alzheimer's disease) tend to also produce greater reactions. One of the most frightening things about some infectious diseases (historically, leprosy or tuberculosis) or diseases that affect the immune system is that they may cut people off from their normal social contacts, or prevent them from enjoying normal activities. Even the treatments that are used may affect how people react. Chemotherapy for leukaemia may result in loss of all hair: a highly visible indication of the individual's condition, even though the condition itself may have produced little in the way of obvious external signs.

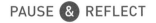

PAUSE & REFLECT

How might the nature of the illness affect a parent's reactions when told that their newborn baby will be intellectually disabled?

THE SITUATION

The size and accessibility of the individual's social support network, their financial and professional situation, and access to health care can all affect how they react to an illness. Other situational factors can include where they live and concurrent stresses in their lives. Reactions to a condition will be quite different if, for example, the individual is temporarily barred from a favourite activity rather than being forced to give up that activity forever. Loss of social status or income due to an illness can produce strong or prolonged reactions. In recent years, we have been learning a great deal about the importance of social support to an individual's health. Those who have more people that they can call on, or who have people who are willing to provide very high levels of support, find coping with illness much easier in general than those who must rely on their own resources.

CROSS-REFERENCE
Social support is discussed in detail in Chapter 13.

THE PERSON

The effects of a particular behaviour on health will not be the same for every person. The impact of a behaviour on the health of a person will be an interaction of factors from the behaviour, the situation and the individual. Personal characteristics that influence the impact of a health behaviour include vulnerabilities (things that make the impact greater) and capabilities (things that lessen the impact).

VULNERABILITY AND CAPABILITY

GENETIC PREDISPOSITIONS

Each person inherits **vulnerabilities** and **capabilities** as part of his or her genetic make-up. That is, the person's internal structure and function can predispose them towards either developing or resisting specific health problems. Examples are numerous: heart disease and its risk factors (such as high cholesterol and high blood pressure), along with many cancers, diabetes, schizophrenia and depression, all have a genetic component. Some genetic predispositions are primarily found within specific families (such as Huntington's chorea), some are found in specific populations (such as thalassaemia) and some are widely distributed.

How—and whether—a specific genetic predisposition results in disease or illness depends on the type of predisposition. Inheriting the gene for thalassaemia from a parent means that a person will develop the condition, regardless of any behavioural or environmental factors. Any other combination of genes will preclude the person from having it. Other predispositions produce only an increase or decrease in the likelihood of disease, given the presence of a particular situational influence. It is relatively rare for people who do not smoke to develop lung cancer, and those non-smokers who do develop the disease have usually been exposed to a similar risk factor, such as air pollution.

In some cases, the genetic predisposition is to the development of a risk factor rather than a disease. An individual may, for example, be predisposed to produce moderately high levels of cholesterol. This is not in itself a disease and is largely symptomless, but remains a risk factor for the development of atherosclerosis, which in turn produces the symptoms of heart disease. The mere predisposition to high levels of cholesterol does not mean that the individual will inevitably have symptoms such as chest pain on exertion or a heart attack. Factors that occur later in life, such as diet, exercise, smoking and alcohol use, will have a large influence on whether the genetic predisposition leads to disease.

Genetic predispositions may influence psychological traits as well as physical ones. Individuals are born with differences in temperament: some may be excitable; others quiet and steady. While it may ultimately be possible to trace these behavioural predispositions back to biological causes, it is often more useful to consider them at the level of behaviour. Certain styles of dealing with anger appear to run in families—even discounting the influence of common learning experiences—and can be used to predict an increased risk of clinical heart disease (Carmelli et al. 1985).

Some theorists suggest that complex patterns of behaviour, such as addiction or substance dependence, may run in families. As yet, the best marker of such proposed genetic predispositions is the presence of addictive behaviour rather any detectable biological characteristics that might lead to addiction.

Vulnerability:
a characteristic or behaviour of the individual that increases the impact of a negative event.

Capability:
a characteristic or behaviour of the individual that protects against a negative event.

IN UTERO ENVIRONMENT

In utero refers to the environment inside the uterus while the foetus is developing during pregnancy. The influence of events—both negative and positive—during this very early stage of development is profound. Something as simple as the presence of a single chemical may cause major damage to the developing foetus. Thalidomide was a tranquilliser given to pregnant women in the late 1950s and early 1960s for treatment of morning sickness. Unfortunately, it

In utero:
the environment inside the uterus while the foetus is developing during pregnancy.

resulted also in the failure of differentiation of the foetal cells that result in the development of arms and legs. If taken during the first third of pregnancy, thalidomide resulted in major birth defects, such as stunted or deformed arms and legs. Until relatively recently, there was little understanding of in utero environment on the infant's health when they become an adult. For example, it was only in 1986 that the *Lancet* published the first of two groundbreaking papers showing that if a pregnant woman ate poorly, her child would be at significantly higher than average risk for cardiovascular disease as an adult. More recently, in a review on intrauterine conditions associated with cancer risk later in life, Grotmol, Weiderpass and Tretli (2006) found evidence that factors acting in utero play a role in the development of cancer in the testis and breast. The exact biological mechanisms for this risk are not clear, but are likely to involve hormonal disturbances, and genetic or epigenetic events.

Foetal alcohol syndrome (FAS):
a syndrome, or group of symptoms, shown by the babies of mothers who drink excessive amounts of alcohol during pregnancy; babies tend to be born prematurely, have low birth weight and an irritable temperament.

Other health influences on the developing foetus have different consequences. **Foetal alcohol syndrome** (FAS) tends not to result in physical deformity (except in certain extreme cases), but babies tend to be born prematurely, have low birth weight and an irritable temperament. They often suffer intellectual deficits, and FAS may be a major cause of intellectual disability (Robinson 2008). Maternal smoking has been linked to low birth weight, susceptibility to delayed respiratory development, and lifelong respiratory problems. The use of illicit drugs by pregnant women, such as marijuana, cocaine and heroin, also have significant impact on the developing foetus. In the case of all of these drugs, the newborn baby goes through a period of withdrawal that can compromise development.

Diseases can also result in major developmental problems for the foetus. The vast majority of deaf and blind babies in developed countries are born to mothers who had German measles (rubella) during the stage of embryonic development when the sense organs are developing. Other known or likely in utero causes of health problems include maternal fever, high blood pressure (which may predispose the baby to high blood pressure in later life), psychiatric illness (although this may be primarily because of the effects on maternal behaviour) and obesity (which may predispose the child to obesity). Good maternal health, nutrition, sleep and emotional stability during pregnancy all provide a head start to the health of the child.

PERINATAL EVENTS

Perinatal: refers to events occurring around the time of birth.

Perinatal refers to events occurring around the time of birth. These can include problems associated with birth itself arising from prolonged lack of oxygen, from passage through the birth canal or as a result of behaviour on the part of health professionals. Drugs given to the mother to relieve pain during labour may influence the baby's alertness, heart or respiratory activity. Similarly, the baby could incur damage caused by forceps or other equipment during birth. Exposure to certain environmental events, such as infections, light and heat, may also have effects.

The influence of breastfeeding in the early days of life on development of the immune system is also significant (Jackson & Nazar 2006). Children who are breastfed not only inherit antibodies from the mother, but also acquire foreign material that encourages the development of their own immune capabilities to protect against diarrhoea, otitis media (infection in the middle ear) and respiratory diseases. Some researchers have suggested that the reason for the increased incidence of asthma in developed countries is that an immune system that is not exposed to a range of microbes at this critical stage will begin to respond inappropriately to environmental triggers, such as dust mite and pollen particles. To some extent, being in too clean an environment may prevent the immune system from developing its ability to distinguish between potential pathogens and benign substances.

PAUSE & REFLECT

There is considerable scientific evidence that breast milk is the ideal food for new babies. The World Health Organization recommends exclusive breast milk to babies for the first six months of life, and yet in many developed countries rates of breastfeeding are declining, particularly amongst young mothers. What range of factors do you think may hinder breastfeeding? What are some of the physical and psychological benefits of breastfeeding for the mother and baby?

Prematurity is another perinatal source of vulnerability. Any baby who is born earlier than 37 weeks' gestation (a normal pregnancy is 40 weeks' duration) is exposed to influences that it may not be physically ready to face. The earlier a baby is born, the more difficulties it will face. Disability occurs in 30 per cent of babies born at 31 weeks and in 60 per cent of babies born at 26 weeks (Tropy et al. 2008). Often there is immaturity of the lungs and the part of the brain that regulates temperature. Where the digestive system is not fully ready, feeding may produce problems. Many of these problems contribute to weaknesses in organ systems that can persist for long periods of childhood—even through the entire lifespan.

EARLY LIFE EVENTS

In the early stages of life, the child is vulnerable to a variety of events that may predispose them to later problems. In addition to injuries and infections, a major category of these events concerns relationships. Postnatal depression in the mother may prevent close bonding between the mother and baby, and predispose the child to depression or other problems in later life. Maternal inability to cope with the skills or stresses of caring for a baby may also lead to bonding problems, irritability in the child and later health problems.

Abuse and neglect represent not only immediate threats to the baby but also long-term threats to cognitive functioning (Gould et al. 2012). It is obvious that deprivation of adequate food and shelter may put the child at risk of developmental delay, but studies in orphanages have shown that emotional neglect, despite the absence of any material neglect, can also lead to failure to develop, and even failure to grow (known as developmental dwarfism). Good, trustworthy caregiving provides a child with capabilities for development of relationships and cognitive skills. Environmental stimulation is also important to the development of intelligence and coping skills.

CROSS-REFERENCE
Later life events are dealt with in more detail in Chapters 3 and 5.

PERSONALITY

There have been many attempts to link personality and health. A major problem with trying to do this is that there is no single agreed definition of personality. In normal conversational terms, it refers to persistent impressions that an individual makes on others (their social stimulus value), which is a very difficult thing to pin down because others may have very different experiences with the individual. Some may see a person only at work, some only at play and some—particularly health professionals—only when they are sick. Another problem is defining 'persistent', as people may act and respond differently according to the circumstances.

One of the oldest attempts to link personality and health involved a personality type called **neuroticism (N type)**, seen as linked to the responsiveness of the autonomic nervous system (Eysenck 1976). The N type described people who tended to develop neurotic symptoms under even relatively mild stress. But there is a problem with this definition, as the judgment about the mildness of stress is made by an observer and does not take account of the individual's appraisal of the situation. A better understanding of the nature of stress as a process in which the individual interacts with the situation (see Chapter 12) calls some of the logic of the N type into question.

The most familiar theory attempting to link health and personality is almost certainly the **type A (coronary prone) behaviour pattern**. This theory (Friedman & Rosenman 1974) proposes that individuals who show a pattern of competitive achievement striving, an exaggerated sense of time urgency, and aggressiveness and hostility are at greatly increased risk of heart attack. Individuals are classed as type A if they show high levels of these characteristics in an interview or on a questionnaire, and type B if they show the opposite. The suggestion was made by Friedman and Rosenman that these types were stable attributes of the individual that persisted over much of the lifespan. An individual could be measured at one point in time and assumed to stay true to type.

A variety of mechanisms has been suggested as to why this type A pattern would be associated with clinical events of heart disease (Steptoe 1981). It could be linked to a pattern of frequent high levels of emotional and/or physiological **arousal** in response to a variety of stimuli, a pattern known as hyper-reactivity that could lead to risky developments in the body, such as surges of adrenaline, periods of hypertension or turbulence in the blood flow through the arteries. Changes in the behaviour of the circulatory system, such as constriction of the blood vessels during tasks, are another possibility.

In general, research attempting to link personality to illness—whether it is neuroticism to anxiety, type A to heart disease, type C to cancer, or some other classification system—is hampered by several problems.

First, there tends to be a lack of evidence about the stability of personality characteristics. For the type A behaviour pattern, gradual changes in level have been noted, particularly where the situation of the person changes (Jones & Lebnan 1988). In many cases, studies may be looking at the effects of long-term (or even fairly short-term) coping strategies (Jones, Copolov & Outch 1986) that do not actually represent typical, or even common, ways of coping for that person. The methods of measurement may be unstable. A particular measurement method or task may produce the kind of behaviour that is expected by the experimenter, or demanded by the task (Jones 1991). The proportion of individuals who are classed as having the type A personality has changed considerably over the last five decades; it also depends on who is doing the measuring.

Second, it is difficult to demonstrate cause and effect. It is very rare to characterise personality types in a large sample in order to show that the personality predated the illness (Jones & Bright 2001). In some cases, the opposite is true—people with an illness are found to have similar personality characteristics; in others the illness and the personality characteristic may result from some common cause. A criticism of the concept of neuroticism is that it is defined in the same way as the outcomes it is linked to.

Third, for personality to produce illness it must logically be through the mechanism of biochemical or physiological change. In most cases, the links between the personality types of interest and bodily responding are fairly unreliable (Allen 1998).

Neuroticism (N type): a tendency to develop neurotic symptoms under even relatively mild stress.

Type A (or coronary prone) behaviour pattern: the idea that individuals who show a pattern of competitive achievement striving, an exaggerated sense of time urgency, and aggressiveness and hostility are at greatly increased risk of heart attack.

Arousal: the activation of the sympathetic nervous system, which produces visceral changes and provides energy for behaviour.

So far, the literature linking specific strategies, response patterns or events to illness look more promising than the personality literature. Along with many other authors, Jones (1991) argued that the type A behaviour pattern is a strategy—that is, a response on the part of the individual to challenges in the environment—and not a personality characteristic. The choice of this strategy may be maintained by the success that it produces; when it stops producing success it is likely to be abandoned (Jones 1985). This strategic view appears to be much more useful in explaining health outcomes than assuming more stable individual personality factors.

EDITH (CONT.)

CASE STUDY

For a long time, Edith has known that she often becomes breathless when she is exposed to animal hair, when she goes outside on a cold day, when she works in the garden and when she is under stress.

While sightseeing on a weekend trip to an unfamiliar country town, Edith experiences a severe asthma attack. She has left her medication at home, something she rarely does. She is aware that she will be much better off if she gets access to medication quickly. Because chemist shops are vitally important to her, every time Edith looks around a street or shopping centre, the chemist shops always seem to stand out. So, as always, she has noticed each chemist shop that she has passed while sight-seeing.

1   What are some of Edith's vulnerabilities and how do they affect her asthma?
2   What are some of Edith's capabilities and how might they affect her asthma?

Points to consider

Edith may well have inherited a genetic predisposition to asthma from her parents. Whether or not she was breastfed, for instance, or her early exposure to the environment (such as dust, plants and environmental pollution) will have influenced the development of her predisposition into an active condition. Her ongoing exposure to the triggers for her asthma will determine whether she will have an attack at a particular time. Her behaviour can modify the triggers: she could remove carpets from her house, for example, or minimise her exposure to them, or she could move to a different climate.

Edith will have a number of strategies for dealing with her asthma, some of which will involve trying to avoid triggers. If such strategies lead to the avoidance of a wide variety of activities or people, they may result in a loss of quality of life. Some of the strategies may have to modify the reaction that Edith has to these triggers. If she has an optimistic approach to life and displays hardiness, her health outcomes are likely to be better.

Edith also will have a variety of illness perceptions relating to the concept of asthma, beliefs about how serious it is, and what the likely course of her condition will be. These perceptions will be modified by her experience, what she is told by health professionals or others, and what she finds out for herself. She will have another set of illness perceptions about her heart disease that will be quite different. As a result of prompt diagnosis and treatment, Edith has a good probability of a successful outcome for episodes of both conditions, which will be a very important part of her illness perceptions. Once her asthma attack has been controlled, she is likely to perceive herself as well again.

PAUSE **&** REFLECT

What are the drawbacks of taking a personality perspective on vulnerability to disease? How could such a perspective harm the rehabilitation of a patient following an episode of ill health? How different might this be if it were a mental health problem?

BEHAVIOURAL STRATEGIES

Individuals select a variety of behavioural strategies for dealing with the environment. These may be selected at any stage in life, but tend to show a certain consistency from early life stages. Those who choose to deal with environmental demands by increased effort powered by increased physiological arousal, for example, may predispose themselves to later development of health problems. When the sympathetic nervous system is activated, the number of circulating platelets—cell fragments that are used to patch damage in blood vessels—in the bloodstream increases, and are stickier. While at any particular moment this is protective in that it helps to deal with injuries to vessel walls, in the long run it can increase the likelihood of atherosclerosis and heart disease.

Other people may choose to deal with the environment by adopting arousal reduction strategies, such as drinking or drug use, that put them at risk of tissue damage and dependency problems. If a child is severely abused or neglected early in life, they may adopt withdrawal as a strategy. This is seen as allowing the child to keep their resources for the task of simply maintaining life. This **conservation withdrawal** is a coping strategy, and may literally be a life-saver in the face of extreme events, but if its use is required very often it can result in severely disturbed coping in later life.

As with conservation withdrawal, any strategy may be protective of or harmful to the individual's health or well-being in some way, especially if it is carried to an extreme or used as the only strategy. Since the early work of Heath (1964), numerous authors have suggested that each individual needs the capability to use a variety of coping strategies if they are to maximise their health and well-being. We need to be able to exert effort when effort will yield results and to withdraw from uncontrollable situations when effort will be wasted. Arousal reduction strategies are very useful, particularly if the stimulus causing arousal is not controllable. Arousal reduction based on control of the ability to relax is especially useful. A great deal of attention is given to this in the discussion of stress management in Chapter 13. Even substance use has its positives, with evidence that a low level of regular alcohol intake may reduce the risks of heart disease, cancer and clinical events.

In general, negative emotional states, including anxiety, depression and hostility, are associated with negative health outcomes (Taylor 2006), and this holds true over a range of medical conditions and diseases. The psychological and physiological factors that are associated with these negative states explain some of this association. Behaviours also need to be included in the explanation, as individuals who are frequently anxious, depressed or angry may not live a healthy lifestyle or adopt healthy strategies. Anxious and depressed people may have trouble getting adequate sleep. Angry people may have difficulty in maintaining relationships with others. All may try to deal with their emotions by self-treatment with alcohol, cigarettes, prescription or illegal drugs, and even with food.

A pessimistic explanatory style may also be stable over adult life and predict a variety of negative health outcomes, including depression and physical illness (Burns & Seligman 1989). This is true, at least in part, because a pessimistic style becomes a self-fulfilling prophecy: if we

Conservation withdrawal: an extreme pattern of withdrawal from interaction with a neglectful or abusive environment by a baby in order to save its life.

CROSS-REFERENCE
How strategies are used to deal with stress is discussed in Chapter 13.

appraise our outcomes as likely to be bad, we are more likely to view them as bad, no matter how a more objective observer might see them. Again, this is more usefully understood as a strategic choice rather than a fixed personality characteristic.

CAPABILITIES AND COPING STRATEGIES

Just as with vulnerabilities, people have more or less stable capabilities and coping strategies. Dispositional **optimism** is a tendency to expect that outcomes in life will generally be good ones, which may affect the health of the individual in a number of ways. People might choose to minimise the significance of minor symptoms, or expect that others will be willing to provide support and therefore be more willing to ask for it. In one study, Scheier et al. (1989) found optimistic people were more willing to tackle their recovery from surgery head on, that they had an expectation that this would lead to a solution, and were less likely to use denial as a strategy. The payoffs came in the form of better physical recovery from illness, a faster return to former activities, and better quality of life after recovery.

> **Optimism:** a tendency to expect that outcomes will generally be good.
>
> **CROSS-REFERENCE**
> Development over the lifespan, and how it affects health and illness, is discussed in Chapters 2 and 3.

This suggests that one significant advantage of being optimistic lies in what it leads the individual to do. Another may lie in experiencing positive emotions rather than negative ones. While an optimistic style is often productive, it is not wise to adopt an unrealistically optimistic approach, particularly where life-and-death decisions are concerned. A critical and objective evaluation of all the issues is likely to be more successful and can protect the individual from making poor guesses about the amount of risk that they face. We might admire the optimism of an elderly individual who decides to try bungy jumping, but if their bone density is low as a result of osteoporosis, this may be a very dangerous decision for their health.

Another proposed capability is **hardiness** (Kobasa 1979). Those who face many stressors but stay healthy had a particular approach to life, including commitment, a belief in their ability to control events, and a willingness to tackle challenges as they occurred. These also do not have to be fixed qualities, but may be strategies applied as needed.

> **Hardiness:** a behaviour pattern of commitment, a belief in ability to control events, and a willingness to tackle challenges as they occur that is associated with continued health in the face of high levels of stress.

PAUSE & REFLECT

What are the vulnerabilities and capabilities of a physically disabled athlete competing at the Paralympic Games?

Beliefs about control appear to be particularly important to the individual in terms of their health outcomes. As you will see in Chapter 12, it is one of the aspects of the individual's appraisal of situations that has a significant role in how stressful those situations are seen to be. Behavioural capabilities may include a predisposition to make stable relationships, which has been found to be protective of health in a variety of ways.

ILLNESS PERCEPTIONS

Each individual will have a personal view or theory regarding their illness that is made up from bodily experience such as symptoms, information from the external environment—such as what they have been told by others, or what they have read or seen on television—and previous experience with illness (Leventhal, Meyer & Nerenz 1980). Views and theories will differ from person to person with the same illness, just as the above factors vary between them. This set

Illness perceptions: personal views or theories that the individual holds regarding their illness, made up from bodily experiences such as symptoms, information from the external environment and previous experience with illness.

of **illness perceptions** will be more important to how the individual reacts than objective facts about the illness.

Perceptions include ideas about what caused the illness, its nature, and its probable course. Leventhal, Meyer and Nerenz (1980) suggest that the individual uses these ideas to guide their coping, including judgments about the seriousness of their illness, and even decisions such as whether they take their medication.

It is useful at this point to know something about the basic processes that are covered by the term 'perception', and how perception works. The next section covers general concepts about perception. If you have already had a background in psychology (for example, if you have taken an introductory psychology course), you may wish to skip to the next chapter.

PERCEPTION

In order to interact with the world around us, we have to collect information about the nature of that world. For example, we use vision to locate objects and identify them, hearing to pick up the communications of others, and touch to soothe a baby. Most of us assume that the information we get from our five senses is a true and complete representation of the world. But is it? How often, for example, have you searched a room for a set of lost keys, only to find that they have been in plain sight all the time? Have you noticed that, in the middle of a noisy crowd, if someone mentions your name you can isolate that one voice from among all others and track what it says? Why does the Moon on the horizon look many times larger than it does when it is high in the sky?

Sensation: the response of receptor organs to stimuli from the environment.

Perception: the conscious experience of objects and events.

In order to understand our interaction with the world, it is necessary to consider the related processes of **sensation** (the response of receptor organs to stimuli from the environment) and **perception** (the conscious experience of objects and events). The study of sensation usually takes place in a psychology, physiology or anatomy laboratory where the structures are fairly constant, and the processes straightforward and observable.

The study of perception is more complex. Although physiological and biochemical processes are part of the explanation of what is perceived, higher mental processes such as memory and cognition are needed to complete the picture. Consider the simple illusion (the Müller–Lyer illusion) in Figure 4.1a. The two vertical lines are identical in length: the images that they make on the retina are the same, but they appear quite different.

Figure 4.1   Müller–Lyer and Ponzo illusions

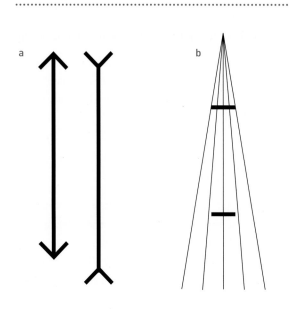

Any attempt to explain this experience must involve psychological concepts. The usual explanation is that the arrow-like markings add context. They cause the vertical lines to be perceived as edges of three-dimensional objects (Gregory 1971). Because of the tendency to perceive size as constant, one of these edges seems closer, and therefore smaller, than the other. The Ponzo illusion (Figure 4.1b) operates in a similar fashion. Because the sloping lines give the impression of depth, the upper horizontal line seems further away, and is therefore scaled up in our perception so that it appears larger than the lower (closer) line.

In the medical context, perceptual illusions can raise problems or provide information. A dramatic experience-based illusion is the phenomenon of the phantom limb. Studies of amputees have shown that, long after a limb has been removed, it still produces a wide range of perceptions. It can be perceived to move, to touch objects and—most distressingly—to cramp or ache. Although it is quite obvious to the patient as well as the doctor that such events within a missing limb cannot be taking place, the fact that they are experienced as real must be accepted, and the symptoms may require treatment. When a patient's perceptions vary from those of others around them, this may be a clue to a sensory problem (that is, damage to the receptor) or to a perceptual one. A blow to the back of the head, where the visual area of the cortex performs the task of integrating the two separate images from the eyes into one, may result in double vision. In the eating disorder anorexia nervosa, sufferers become so obsessed with their weight and body image that they may literally starve themselves to death. In spite of their emaciated appearance to others, their own perception of their body shape is that they are too fat.

BASIC PERCEPTUAL PROCESSES

One of the more remarkable properties of perception is that it serves to make sense out of an enormously complex sensory input. We are able to identify objects when their colour has been changed, when we see them from a new angle, or even when they are reduced to a pattern of disconnected dots. This observation that we are able to perceive more than just the basic sensory stimuli led to the scientific study of how we perceive form, work that began in Germany. Since German contains the useful word **gestalt** (a meaningful grouping or whole), this group of researchers is referred to as the Gestalt School. The Gestalt School was interested in the rules that the brain uses to organise sensory input.

At the most basic level, some of the incoming stimuli are perceived to belong to objects; others are not perceived to do so. The stimuli that are perceived to belong to an object are referred to as the 'figure' and the others as the 'ground'. Note that what is a figure in one instance may be a ground in another, as pebbles may be the ground when we are searching for our shoe on the beach, but the figure when we find one or two pebbles in the shoe. During cricket matches, a sight screen is placed behind the bowler so that the batsman can have it as a plain ground for the figure of the ball instead of having to pick the ball out of a background of spectators. 'Figure–ground' relationships occur in other senses as well, such as when you are able to pick a single voice out of a crowd and track what it is saying. If you hear a significant word from another voice, you can switch your attention to make that voice the figure. The ability to make figure–ground discriminations appears to be innate. Studies of people who were blind from birth but have had their sight restored in adulthood show that they can discriminate figure from ground immediately. Long before they can identify objects by name or purpose without touching them, they can tell what is a figure and what is not.

Gestalt: a meaningful grouping or whole that is perceived.

Other gestalt rules for organising sensation involve the grouping of stimuli. The dots in Figure 4.2a are ungrouped, those in Figure 4.2b are grouped by proximity of the dots to one another, those in Figure 4.2c by continuity, and those in Figure 4.2d by similarity.

The dots in Figure 4.3, however, tend to follow a rule that overrides all of the above: that of simplicity. Even though some of the dots might be grouped by proximity and others by similarity, we still tend to see two intersecting circles, because this is the simplest explanation for the observed arrangement.

Figure 4.2   Gestalt principles

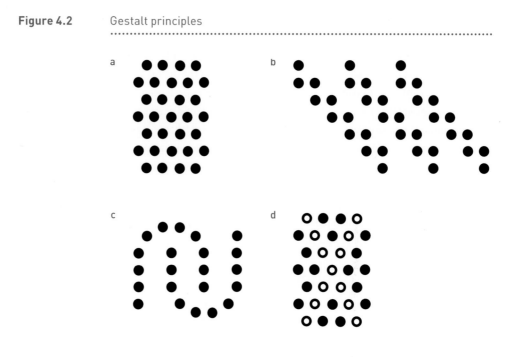

Figure 4.3   The principle of simplicity

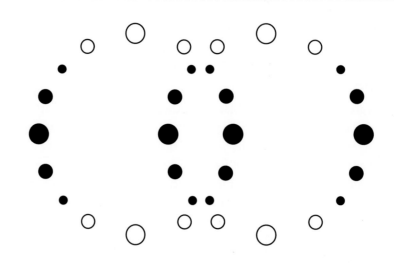

PAUSE & REFLECT

Look again at Figure 4.3 and think about the tendency to simplify visual information. Now imagine that you are a radiographer looking at an x-ray for a break in a bone and that you fail to notice evidence of an old fracture. How could the principle of simplicity be used to explain that failure to perceive?

The movement of objects gives us hints about form as well. Imagine lights attached to several points on the body of a person otherwise covered in black and obscured against a black background. The lights will be perceived as outlining a body when the person moves. At rest these lights will be seen as a random pattern, but as soon as the person moves, the observer will recognise the form as a human body by characteristic patterns of movement.

Consider what happens when someone throws a red frisbee to you. At first, only the leading edge may be visible, giving you a retinal image of a long, flat strip that is fairly small in size. As it gets closer, the image grows in size and may change to an oval shape as the frisbee angles into the wind. As it goes through patches of sun and shade, the light frequencies reaching your colour receptors change. The tendency to see objects as unchanged in spite of changes in sensory input (due, for example, to movement or the brightness of light) is called **perceptual constancy.** We depend on these constancies—size, shape, colour, etc.—to the extent that illusions may be produced by violating them. Special effects in films, for example, can make a person appear to shrink by making the images of the objects that apparently are grouped around them increase rapidly in size.

As well as these processes for perceiving form, there are others involved in perceiving motion. When an object moves, such as the frisbee above, its image changes in predictable ways. The change in its shape is gradual, as is its increase in size. It also obscures different parts of the environment successively. Illusions of movement may occur as well. If we are in a stationary vehicle, and the vehicle next to us begins to move, we may get the momentary sensation that it is our vehicle moving backwards. In the same way, we may get the sensation at night that the Moon is racing through the clouds, when it is actually the clouds that are moving. Since the clouds are part of the ground—the dark sky—it is the figure that is seen to move. It is possible to mimic this apparent movement of stationary objects in the laboratory. The **phi phenomenon** is created when stationary lights are lit in sequence to imitate movement. This effect is used in some neon signs or illuminated scoreboards to grab attention with moving arrows or cartoon-like figures.

Not all of our perceptual processes are innate, and even innate ones can be modified by experience (that is, **learning**). Cultural differences are a good indication of this. People in developed countries tend to have a lot of experience with rectangles—walls, doors and so on. Some of the most impressive illusions are based on distortions from our expectations that walls are rectangles. In some places in Africa, round houses are the standard form, and cultures have few rectangular artefacts. People who live in this kind of perceptual environment are less often fooled by illusions based on rectangles. In the same way, desert-dwelling peoples—including some Indigenous Australians—attend more to detail on the horizon, and are therefore less prone to illusions caused by context. Culture has a strong effect on how we perceive health and illness.

Perceptual constancy: the tendency to see objects as unchanged in spite of changes in sensory input.

Phi phenomenon: the generation of apparent movement by the successive appearance of two spatially separated stimuli, such as the flashing of two lights.

Learning: a change in behaviour that results from experience with the environment.

CROSS-REFERENCE

Culture is discussed in Chapters 14, 15 and 16.

EXPECTATION AND PERCEPTION

Optical illusions are based on images that either give the organism only partial information or provide misleading elements. Perceptual processes normally operate smoothly and consistently in interpreting the world. We are able to navigate without too many accidents, reinterpreting and remapping where problems arise. We expect that the world will make sense, that objects will remain constant, and that sensory data and external events will correspond. Occasionally, we make mistakes because the cues we receive do not fit the reality of the objects we perceive. Most of you will have walked into a familiar room in the dark, reached confidently for the light switch, and found that it was not there. What you have done is to use your expectations about its location and come up with an answer that is not quite right.

Look at the object in Figure 4.4, sometimes called a 'poiuyt' (look at the top row of letter keys on a standard computer keyboard to find the source of this word). Each part of the object makes sense, but the whole does not. It violates our expectations about the systematic representation of objects. Often, illusions take advantage of a **perceptual set**: a tendency to expect to see a particular thing. A perceptual set may be the result of learning in a particular context. When a friend from the United States first arrived in Australia, he used to injure himself on doorknobs because the average Australian doorknob is a good deal higher than the average American doorknob. As there is almost certainly nothing innate about expectations regarding the heights of doorknobs, this must have resulted from learning.

A set may also result from cueing; that is, being led to expect that we will see a particular thing. If we are told that in Figure 4.5 we should see a vase, we are more likely to see the vase and less likely to see the other possible interpretation of this figure—two faces. Expectations can bias our perceptions strongly. When we cannot find our keys, it is probably because they are out of the expected context for them (in the fruit bowl), in a place we are convinced we've already searched, in an unexpected arrangement (with the familiar tag hidden) or even in a logical but unexpected place (still hanging from the door lock).

Perceptual set: the readiness to perceive something in a particular way or using a particular frame of reference.

Figure 4.4   An impossible object

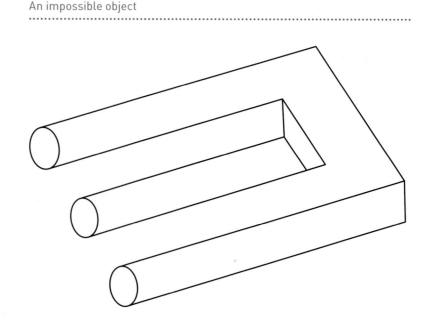

Figure 4.5   A reversible figure

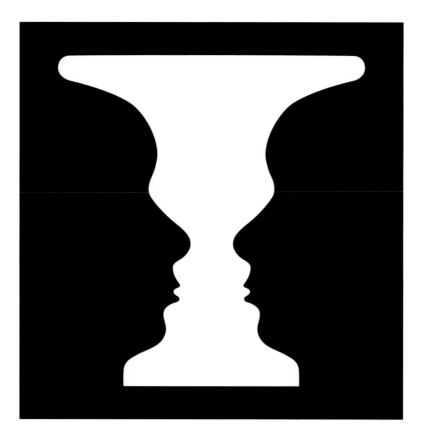

PAUSE & REFLECT

Doctors see a lot of children who have colds, coughs and runny noses. Could this result in a perceptual set? How might this effect the doctor's behaviour?

PERSON PERCEPTION

The perception of other people involves many of the same processes as the perception of objects and is also subject to many of the same errors. We use three main processes for inference about others, processes that are quite similar to perceptual constancies, or sets. We assume constancy over time, across the characteristics of an individual, and across categories of similar individuals.

The first expectation we bring to person perception is that when we meet someone for the first time, we tend to assume that they are giving us a fair sample of their normal behaviour. If that person is drunk, we may assume that they have a drinking problem. This process of **temporal extension** (Secord & Backman 1964)—interpreting the past and future on a sample of behaviour—explains why first impressions are so strong. A second, or third or twentieth contact can never completely erase the first. They can only modify the expectations set up at that time. Gradually, if enough contradictory evidence is obtained, those expectations will change.

The second expectation is that an individual will be consistent within themselves. This assumption of individual consistency will lead us to assume that someone who looks rough

Temporal extension: interpreting the past and future on a single or limited sample of behaviour.

will behave in a rough fashion, that someone with an unusual haircut will be unusual in other ways, or that someone who can perform mathematical wonders will be intelligent. An extreme example of how badly assumptions of consistency can mislead us is the so-called *idiot savant* ('wise idiot', from the French). These are people of subnormal intelligence who can perform tremendous feats in some limited area. Cases have been reported of people who have learnt the perpetual calendar by heart and can instantly tell you which day of the week any given date over a thousand-year period will fall on, but who are unable to tell you what day of the week they go to church. One boy in the USA has memorised the batting averages of every major league baseball player—living and dead—for whom those statistics are available, but is unable to understand how they were calculated, or why. We can even expect consistency from an individual based on their similarity to someone else. If they look somewhat like a friend who is kind, we might assume, without any other information, that the new acquaintance will be kind.

Stereotyping: the assumption that a member of a category of people will share all of the characteristics attributed to that category.

The third process is **stereotyping**, where a member of a category of people is assumed to share all of the characteristics of the stereotype of that category (Allport 1954). Such assumptions include the ideas that fat people are jolly, Chinese are hardworking, redheads have quick tempers or health science students have no leisure interests. It is easy to reject stereotyping as prejudice and to maintain that everyone should be treated as an individual and on their own merits; however, much of our behaviour is based on dealing with categories of people—waiters, pedestrians, women or men, Americans or Indigenous Australians—and having knowledge of appropriate ways to deal with the categories is very useful. Assuming that waiters, say, prefer not to be treated too familiarly and that they like to receive tips will make dealing with most waiters easy and anxiety-free. Imagine how complex life would be if we had to treat each pedestrian as if they shared no common patterns of behaviour, such as where they would cross the road, or whether they would look first. Stereotyping inevitably leads to a breakdown of communications to the extent that it is inaccurate, and may even lead to disaster where it is used to justify discriminatory behaviour. This can influence an individual's access to appropriate treatment when they are ill, among other things.

CROSS-REFERENCE
Inequalities and access to health care are discussed in Chapter 16.

CASE STUDY

SANDI WILLIAMS AND BREAST CANCER

The aim of this case is to consider how a younger woman may react to the experience of a life threatening illness.

Sandi Williams is a 32-year-old mother of two children, Sam (7 years) and Kristie (4 years). Her partner Stewart is a contract builder. Sandi is a partner in the family business: she schedules appointments for Stewart, orders materials and does the accounting for the business. Working from home suits Sandi, especially while the children are so young. Sandi enjoyed breastfeeding both her children and had only stopped night-time feeds with Kristie 12 months ago. From time to time, Sandi was aware of lumps in her breasts. Recently when Sandi first discovered a lump in her left breast, she thought it would pass. When it was still there three weeks later, Sandi decided to see her GP.

Sandi thought the lump was not normal and sought medical attention relatively quickly, but she probably didn't realise the seriousness of her illness. Her GP quickly referred Sandi for a mammogram and a cell biopsy of the lump. On returning to her GP, she was told that the results indicated cancer and that surgery was recommended for removal of the tumour and associated lymph nodes under her arm. These events occurred quickly.

After Sandi was discharged from hospital she said, 'I no longer felt like a woman. I lost my breast, and couldn't have more children. ... [A]ll of a sudden the life I had planned had been taken away from me. When you see your mastectomy scar, it starts under your arm and goes right across your chest. There's no way you can hide that, it's there.... [E]very time you look in the mirror you are reminded of the breast cancer.'

Sandi felt angry that her future reproductive choices had been taken away. She was also distressed by the scarring to her body and other changes as a result of the chemotherapy. At her life stage she was enjoying in her family responsibilities. She was also disadvantaged by the fact she had to attend medical consultations and outpatient treatments by herself without a support person because her husband and other family were either working and/ or caring for the couple's children.

Sandi also found herself supporting others in the family: 'My close family members, including my mother, found it very difficult to accept [the diagnosis] and I found I was counselling them. ... [T]hat was demanding because I had to set aside my own emotions in order to cope with other people's grief.'

The aggressive chemotherapy caused distress. Sandi said, 'I thought I was going to die from the drugs not from the cancer. My mouth was full of painful ulcers.... I was going bald and I lost a lot of weight. I really didn't want my kids to be seeing me like this.'

1   How might Sandi have reacted to the thought of something being wrong when she first discovered the lump in her breast? Consider possible perceptions she may have at this time.

2   How would the speed of the diagnosis have affected Sandi's ability to cope with this event?

3   How did Sandi respond to the recommended treatment?

4   In what ways did Sandi's life stage influence her responses to the breast cancer treatments?

5   How might Sandi's grief reactions about her illness differ from those of an older person in, say, their seventies?

6   What are some of Sandi's capabilities and how might they affect her ability to complete her treatment and move forward?

Points to consider

Breast cancer is the most common cancer diagnosis for women worldwide. The incidence for women under 50 years of age accounts for 25 per cent of all breast cancer cases in Australia (AIHW 2008). However, there is limited understanding about the experiences of young women with breast cancer.

Younger women are more likely to be diagnosed with a biologically aggressive cancer and tend to need a combination of different treatments. Different treatments may result in different physical and psychological consequences. For example, younger women are likely to have heightened concern about body image if surgery is required, and fatigue and nausea from chemotherapy. The treatment regime immediately after diagnosis often causes significant stress.

Young women often go through a 'why me' phase soon after diagnosis. There may be a sense of disbelief quickly followed by anger and fear.

CHAPTER SUMMARY

- Individuals who identify that they are ill—that something is not right with them—experience physical, cognitive, emotional and behavioural reactions.
- The process by which a well person comes to think of themselves as ill is called 'illness behaviour'. Illness behaviour can be thought of as a series of decisions about the individual's experience that may lead them to take on the sick role.
- Taking on this role involves accepting two obligations (to want to get well and to cooperate with appropriate experts) in return for being granted two rights (being excused from normal responsibilities and not being blamed for being ill). If the sick role is accepted for too long, the person may be regarded as showing abnormal illness behaviour.
- Reactions to illness are influenced by characteristics of the illness, the individual and the situation. Each person has a particular set of vulnerabilities and capabilities that may result from genetic factors, which either predispose the individual to the development of future problems or protect the individual from them.
- Genetic predispositions do not guarantee a particular set of health outcomes. Exposure to the environment modifies them. This can happen during development of the baby in the uterus (in utero factors), around the time of birth (perinatal factors) and during life thereafter.
- Vulnerabilities and capabilities can include strategies that are adopted for dealing with life situations, some of which appear to have negative effects (such as hyper-reactivity or negative emotions), while others appear to have positive effects on health (such as optimism, hardiness and positive emotions).
- Illness perceptions arise from the individual's experience and guide the person's behaviour with regard to the illness. These perceptions follow the same principles as other perceptual processes, involving innate and learnt components. As with perceptual illusions, they may not accurately reflect reality.

SELF TEST

1 Jeanelle has been diagnosed with breast cancer. She dreams about turning into a scaly monster, withdraws from her friends, and tells her doctor over and over about how unfair it all is. These reactions:
   a indicate that Jeanelle has a psychiatric disorder
   b would lead her doctor to predict that she will attempt suicide
   c can only be considered abnormal if they go on too long
   d are probably the result of cancer cells lodging in the brain.

2 Marcus is a bricklayer. It can be seen from the x-rays that his wrist is broken. Marcus is relieved when told that the pain he is experiencing is the result of a broken bone because it will allow him to take time off work until it is healed. He feared that his boss would not let him take time off work if his injury was not serious. Marcus is:
   a showing abnormal illness behaviour
   b wanting to claim one of the rights of the sick role
   c trying to avoid one of the obligations of the sick role
   d probably guilty of intentionally injuring himself.

3 Which of the following examples would be seen as inconsistent with the sick role?

   a Marian follows her doctor's directions very carefully.

   b Pyotr goes to bed with a migraine headache, even though it is his turn to cook dinner.

   c After having chest pains, Eric checks himself out of hospital because he feels OK.

   d After Eric has chest pains, his boss sends him home from work.

4 In which of the following situations would it be best not to use optimistic thinking?

   a dealing with rejection

   b making a life or death decision

   c dealing with a chronic illness

   d going for a job interview.

5 Evidence that health-related personality type behaviour patterns are more usefully seen as strategies includes all of the following except:

   a personality is largely determined by genetics and does not change

   b the distribution of behaviour patterns in a group changes over time

   c different tasks and situations can produce different patterns

   d individuals do not show the same patterns of behaviour at all times.

FURTHER READING

Coyne, E., Wollin, J. & Creedy, D. (2012) Exploration of the family's role and strengths after a young woman is diagnosed with breast cancer: Views of the women and their families. *European Journal of Oncology Nursing*, online: http://dx.doi.org/10.1016/j.ejon.2011.04.013.

Dietz, D.M., LaPlant, Q., Watts, E.L., Hodes, G.E., Russo, S.J., Feng, J. et al. (2011) Paternal transmission of stress-induced pathologies. *Biological Psychiatry*, 70(5), 408–14.

Swarmy G.K., Østbye T. & Skjærven R. (2008) Association of preterm birth with long-term survival, reproduction, and next-generation preterm birth. *JAMA*, 299(12), 1429–36.

USEFUL WEBSITES

Asthma Foundation:

www.asthmafoundation.org.au

Heart Foundation:

www.heartfoundation.org.au

Living with breast cancer (Cancer Council NSW):

www.cancercouncil.com.au/breast-cancer/living-with-breast-cancer/

The Illness Perception Questionnaire:

www.uib.no/ipq/index.html

UNDERSTANDING REACTIONS TO CHRONIC CONDITIONS

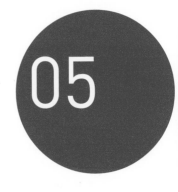

CHAPTER OBJECTIVES

By the end of your study of this chapter, you should be able to:

- define and give examples of chronic conditions
- discuss the prevalence of different chronic conditions
- outline the emotional, physical and social challenges faced by individuals who have a chronic condition
- describe common reactions to living with a chronic condition
- explain factors that may influence positive coping
- apply self-care models to explain varying ways of managing a chronic condition
- describe practical interventions and care programs for people with chronic conditions.

KEYWORDS

acceptance
affective support
chronic condition
chronic grief
cognitive responses
collaborative model
compassion fatigue
controllability
disability
efficacy beliefs

helplessness
instrumental support
medical model
optimism
perceived benefit
prevalence
psychosocial interventions
self-agency model
self-care

CHRONIC CONDITIONS

Chronic conditions are permanent, incurable and irreversible. While such conditions do not cause death, they do require ongoing lifetime attention and care. The prognosis for many chronic conditions may be unclear and treatment and/or management prolonged. The condition may interfere with activities of daily living and be accompanied by persistent emotional distress. Some individuals may cycle through periods of relatively good health, and then relapse, with associated fluctuating emotions (Imao 2005). Living with a chronic condition is often associated with a sense of loss and may have more ramifications for quality of life than other life stress.

Chronic condition: a medical condition that is permanent, incurable and irreversible.

Chronic conditions commonly reported in Australia include vision problems (such as short- or long-sightedness as well as loss of sight), allergies, back pain, arthritis, mental conditions, hypertension, asthma, deafness and diabetes (AIHW 2010). Other chronic conditions include epilepsy, renal problems, sickle cell anaemia, HIV/AIDS, tuberculosis, tinnitus, respiratory disorders (such as chronic bronchitis) and colitis. Chronic conditions, such as some forms of cancer, may be life-threatening; some, such as dementia and vision impairment, may require help with daily activities over a long period of time; and some are painful—but all demand adaptive behaviours on the part of the individual. Other chronic conditions are ambiguous, with vague symptoms that are hard to diagnose, including interstitial cystitis, chronic fatigue syndrome, fibromyalgia, irritable bowel syndrome, Crohn's disease and coeliac disease. These conditions require people to be persistent in their attempts to obtain an accurate diagnosis and this frustration and uncertainty adds to the emotional burden of living with a chronic condition (Johnson & Johnson 2006).

Chronic conditions also can cause **disability**, depending on the extent of its impact on daily life. It is important to understand that disability is neither inability nor sickness, as almost everyone will have at least one disability at some point in their life (AIHW 2010). The general public, governments and health professionals may have different views in regard to how disability is perceived, labelled and discussed. Negative perceptions by health professionals may marginalise individuals with a disabling condition and create obstacles and barriers to the access and provision of services. In fact, disability is as much about environmental obstacles and challenges as it is a medical condition (Kearney & Pryor 2004).

Disability: a characteristic of the body, mind or senses that affect a person's ability to engage independently in some or all aspects of day-to-day life.

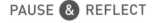

PAUSE & REFLECT

What are your personal beliefs about people with a disability?

The words used about people influence attitudes. Previously, it was acceptable to describe individuals with a mental or physical disability as 'retarded' or 'handicapped'. These terms are no longer acceptable because they imply that the person is somehow completely incapable. Even the term 'disabled' should not be used because it suggests that the whole individual is disabled and that they have no abilities. Although less fluent, the term 'individual with a disability' is more accurate and less limiting.

PREVALENCE OF CHRONIC CONDITIONS

As discussed in Chapter 1, **prevalence** is the number of existing and new cases of a specific disease present in a given population at a certain time. Many people are afflicted by a chronic

Prevalence: the number of existing or new cases of a specific disease present in a given population at a certain time.

Incidence: the rate at which new cases of a specific disease occur in a population during a specified period.

condition, and this high prevalence accounts for the bulk of health care expenditure and mortality in Australia (AIHW 2010). Individuals living with a chronic condition form a large health-care consumer group. Just under one in five Australians (18.5 per cent) reported a disability in the National Health Survey 2007–08. A further 21 per cent had a long-term health condition but it did not restrict their everyday activities at that time (ABS 2009b). The **incidence** (that is, the rate at which new cases occur in a population during a specified period) of disability also increases with age. Almost ninety percent of people aged 90 years and over have a disability, compared with 3.4 per cent of those aged four years and under (ABS 2009a). Disability is not inevitable in older age but it does become more common, with conditions such as dementia, back pain and arthritis being leading causes that severely limit activities of daily living (AIHW 2010). Ageing can also accelerate the level of impairment associated with a chronic condition.

Most chronic conditions of childhood, unlike those of adults, are not preventable by lifestyle changes. Surprisingly, at least 10 per cent of adolescents live with a chronic condition. Some conditions are characterised by increasing incidence (for example, type 1 diabetes) or improving survival rates (for example, cystic fibrosis), while other conditions such as cancer or mental illness are concerning because the outcomes are poorer for adolescents compared with adults. Young people with chronic conditions are doubly disadvantaged. Sawyer et al. (2007) reported that adolescents with a chronic condition engaged in risky behaviours as often or more often than their healthy peers, but had the potential for greater adverse health outcomes from these behaviours. For young males, the risk of disability lies more frequently in injury from accidents, whereas in the middle years of adulthood the risk factors tend to be work-related injury or conditions such as arthritis, cardiovascular disease, hearing problems and psychiatric conditions (AIHW 2010).

Gender also appears to be associated with certain chronic conditions. Arthritis is a group of conditions characterised by inflammation of the joints causing pain, stiffness, disability and deformity (AIHW 2010). Worldwide, osteoarthritis (degenerative disease of the joints) is the most common musculoskeletal disorder. It affects 1.6 million Australians, with females more affected than males (AIHW 2010). Similarly, osteoporosis (low bone density) is a disease that mainly, though not exclusively, affects postmenopausal women. Although it is preventable, osteoporosis is called a silent disease because symptoms often don't become evident until a major incident (such as a fracture) occurs. Women across all age groups are also more likely to be diagnosed with depression. This is not to say that gender is predictive of certain chronic conditions developing. Rather, this relationship is more likely to reflect that women live longer than men and so proportionally there are more women with degenerative conditions such as dementia or arthritis. Similarly, it is well known that women are more likely to express their distress and seek professional help than are men and so are more likely to be diagnosed with symptoms of depression or any other condition.

IMPACT ON DAILY LIFE

Living with a chronic condition or acquired disability can have disruptive effects on many areas of functioning and require positive and persistent coping strategies. The sense of loss may be more debilitating than the condition itself. People with a chronic condition may not require acute medical interventions beyond the primary diagnosis and treatment, but this does not mean that they are free to live an unrestricted life. Chronic conditions affect work, social life, relationships and recreational activities, as well as family, friends and the community. Individuals are faced with managing their condition every day. Some chronic conditions limit movement and the person may require daily assistance with activities such as hygiene, walking or communication. Much of this assistance is provided by informal sources such as family, friends and neighbours (AIHW 2010). Individuals not only live with the physical symptoms of their condition (such as pain for arthritis sufferers), but may also endure ongoing fatigue, depression and sleep disturbances. They also often suffer financial stress from treatment costs and loss of income.

BEN FELDMAN AND MULTIPLE SCLEROSIS

CASE STUDY

The aim of this case study is to explore the experience of living with a chronic condition.

Ben Feldman is a divorced 42-year-old mechanic who owns a busy mechanical repair outfit. He has two school-aged children from his marriage and has custody every second weekend. Recently, Ben experienced tingling in the fourth and fifth fingers of his left hand and began to feel uncoordinated when working on a motor. It was as if he had lost feeling in his hands. He went to his local general practitioner who identified some minor neurological changes (intermittent tingling and slight loss of strength). The doctor thought there was nothing to worry about and the symptoms disappeared after six weeks. When the symptoms reappeared the following year, Ben was referred to a neurologist for a comprehensive assessment. The MRI revealed abnormal changes in his brain and spine. A detailed history identified that symptoms had been evident for the past five years. Ben was diagnosed with multiple sclerosis (MS) and began intramuscular injections every second day, which needed to continue even when he no longer had symptoms.

1   What might Ben's immediate reaction be to his diagnosis and treatment?
2   Which areas of Ben's life might be affected by the symptoms of his condition?

Multiple sclerosis (MS) is a chronic and highly disabling condition. The myelin thickness (covering) around nerves is reduced, and results in muscle weakness, balance problems and spasticity (Gallien et al. 2007). Although MS usually affects young women, 30 per cent of sufferers are men. The degree of disability depends on which nerve myelin is affected and the course of the disease: relapsing, remitting or progressive. Fatigue is one of the symptoms most frequently reported. Therapy for MS involves supportive care, management of symptoms, and disease-modifying drugs that may delay progression and reduce the number of exacerbation (deteriorating) episodes (Taylor et al. 2007).

Psychological responses to a chronic condition vary, but it is common for individuals to feel helpless, anxious and depressed. At times they may also feel resentful that this is happening to them. As the condition continues the person may feel inferior to others, guilty for being a burden to their family, fearful of the future, discouraged by the continuing decline in their health, and lonely because of social isolation.

Feelings of anxiety may be associated with a lack of knowledge about the condition and its long-term implications. While some conditions have a relatively stable course, others involve cycles of exacerbation and remission, with all the associated fluctuations of emotion. Responses may be akin to mourning, since the individual experiences several losses—including loss of bodily functions—and a wide range of social limitations. As discussed in Chapter 3, stages of mourning include shock, denial, emotional confusion, attempted resolution and acceptance or closure. Individuals are unlikely to progress through these stages in a neat, linear fashion; stages tend to overlap, occur in parallel and recur (Imao 2005).

Chronic grief:
unresolved grief characterised by an impaired ability to recall personal life details, imagine future events and plan for the future.

Living with a debilitating chronic condition may lead to complicated or **chronic grief**. Maccallum and Bryant (2011) observed that individuals suffering chronic grief had difficulty recalling positive personal life details and imagining future events. The ability to picture the future is important for effective planning of day-to-day activities, evaluating future outcomes, judging likelihood of success and deciding on a particular course of action. Imagining specific details of events in the future can affect whether a person takes action or not. For example, individuals who develop specific plans about where and when they intended to start a particular health-related behaviour (such as going for a morning walk in the park) are more likely to do it. Individuals living with a chronic condition are faced with many new and challenging situations. Difficulty imagining specific future events may impact not only on day-to-day tasks, but also on the degree to which these individuals are able to develop new roles and aspects of their identity.

Positive emotions also play a role in living with a chronic condition. Humour, hope and courage were found to be key factors for rural women learning to live with a chronic condition. For these women, humour was the most frequently used strategy (Sullivan, Weinert & Cudney 2003). For others, reflecting on a sense of purpose and meaning of the experience was helpful.

CROSS-REFERENCE
The broader issues of coping with stress are addressed in Chapter 13.

Individuals with a physical disability as a result of their chronic condition also suffer a number of other life stressors and limitations, including poor employment prospects and low income. Many have to pay for a carer, or their family may need to pay for respite care. A physical disability may isolate a person, making it difficult to form friendships and intimate relationships, which in turn can contribute to emotional issues such as depression. Some people who are socially isolated and dependent on others can also be at increased risk of abuse from carers, particularly family members under stress (Piotrowski & Snell 2007).

Chronic conditions also have ramifications for family or other carers. Consider, for example, the roles and responsibilities of parents not only caring for a child with a chronic condition, but also managing the child's developing understanding of their illness (as discussed in Chapter 2). Parents' attitudes often define the situation, including whether they focus on illness and vulnerability, or normalcy and capability (Creedy et al. 2005). They have to carry out many tasks to manage the condition, such as administering medication, developing a consistent parenting philosophy, and having a family routine that is as normal as possible and allows some fun. Finally, there are future implications and expectations about the impact on the child and the family. A picture emerges of what it might be like to care for a child with a chronic condition or disability, including how parents can shape the child's identity as someone who is sick or someone who copes, and demands on parents to be knowledgeable and capable about treatments, and to work together and have an integrated care strategy. Other issues include how the child's condition might dictate to or dominate family life, and the parents' concern for the child's future. At the other end of the age spectrum, the burden of caring for ageing parents is increasingly falling to their middle-aged children.

Compassion fatigue: a deep physical, emotional and spiritual exhaustion related to repeated exposure to another's suffering.

Having a close relative or friend involved in care can have positive or negative implications on the person's experience of living with the condition, in terms of both following treatment advice or engaging in other health promoting behaviours. However, providing care for someone with a chronic condition can take its toll on family or other caregivers. Those providing long-term care for individuals with a chronic condition can suffer **compassion fatigue**, which is one cost of caring for an individual who is not going to recover completely (Day & Anderson 2012). Compassion fatigue is a deep physical, emotional and spiritual exhaustion related to repeated exposure to another's suffering and can lead to depression, anxiety and burnout.

PAUSE & REFLECT

Imagine that you have just been diagnosed with a chronic condition such as diabetes, asthma or epilepsy. How would you feel? Would one type of chronic condition be better or worse than another? Why?

BEN (CONT.) CASE STUDY

Initially, Ben found it difficult to think of himself as sick, and he was resentful about the need to have the second daily injections. A year after his diagnosis, the symptoms reappeared for three weeks. This episode unsettled Ben. The reality of his condition became obvious to him in a way that he had not thought about before. He was worried about his future: his health, his business, his ability to see his children, and how his new partner Dianne would cope being in a relationship with 'an invalid'. These thoughts kept going around in his mind and contributed to sleeplessness and, subsequently, depression.

His doctor prescribed antidepressant medication, but after a week Ben didn't feel any different and so stopped taking it. His schedule of injections was also changed to weekly to reduce the likelihood of drug fatigue. Fortunately, Ben's brother, who is also a mechanic, agreed to join the business and now manages the repairs. Ben continues to be involved by doing minor work and and taking care of the bookwork. He can cope with routine tasks but becomes frustrated easily and he is having difficulty with problem solving due to changes to the frontal lobe of his brain. He wonders how he will cope when he has another episode.

1   What other day-to-day difficulties might Ben and the people in his life face?
2   How might Ben's children respond to changes in him? What might they understand about his condition?

VARIATIONS IN INDIVIDUAL COPING

Psychological responses and problems associated with chronic conditions are not always similar. It is incorrect to assume that people living with a chronic condition or disability all experience or cope with the condition in the same way. Individuals may respond with either problem-focused coping or emotion-focused coping, or both (as discussed in Chapter 4). Whether individuals cope well with their condition relies on a range of factors, including the type of condition, how they rate their health, the way they think about their condition, their belief in their ability to cope (their optimism) and the controllability of the condition.

A diagnosis of HIV/AIDS has a profound psychological impact, with complex stressors and multiple symptoms along with potential discrimination and loss of social support. Cancer is a particularly frightening diagnosis for the person who may have to face the possibility of death

CROSS-REFERENCE
Individual differences in vulnerability are discussed in Chapter 4.

Cognitive responses:
how a person views
their condition.

CROSS-REFERENCE
The discussion of
cognition and health
continues in Chapter 7.

Helplessness:
a negative, maladaptive
response to a condition
that has long-term,
adverse implications
for psychological and
physical health.

Acceptance: a more
neutral or middle-
of-the-road reaction
to a condition that
diminishes the negative
meaning of the condition
and thus represents a
decrease in negative
thinking.

Perceived benefit: a
positive response to
a condition that adds
optimistic meaning
through increased
positive thinking.

Efficacy belief: the
belief by a person that
they can carry out
required treatments.

Optimism: a tendency
to expect that outcomes
will generally be good.

Controllability: the
level of control over a
condition; it can be both
actual and perceived.

and an unpleasant and difficult treatment regime that has debilitating side effects (Petrie, Broadbent & Meechan 2003). As identified in the case study of Ben Feldman, MS is a progressive disease that produces a wide range of symptoms that the person cannot predict or regulate. The condition, which causes the individual to deteriorate over time, affects several life domains, including work, family, relationships and sexual functioning.

Cognitive responses, or the way a person views their condition, has received considerable attention in research. A large study by Finnegan, Marion and Cox (2005) showed that people's views about their health ranged from excellent to poor, even though all had a diagnosed chronic condition. When faced with the long-term stress of a chronic condition, individuals can react in favourable and unfavourable ways. These responses represent reliable and stable patterns and can be classified into three common cognitive evaluations of what is an inherently life-changing situation (Evers et al. 2001).

The first type of response is **helplessness,** which emphasises the negative aspects and meaning of the condition as unmanageable, uncontrollable and unpredictable. This cognitive pattern is associated with increased functional disability. The second type of response is **acceptance**, a more neutral or middle-of-the-road reaction that diminishes the negative meaning of the condition and decreases the amount of negative thinking. It consists of accepting the condition and learning to tolerate or live with it. **Perceived benefit** is the third response. It adds optimistic meaning to the condition and increases the likelihood of positive thinking and coping. Individuals who think this way may see the condition as an opportunity to reassess their life and priorities, such as spending more time with their families or slowing down at work. Acceptance and other adaptive thoughts are associated with less focus on disease-related activity, fewer physical complaints and more positive mood (Evers et al. 2001).

Efficacy beliefs play a key role in coping. Fear remains high if the person doesn't believe the recommended treatment is effective (response efficacy) and if the person doesn't believe they can carry out the treatment (self-efficacy). In a study of young people with type 1 (insulin-dependent) diabetes, Lawson et al. (2005) found that many participants reported high anxiety about the future and had low perceived control of their condition. Rather than taking action to manage the condition and address threats to their physical well-being, they took action to reduce their perceptions of fear (including smoking marijuana, drinking alcohol, taking tranquillisers and other drugs, listening to music or otherwise distracting themselves).

Optimism is another factor that determines how well or poorly individuals cope. In a longitudinal study on the effect of living with diabetes or multiple sclerosis on optimism, Fournier, Ridder and Bensing (2003) found three types of optimistic beliefs: positive outcome expectancies (an expectation that things will turn out well), efficacy expectancies (the belief that a range of difficult situations can be coped with) and optimistic bias (a tendency to unrealistically expect only positive things will happen). Importantly, individuals with positive outcome and efficacy expectancies were more likely to exhibit more adaptive responses to this chronic condition; they tend to accept the health risks and take positive action to cope.

Controllability is also associated with coping and can be both actual and perceived. If the individual believes that they are able to control symptoms, they are more likely to adjust, enjoy life and avoid depression. Medical knowledge tells us that some diseases are more manageable than others. Controllability of MS, for example, is low, whereas type 2 diabetes mellitus can be controlled through diet, exercise and insulin. A person with type 2 diabetes, therefore, is likely to perceive high levels of control over their condition and to actually demonstrate their control on a daily basis.

Perceptions of control can also be influenced by the unique characteristics of specific conditions. Asthma and epilepsy, for example, are two chronic conditions that can have dramatic and severe episodes interspersed with periods of relative symptom-free health. Epilepsy, however, is associated with a lower quality of life in young people, partly because a seizure is more dramatic and unpredictable than an asthma attack. When compared with other young people with asthma, adolescents with epilepsy experienced more anxiety and less happiness, along with social withdrawal and negative attitudes towards the condition (Stanton, Revenson & Tennen 2007). Gender differences were also identified, in that girls generally fared worse than boys.

MODELS OF SELF-CARE

Self-regulation, which was first introduced by Leventhal, Meyer and Nerenz (1980), is a useful theoretical perspective for understanding how a person manages their chronic condition. **Self-care** or self-regulation in the context of a chronic condition relates to the action taken by a person to improve their health and limit the negative effects of the condition. There is a strong and growing body of evidence that self-regulation has many benefits for individuals living with a chronic condition, including improved health status and better quality of life. Individuals who are able to regulate their thoughts and feelings are more likely to proactively approach their problems and develop certain thoughts and beliefs that guide how they respond to the condition in order to manage it. Self-regulation is modified by feedback; for example, blood glucose levels in the case of diabetes or peak flow measures of lung capacity for a person with asthma. These measures provide immediate feedback to a person about how well they are managing their condition and motivate them to keep up the good work or make some changes in their lives. Coping strategies may include short-term and immediate action to manage the physical symptoms, such as taking preventative medicine to avoid serious asthma attacks, or long-term action such as maintaining a low-dust environment in the home. Coping also includes learning how to engage with the health system for care, obtain support from health care services and organisations, and seek out information.

Timely and accurate feedback can help individuals to manage or regulate their condition more effectively. In the case of diabetes, testing blood glucose levels gives immediate feedback about whether more insulin is needed. Other self-management behaviours, such as diet and exercise, require persistence before longer-term impact is observed. Since this feedback is not immediate, individuals are less likely to carry out this aspect of regulating their condition (Petrie, Broadbent & Meechan 2003). There many models of self-care or self-management for chronic conditions and we discuss three here: the medical model, the collaborative model and the self-agency model.

The **medical model for managing a chronic condition** is prescriptive. It focuses on patients' compliance with or adherence to medical management instructions about medication and testing routines as directed by health care practitioners (in most cases, the general practitioner). In this model the individual is objectified as the patient, the health practitioner is the authority, and the person isn't given much credence. The doctor manages the disease process, with the patient compelled to trust the doctor's medical knowledge. In this situation, the focus is on medical criteria with little thought given to how the condition affects other aspects of day-to-day life and how to cope with it (Koch, Jenkin & Kralik 2004).

Self-care: the management by health care practitioners of their own personal resources, including their time, energy and physical health.

Medical model for managing a chronic condition: a model that is prescriptive and focused on patients' compliance with or adherence to medical management instructions.

Collaborative model:
a model in which patients are active participants, in partnership with health care providers, in regulating and managing their chronic condition.

A less paternalistic model of care sees patients as active participants in regulating and managing the chronic condition (Petrie, Broadbent & Meechan 2003). This **collaborative model** of self-management is about a partnership between the person and health care providers. The management of the chronic condition is seen as a combination of biomedical knowledge and patient experience. This model is often reflected in services offered by community-based clinics, where people can learn about a range of strategies to manage their day-to-day life as well as medical management involving medication and monitoring (Koch, Jenkin & Kralik 2004). A variation of this model is 'supported self-care', which aims to empower individuals, views patients as experts, and ultimately reduces demand on health care resources (Wilson & Mayor 2006). The role of the health professional in this model is to identify existing strengths and skills of the person and to work towards using these abilities more effectively. Although programs based on this model aim to reduce health care costs, the evidence for this is mixed (Richardson et al. 2005).

Self-agency model:
a model in which individuals take charge of their condition, identify their responses and manage their lives accordingly.

CROSS-REFERENCE
Part 4 of this book looks at other aspects of agency.

The **self-agency model** requires individuals to take charge of their condition, identify their responses to the condition and manage their lives to create order, control and discipline. Although individuals with a chronic condition are required to regularly take medication and follow the recommended regime of care, this model also involves self-monitoring and developing lifestyle habits to accommodate the condition. People are also able to exhibit strategic cheating or non-compliance. It is possible for a person with diabetes, say, to be less strict with their diet and medication in a well-thought-out fashion, such as when they need to make compromises in their diet for work or a social event. In the self-agency model, individuals choose when to call upon professional health expertise. People who have lived with their condition for a long time often develop a great deal of expertise about managing their lives and their condition. The knowledge and skills of the health care providers are added to their own (Koch, Jenkin & Kralik 2004). The self-agency model was identified in one study in which individuals with diabetes did not attend diabetes clinics (Lawson et al. 2005). Labelled 'patient as expert', these people were independent, with high self-efficacy beliefs and high controllability perceptions. They did not need a great deal of outside help and felt no need to attend clinics.

PAUSE & REFLECT

There are different models of self-care. What factors could determine whether individuals with a chronic condition and health care practitioners prefer one model over another?

CASE STUDY

BEN (CONT.)

One of Ben's friends looked up MS on the internet and gave him a lot of information about it. Some of it was very confusing and technical, especially in regards to 'exacerbation' of the condition. Ben and Dianne went back to his doctor to try to get a clear, simple explanation of the long-term consequences of the condition. The doctor spoke to Ben and Dianne about MS and suggested that he attend the MS clinic at the local hospital, as well as book in for an information session there. The doctor also recommended that Ben take Dianne with him.

When Ben's children came over for the weekend, his daughter, Hayley, who started high school this year, said that she was reading a biography on the First Lady of the United States, Michelle Obama. Mrs Obama reported that her father had MS that started in his mid-thirties, but unfortunately the book did not go into much detail about how it affected her childhood. Hayley did not realise that MS affects a lot of people around the world. She was beginning to notice some physical changes in her dad, and he sometimes became angry over little things that would not have bothered him before. She was worried about him and wondered what she could do to help.

By going to the information session, Ben and Dianne started to get some understanding of what having MS really meant. He was struggling with the regular injections and found it hard to cope with functional changes to his dexterity in his hands and balance, as well as his mood swings. He sometimes felt quite well and wondered if the injections were really necessary and if the doctor's dire warnings about what might happen to him were just scaremongering. Ben believes that his MS isn't that bad. Surely nothing really serious would happen to him?

1   How might Dianne benefit from going to the clinic as well?

2   How would you describe Ben's coping at this stage?

3   What sort of support does Hayley need right now? How can she best support her dad?

PRACTICAL CARE AND INTERVENTIONS

By definition, chronic conditions do not have a cure. Therefore, health care tries to help the person to adapt, be resilient and obtain the best quality of life they can. Helping people with a chronic condition requires a shift in thinking from the acute-care model to a flexible, long-term approach (Sullivan, Weinert & Cudney 2003). Rehabilitation and other health interventions should be focused not only on physical health, but also on engaging or re-engaging with day-to-day life and the broader society in the form of work, community groups and so on.

The aim of interventions for those with a chronic condition or disability is to achieve a satisfying, hopeful life in which contributions can be made and valued. This requires the support of people who will stand by and believe in the individual. Life-long coping requires persistence and patience since there will be many small gains and just as many setbacks. People with a chronic condition need a range of different supports. One study of people with vision impairment found that **affective (emotional) support** (such as communicating positive feelings and providing constructive feedback and advice from family, friends and others) was more useful than **instrumental support** (such as physical assistance or checking up on them) (Reinhardt, Boerner & Horowitz 2006). Affective support helped reduce symptoms of depression and helped individuals to adapt. Instrumental support did not have such positive effects, even though the individuals recognised that they needed physical help with their condition.

Health care providers working with people with chronic conditions may be part of a multidisciplinary team of nurses, physicians, psychologists or other mental health workers, pharmacists, occupational or physical therapists, and members of the clergy or other spiritual support people. This multidisciplinary approach can be illustrated in the case of cerebral palsy. Cerebral palsy results from damage to the brain prior to or during birth. There are physical

Affective support:
communicating positive feelings and providing constructive feedback and advice.

Instrumental support:
the act of giving physical assistance.

consequences, such as muscular impairment, that affect physical coordination, speech and movement. There are risks of secondary physical problems such as bronchitis, and emotional problems such as depression and anxiety. An integrated disciplinary approach involving doctors, nurses, psychologists, dieticians and physiotherapists is required because the condition adversely affects mobility, self-care and learning, and limits social roles and participation in education, work and relationships (Kearney & Pryor 2004).

HEALTH PROMOTION

The concept of health has traditionally been defined as the absence of disease (as discussed in Chapter 1), making it difficult to conceive that people with a disability might otherwise be healthy. The health of individuals with a chronic condition varies as much as it does among people without any such condition. Health is a dynamic entity that oscillates from good to poor throughout life. This is true for all people, including those with a chronic condition. Someone with a spinal cord injury who eats well, exercises and maintains the right weight could be considered at the higher end of the health continuum, whereas another individual with the same disability might eat poorly, be overweight and bed-ridden, and thus at the lower end of the scale.

CROSS-REFERENCE

Health promotion strategies are discussed in Chapter 16.

Health promotion and disease prevention are crucial for people with chronic conditions, not only to improve wellness and functioning but also to prevent secondary conditions such as obesity and osteoporosis. However, people with disabilities may experience difficulty accessing general health monitoring and screening services. Clinics may not be set up to easily accommodate people with wheelchairs, and patients may not be able to stand or manoeuvre themselves to fit in with standard equipment such as mammogram machines or examination tables. They also may need longer appointment times and more help from additional staff during examinations. During adolescence, a young woman with a chronic condition may not be interested in long-term disease prevention for conditions such as osteoporosis or diabetes; however, education at this stage is vital to take preventative action as these conditions are more likely to appear earlier in women with disabilities (Piotrowski & Snell 2007).

PSYCHOSOCIAL INTERVENTIONS

Psychosocial interventions:

psychological, social and educational strategies that aim to minimise the adverse emotional and social impact of a condition on individuals and their families.

Psychosocial interventions aim to address the psychological and social consequences of living with a condition. Emotional support and information are required to help reduce the initial confusion and shock associated with diagnosis, and, in the longer term, help individuals and their families to avoid negative emotional symptoms. Accurate information improves patients' coping because they are able to develop a realistic view of their capabilities. Psychosocial interventions also need to focus on practical aspects of living with, and managing, the chronic condition. In the case of asthma, for example, understanding factors that trigger an attack, treating symptoms quickly, and staying calm and optimistic means fewer attacks, fewer visits to hospital outpatient departments, fewer days off work and better overall quality of life (Petrie, Broadbent & Meechan 2003).

Attention should also be given to challenging false beliefs and reframing possible negative thoughts about the condition as being an unmanageable or uncontrollable burden. Some psychosocial interventions should aim to strengthen individual self-efficacy beliefs regarding coping with adversity, and to encourage more positive reappraisal (Karademas, Karvelis & Argyroupolou 2007). People who are positive and optimistic about their condition are more likely to rate their health as better and have lower health care costs than those with less positive views (Cross et al. 2006). Providing cancer sufferers with access to support groups and education about stress management and coping skills, for example, means they can stay focused on engaging with life, suffer less distress and depression, and cope better with treatment (Carver 2005). Provision of psychosocial interventions has been associated with increased satisfaction with treatment, closer adherence to the treatment plan and better quality of life than might otherwise be possible (Petrie, Broadbent & Meechan 2003). Further, psychosocial approaches may assist the individual to find positive meaning in the situation.

BEN (CONT.)   CASE STUDY

Three years have passed and Ben is recovering from a recent episode in which he experienced severe muscle spasms. He often gets tired, and has needed to make substantial changes to his work and home routines. As the disease has progressed, Ben has experienced other symptoms including muscle spasms, sensitivity to heat and sexual problems. By mid-afternoon he feels exhausted and is unable to concentrate. He tries to avoid heat as his symptoms seem worse after a hot shower or when he is close to a hot car engine at work. During this last episode, Ben complained of feeling 'light-headed' and felt as though everything was spinning. The doctor later explained that these symptoms are caused by damage to the nerve pathways that coordinate vision and other inputs into the brain that are needed to maintain balance. He has vision problems with blurring in one eye.

He has suffered other depressive episodes and, with Dianne's encouragement, he is taking his prescribed antidepressant medication. Ben and Dianne are attending sessions at the MS clinic at the local hospital every month. There Ben met some other men with MS and they have formed a men's support group. He also learnt some useful tips on coping with fatigue and maintaining a good level of physical well-being. His business is still operating with the help of his brother.

1   What else might Ben be able to do to improve his situation?
2   What are some of the physical and psychosocial issues Ben will face as he gets older?

PAUSE & REFLECT

Negative beliefs and attitudes make it more difficult for individuals to adjust to their condition. What might be some of the challenges to developing positive beliefs and attitudes?

Psychosocial interventions should also be offered to the family in order to promote coping and build capacity. An Australian study of young women with cancer and their families found that family members played an essential role in providing emotional support, but they also struggled to adapt to their changing circumstances (Coyne, Wollin & Creedy 2012). Families who have a member with a life-threatening condition often need help to deal with conflict, and to learn how to avoid overprotective or oversolicitous behaviours that may disempower the person they are trying to support.

There is considerable research that shows that providing psychosocial interventions to people with chronic conditions can be effective. Interventions include stress management, relaxation training, cognitive reframing and enhancing self-efficacy beliefs. Such interventions improve individuals' ability to monitor their condition, take corrective and preventative action, and reduce the distress, anxiety and depression that may accompany their condition.

CASE STUDY

LINDA NOVESKA AND OSTEOARTHRITIS

Linda is 62 years old and lives in a small rural community in South Australia. She was diagnosed with osteoarthritis five years ago, but recognises that she had signs of arthritis many years earlier. Her joints have become stiffer and harder to move over time and she notices grating sounds when she moves. On a usual day, Linda finds it hard to move when she first wakes up in the morning. The stiffness usually lasts for 30 minutes or so. It improves as she goes about her daily activities that 'warm up' her knee and ankle joints. However, later in the day, the pain gets worse when she is more active and feels better when she is resting. On some days, the pain is still present when she is resting. Overall, the pain is persistent, even at night.

Linda was an enrolled nurse in a nursing home for 20 years and realises that all that physical work played a role in the development of her arthritis. She currently receives a disability pension through her superannuation fund. Her mother who died seven years ago at the age of 74 also had arthritis. Linda is divorced, and her children are married and have families of their own to care for. Although Linda knows that her children do care, the discomfort and pain of arthritis is invisible to anyone who doesn't have it, and they cannot appreciate the restrictions it places on her. If she says 'I can't' or 'My legs hurt' or 'I'm having one of my bad days', she knows her children and grandchildren understand but still are disappointed or impatient.

Linda said that she was upset after finally being diagnosed with arthritis. Within three years she needed to resign from work due to incapacity. She then realised that she needed to accept her diagnosis and started thinking about how to adapt her life.

Linda knows that osteoarthritis cannot be cured, and that it will most likely get worse over time. However, she is trying her best to stay positive and control her symptoms. She reminds herself: 'It just helps to put this in its place. You have arthritis—it does not have you.' She knows that she will eventually need to have both knee joints replaced, but this major surgery is performed in Adelaide. She will need to find accommodation in the city and then have a lot of help during her post-operative recovery and rehabilitation. Meanwhile she does a range of things that cannot make the arthritis go away, but can help delay surgery. Linda was 22 kilograms overweight, but has now lost 16 kilograms in an effort to reduce wear and tear on her hip, knee and ankle joints. She takes over-the-counter pain medication and her doctor recommended nonsteroidal anti-inflammatory drugs (such as aspirin or ibuprofen).

If the pain is continually present, Linda has corticosteroids injected into the joint to reduce swelling and pain.

Linda lives an hour from the closest hospital, and she finds that driving that distance while in pain drains all her energy before she even arrives. However, Linda does volunteer work on the days when the pain is not too bad. She helps to make craft for Red Cross. She said, 'Coming out of the spin cycle of dwelling on the pain and letting it dominate my thoughts helps me cope.'

1   What might Linda's reaction be to her initial diagnosis and treatment?
2   What are some of the positive and negative effects of family attitudes on the person with a chronic condition?
3   How could Linda be assisted in coming to terms with her condition?
4   How would you describe Linda's response to her condition? Has her response changed over time?
5   What might be some of the warning signs for Linda and her family that she is depressed?
6   What are some other possible activities that someone like Linda could be involved with?

Points to consider

The challenges and problems associated with chronic conditions are felt more strongly by those living in rural areas due to social isolation. There are also fewer health care resources for rural residents who may have to travel long distances to obtain treatment. The lack of local support groups may contribute to feelings of isolation. Access to the internet can address some of these restrictions.

CHAPTER SUMMARY

- Chronic conditions such as asthma, epilepsy and diabetes are long term and irreversible, and require ongoing management.
- Individuals with a chronic condition have to make many adjustments to the physical, emotional, social and financial challenges of their situation. The extent to which such individuals can engage in day-to-day life varies; however, it is incorrect to assume that they are not able to carry out most activities.
- Chronic conditions are prevalent, particularly among older people. This prevalence is expected to increase, which will place a heavy burden on health care systems and informal carers alike.
- The onset of a chronic condition or acquired disability can signify many life changes, including grief and loss, ongoing emotional ups and downs, and the need to deal with the usual demands of daily life, along with those imposed by the condition. Other factors include financial stress and the impact of the condition on family and friends.

- Cognitions play a significant role in how well individuals cope. Responses include feelings of helplessness, acceptance and positive benefits. Self-efficacy beliefs and optimism contribute to positive coping.
- Self-regulation and self-care is essential for understanding and managing chronic conditions.
- Different models of self-care may marginalise the individual's role (medical model), see it as a partnership (collaborative model) or place the individual actively at the centre (self-agency model).
- Care implications are long term. They involve managing the physical symptoms, but, just as importantly, promoting overall quality of life through diet and exercise planning, avoiding secondary conditions, dealing with negative emotions and cognitions through stress relief, reframing negative cognitions, and promoting efficacy and optimism.

SELF TEST

1 A chronic condition is one that is:
   a terminal
   b curable
   c permanent
   d reversible.

2 Which of the following is the correct terminology?
   a the handicapped
   b individuals with a disability
   c disabled people
   d non-able-bodied people

3 In terms of emotional responses to chronic conditions, which of the following statements is true?
   a There is no role for positive emotions.
   b The person is likely to feel the same emotions throughout the term of the disease.
   c There are no feelings of grief or loss.
   d The person is likely to feel anxiety and/or depression.

4 Three generic cognitive evaluations of a chronic condition are:
   a helplessness, acceptance and positive benefits
   b helplessness, acceptance and resentment
   c resentment, acceptance and positive benefits
   d helplessness, acceptance and self-rated health.

5 The self-agency model of care sees individuals:
   a taking charge of their own condition
   b identifying their own responses
   c planning and managing their lives
   d all of the above.

FURTHER READING

Audulv, A., Asplund, K. & Norbergh, K. (2012) The integration of chronic illness self-management. *Qualitative Health Research*, 22(3), 332–45.

Day, J.R. & Anderson, R.A. (2012) Compassion fatigue: An application of the concept to informal caregivers of family members with dementia. *Nursing Research and Practice*, Article ID 408024, doi:10.1155/2011/408024.

Holgate, S.T., Komaroff, A.L., Mangan, D. & Wessely, S. (2011) Chronic fatigue syndrome: Understanding a complex illness. *Nature Reviews. Neuroscience*, 12(9), 539–44.

Maccallum, F. & Bryant, R. (2011) Imagining the future in complicated grief. *Depression and Anxiety*, 28(8), 658–65.

Sawyer, S.M., Drew, S., Yeo, M.S. & Britto, M. (2007) Adolescents with a chronic condition: challenges living, challenges treating. *The Lancet*, 369(9571), 1481–9.

USEFUL WEBSITES

Arthritis Australia:
www.arthritisaustralia.com.au

Arthritis Foundation:
www.arthritis.org

Living with MS (National Multiple Sclerosis Society):
www.nationalmssociety.org/living-with-multiple-sclerosis/index.aspx

What is MS? (YouTube):
www.youtube.com/watch?v=qgySDmRRzxY

PART 2

HEALTHY AND RISKY BEHAVIOUR

WHY DOES UNHEALTHY BEHAVIOUR CONTINUE?

The media are full of information about health. Information about the risks of smoking has to be included on the packaging of tobacco products. Almost every issue of every popular magazine discusses weight in one way or another. So, why do people still continue to do things that are bad for them? And, more importantly, why does it seem to be so hard to do things that are good for you? In Chapter 6, health and risky behaviours are discussed, and concepts from learning and memory are used to help understand these behaviours.

Agency: what or who is responsible for the modification of unhealthy behaviour.

A critical part of the answer to these questions has to do with what or who is responsible for those things happening. The word for this is '**agency**'. In the case of experimental animals in the laboratory, such as Pavlov's dogs or Skinner's rats, the experimenter has control over the stimuli that trigger behaviour—and/or the costs and gains of those behaviours—which makes the experimenter the agent for change.

For health behaviour, the agents are complex. Usually, we believe that it is the individual who needs to become the agent for their own change. Not surprisingly, whether this happens is dependent on what the individual is thinking—their cognitions. A very simple statement of this part of the equation comes from Bandura (1998: 624): 'Unless people believe they can produce desired effects by their actions, they have little incentive to act.' People also need to believe that action will make a difference. These outcome expectations can come from a number of sources. Chapter 7 deals with cognitions, particularly beliefs about health and the influence they can have on health behaviours.

An understanding of how behaviours are acquired, and why they continue, provides a basis for thinking about how to modify them. Chapter 8 examines the principles of behaviour change, attempting to link the two previous chapters to solutions. The control of the stimuli that trigger behaviour, and the reinforcements that support those behaviours and keep them occurring, are discussed—along with the impact of cognitions on how health behaviour can be modified.

The most significant modifiable influence on health is now considered by health professionals to be overweight and obesity. However, the issues associated with the obvious side of the problem—the direct health risks of obesity—are complex, and involve much more than just how many kilojoules an individual consumes. Clearly, how many of these kilojoules are used as fuel during physical activity is also important. However, there are a variety of other issues involved— for example, habits, beliefs, culture, self-image and self-esteem—that also need to be considered if we are to understand weight as a health issue. Chapter 9 is devoted to a detailed consideration of this one critical area of health behaviour.

06 UNDERSTANDING HEALTH BEHAVIOUR

CHAPTER OBJECTIVES

By the end of your study of this chapter, you should be able to:

- understand how the behaviour and lifestyle of the individual can influence health and illness
- recognise the differences between behaviours that improve health and those that minimise harm
- apply the basic principles of learning and memory to explain the development and maintenance of behaviour.

KEYWORDS

aversive conditioning
avoidance learning
classical conditioning
confabulation
habit
health behaviours
learning
learnt helplessness
lifestyle disorders
memory
neuroplasticity

phobia
punishment
reinforcement
risky behaviours
risk-reduction behaviours
secondary gain
shaping
stimulus
stimulus generalisation
synaptic cleft
unsafe sex

THE RELATIONSHIP BETWEEN BEHAVIOUR AND HEALTH

Chapter 4 looked at the effects on behaviour of health, illness and disease. This chapter looks at the other side of the coin: the effects of behaviour on health, illness and disease. Due to extraordinary progress in biomedical sciences and in public health, patterns of health and illness in the world have changed enormously over the last century. Infections such as poliomyelitis, smallpox, influenza, venereal diseases and diseases of childhood are no longer the main killers in developed countries. Their place has largely been taken by **lifestyle disorders**, so-called because they arise from, or are strongly influenced by, the behaviours (or habits) that characterise a person's lifestyle (AIHW 2008). Heart disease, cancer and cerebrovascular disease (stroke) are now the major killers in all of the developed and much of the developing world.

Lifestyle disorders: diseases in which behaviours of the individual over a prolonged period of time influence the development or course of disease, such as heart disease, many cancers and stroke.

PAUSE & REFLECT

How do we know that lifestyle disorders are the major causes of disability and death? Review the section 'Measurement of Health and Illness' in Chapter 1 if you are not sure.

A consequence of this change is that prevention of illness and reduction of suffering is no longer simply a matter of medical science producing a vaccine, or a doctor providing treatment of physical symptoms. A large proportion of the morbidity and mortality associated with lifestyle diseases is preventable. Taylor (2006) has estimated that 25 per cent of all cancer deaths and a large proportion of deaths from coronary heart disease and stroke could be prevented by modifying just one behaviour: cigarette smoking. Access Economics (2008) has estimated that 20–25 per cent of diabetes, cerebrovascular disease, osteoarthritis and cancer are caused by obesity. In fact, overweight and obesity have passed smoking as the number-one modifiable risk behaviour in developed countries, so a separate chapter has been devoted to weight and the related issues of diet and exercise (see Chapter 9). Modification of eating habits, alcohol consumption, exercise, leisure pursuits, sexual behaviour and even minor habits (such as slouching or nail-biting) could also improve quality of life, extend life expectancy and reduce the risk of ill health.

CROSS-REFERENCE The influence of gender on health is discussed in detail in Chapter 14.

RISKY BEHAVIOURS

A number of behaviours produce a risk to the health of the individual. In some of these, the risk is a direct result of the behaviour (for example, smoking damages tissue), while others are more indirect in their effects (for example, driving while angry increases the risk of accidents and has a subsequent health impact). French et al. (2010) provide a detailed survey of the impacts of a variety of hazardous behaviours. Important **risky behaviours** include cigarette smoking, alcohol and problem drinking, illegal drugs, risky sexual behaviour and dangerous activities. These are now discussed in more detail.

Risky behaviours: behaviours that increase the chance of ill health for the individual.

CIGARETTE SMOKING

Approximately 15 per cent of adult Australians are smokers (AIHW 2011a), continuing a trend for the proportion of the population who smoke decreasing for several decades. Smoking is difficult to eliminate in existing smokers because the nicotine in tobacco is highly addictive. In addition, cigarette manufacturing and sales make large contributions to the economy and to taxation revenue of governments, so that the process of controlling smoking by regulation has been difficult and slow.

Restriction of the areas where smoking can take place has progressed worldwide, and now may include public buildings, indoor spaces such as restaurants and hotels, and even cars where children are present. Although the main aim of such restriction has been to reduce 'passive' exposure to second-hand smoke for non-smokers, the effects of making smoking appear to be antisocial have had an impact on smokers as well. In most developed countries, cigarette packages now must contain health warnings, and even graphic pictures of health problems associated with smoking. In 2012, the Australian government was considering a requirement for all cigarettes to be sold in standard plain packaging. The large number of harmful substances in tobacco smoke are risk factors in many illnesses, the major risks resulting from smoking's effects on the cardiovascular and respiratory systems.

JAMES CHO AND SMOKING

CASE STUDY

The aim of this case is to look at a risky behaviour and examine the reasons for its development and maintenance.

James Cho is 40 years of age. He smokes between 25 and 30 cigarettes a day. His father smoked prior to his death at age 57 from a heart attack, but his mother does not. James had his first cigarette at the age of 12, when he and some boys from school obtained cigarettes from the older brother of a friend. By the time he was 15, James was smoking regularly on the way to and from school with this same friend. At first, he just smoked because other people that he liked did. Soon, he came to enjoy the experience of smoking, and found he could use cigarettes to calm down when he was tense, or wake up when he was tired. Even though he realised it was bad for him, when he tried to do without smoking he felt irritable and restless.

1   Why might James have been attracted to smoking in the first place?
2   Why does James's past experience of the positive aspects of smoking (peer pressure, pleasure and regulation of mood) appear to outweigh the negatives (coughing, financial costs and knowing that smoking certainly had something to do with his father's early death from heart disease)?

ALCOHOL AND PROBLEM DRINKING

Although there is evidence that moderate alcohol consumption—one to two standard drinks a day—has some health protective effects, overuse and abuse of alcohol have major negative impacts on health, partly as a result of direct effects on tissue in the body that give rise to liver, kidney, gastrointestinal and nervous system problems. Problems also occur as a result of indirect effects on behaviour of drinkers, such as accidents, violence and other unhealthy habits that tend to go with alcohol abuse, such as smoking. While the direct effects take time to occur, the indirect consequences result from alcohol's effects on the drinker, and occur even in new drinkers. Binge drinking and its associated accidents and violence are big risks for young drinkers, such as university students (Taylor 2006). While it appears that the proportion of the Australian population who drink regularly is decreasing, the evidence regarding risky levels of drinking is less clear (AIHW 2011a).

ILLEGAL DRUGS

Although fewer people use illegal drugs than use tobacco and alcohol, the level of health risk and the likelihood of associated consequences are quite high. These drugs include marijuana, cocaine, opiates (such as heroin), amphetamines and a variety of so-called party or designer drugs such as ice and ecstasy. Like alcohol and tobacco, these have direct physical risks and indirect behavioural risks. Unlike the decreases in use of tobacco and alcohol noted previously, it would appear that use of illegal drugs in increasing slightly among younger adults (AIHW 2011a).

There are potential problems associated with one-time use of all of these substances. They may vary considerably between substances, however, and do not just include increased likelihood of accidents or undesirable behaviour such as unprotected sex. One so-called party drug is GHB (gamma-hydroxybutyrate), which has received a lot of attention in media in recent years due to the hospitalisations and deaths that have followed its use. The major problem with one-off use is that: 'There's a very fine line between the amount of GHB required to get someone intoxicated and how much will put them in a coma' (Australian Government National Drugs Campaign 2010). Varying risks exist for the one-off use of other recreational drugs, but a major problem is that many people mix them with other drugs such as alcohol or prescription drugs, which can greatly increase the risks.

Even mixing these drugs with 'energy drinks' containing high levels of caffeine, taurine and/or guarana can be dangerous, because the combination can lead to overexertion and dehydration. Some people mistakenly believe that because these energy drink ingredients are legal and 'natural', they pose no risk. However, all of them—on their own or in combination—have been linked to physical and psychological problems (particularly when used to excess) and even deaths (Arria & O'Brien 2011).

With repeated use, all of the mentioned illegal drugs pose some risk of addiction or psychological dependence. These are complex topics, and will not be dealt with here. Chapter 8 includes discussion of opponent-process theory and its application to addiction.

Unsafe sex: having sex without using contraceptive devices such as condoms, not finding out about a partner's sexual history and/or having multiple partners.

RISKY SEXUAL BEHAVIOUR

The two most obvious risks of sexual behaviour are unwanted pregnancy and sexually transmitted infections (STIs). Both of these risks are associated in the public mind with what is termed **unsafe sex**, a term that covers not using contraceptive devices such as condoms, not finding out about a partner's sexual history, and having multiple partners.

The most dangerous STIs have changed with both advances in biomedical science and changes in behaviour. Many STIs, such as syphilis and gonorrhoea, can now be easily cured if detected early and treated, which in fact appears to have led some people to ignore their existence and to overlook symptoms when they occur. Other STIs, such as genital herpes, have become more important health issues because they are not curable. Others, such as HIV, are important because symptoms are often silent, so the carrier does not realise that they have the STI or that they can pass it on to others.

The major change in risk associated with an STI in recent times has been the development and distribution of vaccine against human papillomavirus (HPV) for girls who are not yet sexually active. Due to a strong link between HPV and later development of cervical cancer, this program should produce a major reduction in cervical cancer rates in the future.

DANGEROUS ACTIVITIES

A number of activities expose the individual to a higher than normal risk of injury. Soft tissue injuries—such as bruising and muscle strains, broken bones, and tendon and cartilage damage—are not uncommon in sports such as football, tennis and skiing. Some sports, such as boxing, have very much higher risks. Indeed, there are a number of sports that the medical profession believes have risks that are so high that they should be banned, with boxing being at the top of the list. Steps can be taken to make some of these activities less dangerous; for example, proper equipment and training are important. The wearing of crash helmets and proper clothing by cyclists and motorcyclists has greatly reduced serious injuries and deaths in these pastimes.

The major cause of untimely death and injury for young adults is automobile accidents. It is often a combination of a willingness to take risks and the circumstances under which young people are likely to drive—at night, in groups, when tired or after consuming alcohol or other drugs—that lead to the most serious accidents.

The next section looks at behaviours that either reduce risk or actively encourage health.

PAUSE & REFLECT

How many other examples of risky behaviours with regard to health can you think of?
Do you have any risky behaviours?

HEALTH BEHAVIOURS AND RISK-REDUCTION BEHAVIOURS

Two types of behaviour are directly related to improvement in a person's state of health and well-being. **Health behaviours** are those that promote health, such as eating the right foods, getting enough sleep, relaxing and exercising sensibly. **Risk-reduction behaviours** refer to actions that reduce the occurrence of unhealthy behaviours such as smoking, drinking alcohol in excess and unsafe driving. Sometimes these are categorised as preventive behaviours, but as many of them involve simply avoiding the risky behaviour in the first place, the term 'risk reduction' is preferred here. Many direct associations have been demonstrated between health behaviours and risk-reduction behaviours and health outcomes, not just in terms of the targeted problems but also in terms of the sense of overall well-being and the ability to cope with other life events.

health behaviours: behaviours that are carried out specifically to promote the health of the individual.

Risk-reduction behaviours: the avoidance of unhealthy behaviours specifically to protect the health of the individual.

It is useful to think in very broad terms about both of these types of behaviour. As well as the behaviours themselves, health behaviour can involve the pace at which behaviours are carried out or the emotional state of the individual while carrying them out. Road rage has received a lot of media attention in recent years. The risks associated with driving are greatly increased if we are in a competitive and aggressive state of mind while driving. This state of mind leads us to taking unnecessary chances, and then blaming other drivers for any behaviour that affects us as a result. Such behaviour leads to anger. The biggest risk of driving while angry is not that we will actually get out of our car and murder someone, but that our judgment while behind the wheel will be impaired, resulting in dangerous behaviour. Angry people are much more likely to put themselves in situations where the margin for error is small, which results in both a greater likelihood of accidents and a greater chance that those accidents will be serious. A risk-reduction strategy in this area might involve dealing with the connection between anger and driving. Since we often drive aggressively when we are late or under time pressure, road rage could be dealt with by changing a driver's approach to time management.

PAUSE & REFLECT

Since angry drivers cause more than the expected rate of accidents, should this be taken into account when issuing driver's licences? Can you think of other risk-reduction strategies that might be more workable than this?

Habit: an activity that has become relatively automatic through prolonged practice.

When a behaviour is practised regularly it becomes a **habit**, is more likely to occur, and becomes relatively automatic (that is, it occurs without awareness). Habits are learnt and remembered. Even minor habits can have an effect on health and well-being. Snacking while we watch television, for example, can have disastrous effects on an otherwise healthy diet. Chairs in school and university classrooms tend to be designed to be stackable, attractive or indestructible rather than to encourage good posture. As a result, they may encourage slouching for comfort, which leads in the short term to back, neck or joint pain. If bad posture becomes a habit, it can lead to chronic pain, or affect joint health or the operation of the digestive system. Biting fingernails can lead to infections and even loss of sensation or function. To understand habits and to begin to think about their modification, some understanding of basic concepts of learning and memory is necessary.

THE BASIS OF LEARNING AND MEMORY: THE CHANGING BRAIN

Until recently, it was believed that the number of cells in the brain was fixed fairly early in life, and that its structure then remained fairly constant throughout life. It can be difficult to understand how learning and memory take place if the brain is so fixed. Research in a variety of areas has now made it clear that the brain is much more changeable than was formerly understood (Doidge 2008).

The basic neural processes that allow us to throw a ball, remember what we had for breakfast or walk without falling over seem so automatic to us that we rarely consider how remarkable they really are. However, if we were to lose some of our abilities—perhaps as a result of damage received in an accident—it would seem an enormous loss. Imagine the difficulties experienced by someone who suffers from dementia, gradually losing more and more of the basic information that allows them to function in the situations they encounter. It is little wonder that those sufferers often experience frustration, anger and anxiety. But how does the biological machine that each of us occupies accomplish these enormously complex mental tasks? And equally important, what can be learnt from the structure and function of the nervous system that will help with the understanding of human behaviour?

INTERCONNECTEDNESS OF THE NERVOUS SYSTEM

The nervous system can accomplish so much—from movement, to thought, to emotion—largely because of its incredibly high level of interconnectedness. Each of the billions of individual neurons may have between 1000 and 10,000 synapses, and be connected to up to 50,000 other neurons. In such a structure, any one neuron is unlikely to exert very strong control over any other neuron all by itself. Each time a neuron fires, it communicates widely and often not very deeply. However, neurons are not spread randomly into a sort of homogeneous pudding of cells. Often cells run in common patterns. They may form bundles that run from one location to (or at least in the general direction of) another. These bundles are nerves, and the information they transmit depends not on the individual neuron but on the preponderance of the action of many neurons. Some neurons may share many synapses with other single neurons; for example, because they are close to one another physically and going in the same direction.

The way in which a particular neuron responds to information from other neurons can be seen as having parallels with the process of polling. It is the total sum of the information received that determines the rate of firing of the neuron. Imagine the behaviour of a television quiz show contestant when the presenter asks, 'Would you like to continue or stop now?' If you have ever seen a quiz show, you will know that at this point the people in the audience *always* start shouting advice. Some will shout 'yes' and some 'no', and some will shout totally incomprehensible or irrelevant things, or say nothing at all. Although the contestant already has a preference for stopping or continuing, this audience advice will have an effect—particularly if it is unanimous. If everyone in the room shouts 'no', it is likely to make the contestant hesitant to say 'yes', no matter how much they want to. In a similar way, the neuron responds to the preponderance of incoming information—that is, excitatory ('yes') minus inhibitory ('no')—by varying its firing rate. The television contestant is also likely to be most influenced by those who yell loudest, or they may look to family or friends in the audience for advice. Similarly, the neuron responds more strongly to strong input, which may come from particularly excited neurons, or neurons with which it has a large number of synapses all giving the same information. Each time the neuron fires it has to pause a bit, although this is actually a very short time, measured in microseconds, as the rate of firing can be quite high. This allows it to build up its resources for another firing. This is a gradual process, and during this time it will only respond if the input is strong. The stronger the input, the closer the neuron will come to firing at its maximum possible rate.

The influence of one neuron on another does not cease as soon as firing takes place, because the message is carried by neurotransmitters that remain in the gap between the neurons (the **synaptic cleft**) for greater or lesser periods of time. These may influence neurons after the incoming neuron has stopped signalling, and it takes time for the receiving neuron to free up its receptors by breaking down or releasing the neurotransmitters. Less normal events may

Synaptic cleft: the tiny space between two nerve cells, across which they communicate using neurotransmitters.

occur as well. As an extreme example, heroin or other drugs introduced into the body can block receptor sites that are intended for neurotransmitters, and so interfere with normal transmission. Substances may be introduced that break down a neurotransmitter before it can lock into receptor sites, thereby reducing the amount of that neurotransmitter in the synaptic cleft. Other substances may prevent the breakdown or re-uptake of a neurotransmitter and thereby increase the amount present. These principles underlie a great deal of the drug treatment that is used by doctors for things as divergent as high blood pressure, depression, cancer and impotence. As you will see in the following sections on learning and memory, firing changes the neuron, with information being permanently stored through actual physical change in the structure and interconnections of the neuron. The effect of all of this action is that the influence of information spreads widely. It becomes associated with other information—and the more similar the information, the more closely associated it becomes.

Particular input tends to be dealt with primarily in certain locations because of the structure of the nervous system, but because of the high degree of interconnectedness it is also communicated to other brain locations. Following damage to the preferred location, this communication can allow another—usually neighbouring—area to take over a function, although this may take a great deal of retraining. This principle of **neuroplasticity** suggests that functions within the brain that are lost through injury or illness are not gone for good, but can be recovered through appropriate retraining. This notion that functions can be replaced through training forms the core topic of Doidge's best-selling book, *The Brain that Changes Itself* (2008). However, it also highlights that the basis for all learning and memory lies in physical changes to the brain.

Because the brain is a constantly developing organ, the earlier in life that damage occurs, the more rapidly functions can be transferred to nearby areas. For example, children who lack the usual number of cells in the language areas of the brain—because of developmental problems or injury—may develop language in a normal way and at the usual times, using other brain areas. For adults, however, relearning language skills after damage may be a very slow process because it involves retraining rather than the initial training of brain cells. Special treatment procedures (Doidge 2008) have been developed that offer hope that this retraining can be speeded up, and can reach a wider range of lost functions than previously believed.

Neuroplasticity: the brain's ability to reorganise itself by forming new neural connections throughout life.

CASE STUDY

JAMES (CONT.)

Clearly, James had learnt a great deal about smoking before he ever had a cigarette himself. He learnt from observing his father that smoking is something that adult males do, and that a person that he is close to and admires does. He also learnt a lot about smoking—though not about its disadvantages—from movies and television, and from observation of others around him. His friends contributed to his knowledge about smoking and his attitudes towards it. They also changed the availability of cigarettes. All these sources indirectly taught James about how he should feel about the bodily effects that resulted from smoking. He had to learn that the bodily effects were pleasant—since most people feel ill the first time they inhale cigarette smoke. As he continues to smoke, he begins to associate other experiences—such as parties and breaks with friends—with smoking.

1   Learning about smoking from parents and friends is just one of the factors that contribute to smoking in young people. Could there be other forms of learning involved in James's smoking?

2   How do experiences of one kind (in this case, smoking) become associated with experiences of a completely different kind, like socialising, drinking alcohol or taking breaks?

LEARNING

Why do some people develop an irrational fear of flying? Why do you get very hungry exactly at the end of your one o'clock class? How do we gain the skills that allow us to survive in a complex environment? Why do we do things that we know very well are bad for us? All of these responses depend on learning. Learning is such a basic process that it is hard to come up with a good working definition. Probably the clearest way to think about **learning** is that it is a change in behaviour that is a result of one's experience with the environment. This would exclude the instance of a child who could not roll over at three months of age being able to do so at four months (the result of maturation), or of a rat working harder to get food when it is hungry than when it is not (the result of change in internal state over time). However, if someone threatens to hit you if you do not shut up, and you shut up, that is learning. It is perhaps easiest to understand the nature of learning by looking at some of the simplest models of learning.

Learning: a change in behaviour that results from experience with the environment.

CLASSICAL CONDITIONING

Probably the most famous experiments in psychology are those involving Pavlov's dogs (Rathus 1997). What is generally remembered about this—and parodied in cartoons—is that Pavlov taught his dogs to salivate to the ringing of a bell. However, what is of most importance of the understanding of learning is that, through experience, an already existing response to the presentation of food (salivating) became connected to a previously irrelevant stimulus (bell). This kind of learning is called **classical conditioning**.

For classical conditioning to take place, you must have an unconditioned response (UR) that reliably follows an unconditioned **stimulus** (US) whenever it occurs. Examples of stimulus–response pairs that fit this model are such reflexes as blinking your eye (UR) when air is puffed into it (US), or the knee jerk (UR) that follows the knee being tapped by a hammer (US). Learning occurs when an irrelevant stimulus is paired with the US; that is, presented at roughly the same time. Any initially irrelevant stimulus will do. It is not the nature of the stimulus that matters, only its pairing with the US. After this pairing has occurred a few times, the irrelevant stimulus will have become a conditioned stimulus (CS). If the CS is now presented without the US, it will produce a response that looks like the UR. This response is called the conditioned response (CR). Although it looks like the UR, it will be weaker, and if the CS is presented repeatedly without the US, the CR will gradually fade away or extinguish.

You can see how a **phobia** might develop through classical conditioning. A child will quite typically react with distress (UR) when startled (US). Suppose the child meets a strange dog (CS) and, not being afraid of it, begins to play with it. Worried about the child's safety, the child's parent suddenly shouts at the dog (US), startling the child and producing distress (UR); the dog

Classical conditioning: a learning process through experience where an already existing response to the presentation of food (salivating) becomes connected to a previously irrelevant stimulus (bell).

Stimulus: any change in physical energy that activates a receptor, and activates or alerts an organism.

Phobia: a strong, persistent and irrational fear of some object, person or event.

runs off. If this sequence is repeated, the child will begin to show distress (CR) to the presence of strange dogs (CS).

One characteristic of classically conditioned responses is that they generalise to other stimuli that are similar to the CS. The strength of the response to a new stimulus will be directly related to how similar it is to the original CS. In this case, the child's conditioned fear of dogs could generalise to all small furry animals.

PAUSE 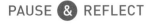 REFLECT

When an individual, such as a member of a sporting team, acts badly, we may think that other members of the team will do the same. How can **stimulus generalisation** help to understand this process?

Stimulus generalisation: the principle that a conditioned response will tend to occur in the presence of stimuli similar to the original conditioned stimulus.

Why does the phobia not extinguish over time? If the child was placed in a situation where encountering strange dogs was unavoidable, and a parent was not present to produce the UR of fear by producing the US of screaming, then it probably would. Phobias are frequently maintained by avoidance behaviour. Each time the child has an opportunity to interact with strange dogs, it is likely to choose instead to avoid them. This avoidance learning represents another kind of learning called operant conditioning.

OPERANT CONDITIONING

Classical conditioning on its own could hardly explain all learning, especially the learning of complex or novel behaviours. A different kind of conditioning occurs in trial-and-error learning situations. Suppose a hungry rat is placed in a new enclosure. It will scramble around doing a variety of things until it discovers food, or until it is removed from the enclosure. In fact, the hungrier the rat gets, the more vigorously it will scramble around and the greater the variety of things it will do. If it finds some food, the behaviours that occurred at about that same time will be learnt; that is, they will become more likely to occur in future when the rat is hungry. Over repeated trials, any random behaviours—those that actually had nothing to do with the food—will be likely to stop occurring (or extinguish). The only behaviours that will really stick will be those that operate to produce the desired outcome (thus, operant conditioning). The rat's behaviour will become more precise and faster as the correct responses are stamped in and the incorrect ones are stamped out. These behaviours become habits and may occur automatically, which describes a fairly typical study in operant conditioning, as developed by Skinner (1938), who created much of the theory surrounding our current understanding of operant conditioning.

Reinforcement: a consequence or outcome that in conjunction with a behaviour makes that behaviour more likely in future; this may be the beginning of a pleasant consequence (positive reinforcement) or the ending of an unpleasant consequence (negative reinforcement).

Originally, discussions of operant conditioning used common language terms (such as 'reward') to describe what was happening, but these can prove to be confusing. What is rewarding to one rat (for example, a food pellet) might not interest another, and its effect on a given rat when it is hungry is quite different from when it has just eaten. The concepts become clearer if events are described in terms of their effects on behaviour. **Positive reinforcement** is when the occurrence of a consequence or outcome in conjunction with a particular behaviour makes that behaviour more likely in future (such an outcome might be food, money or sex). The consequence is called a positive reinforcer or a positive reinforcement. **Punishment** is when the occurrence of a consequence makes a behaviour less likely (for example, an electric shock or a bad grade). Putting an end to a pleasant state (such as turning off the television or being

Punishment: a consequence or outcome that in conjunction with a behaviour makes that behaviour less likely in future.

awakened from a nap by being yelled at) is also punishment because it reduces the likelihood of the target behaviour.

Note that the termination of an unpleasant state (such as turning off an electric shock or allowing the organism to avoid it) can also serve to increase the likelihood of a behaviour. To emphasise its special characteristics this is sometimes called **negative reinforcement**. Note that it is reinforcement because it increases the likelihood of a behaviour. Do not allow the word 'negative' to lead you to confuse it with punishment.

When the behaviour to be learnt is complex—for example, if you wanted to train a rat to dance—it would make little sense to wait around until a random moment when the rat just happened to put on tap shoes. A faster solution is **shaping**. To begin with, the animal would be reinforced for any behaviour that looked like dancing, and then for progressively closer approximations of the particular step we wanted it to do. Parents often use shaping to teach their children things such as writing their name. At first, the children are praised for holding the pencil properly, then for scribbles that look like writing, then for individual letters, then for groups of letters, and so on until they are actually writing. Most of what we learn is complex behaviour that probably results from shaping arising from our experiences with the environment.

Learning without reinforcement or punishment is also possible and is discussed later in the chapter.

Negative reinforcement: the termination of an unpleasant state that can serve to increase the likelihood of a behaviour.

Shaping: teaching a complex behaviour by reinforcing, one at a time, the series of steps that make up the behaviour.

PUNISHMENT

The impact of punishment on behaviour is more complex than that of positive reinforcement (Walters & Grusec 1977). Treatment approaches based on punishment of unwanted behaviour—called **aversive conditioning**—frequently produce unexpected outcomes. One treatment for alcoholics involves the taking of a substance (Anatabuse) that makes the patient violently ill if they subsequently drink alcohol. The expected result is that an aversion to the taste of alcohol should be classically conditioned, but the actual result tends to be a very high drop-out rate from therapy—unless the patient has an intact family that is highly supportive of the treatment. One way of viewing this is that patients find it easier to acquire an aversion to the treatment than to alcohol. This is an example of **avoidance learning**. When the individual avoids a punishment, the behaviour that leads to avoidance gets reinforced.

Another drawback of punishment is that it may generalise; that is, its effects may spread to similar stimuli so that desirable behaviours disappear along with the undesirable. If a child is punished for being noisy in class, that child may withdraw into not only quiet but also passive behaviour. While no longer acting up, the child may also no longer ask questions about things they have not understood. The loss of positive interaction with the teacher and other children may handicap the child's learning. Punishment also generalises to the punisher, so that the child may come to dislike the teacher, the class or school in general.

Reinforcement works in two ways. The right behaviour is stamped in and the wrong behaviour—which is not reinforced—extinguishes. While punishment stamps out the wrong behaviour, it provides no information about the right behaviour, which may therefore extinguish. Because of this, aversive conditioning needs to be paired with reinforcement of the right behaviour. Treatment for alcoholics is likely to be more effective if adaptive behaviours are taught and reinforced, as well as drinking being punished. Alcoholics Anonymous, as an example, encourages alcoholics to call for company when they are tempted to drink, an act that reinforces

Aversive conditioning: the use of punishment to decrease the occurrence of unwanted behaviour.

Avoidance learning: the learning of a response that will allow the individual to escape punishment, often fear; it is reinforced by a reduction in the level of fear experienced.

non-drinking behaviour and puts the focus on interpersonal rather than internal events. The elimination of aggressive behaviour by punishment usually works best when accompanied by training in appropriate assertive behaviour—using positive reinforcement—as a better alternative.

LEARNING WITHOUT REINFORCEMENT

Learning is based on the development of associations between stimuli and responses. Conditioning theories account for much of this development, but not everything that fits the definition of learning can be explained in conditioning terms. Can you recall the slogan from a particular bread commercial? Can you hum the Coca-Cola or Pepsi jingle? It is hard to see how you could have been reinforced for acquisition of these behaviours.

It is easier to account for events such as these if we consider the complex mental activity going on inside us. We have elaborate mental networks of expectations about the workings of the world, sometimes termed 'schemas'. These schemas can be affected by conditioning, but other things affect them as well. If you place a non-hungry rat in a maze, it will explore (possibly out of curiosity). If you then place the same rat in the same maze when it is hungry, you will see clear evidence that it has learnt something about the arrangement of the maze from its previous experience with it, which the rat only calls into play now that it is hungry. This latent learning (Tolman 1932) indicates that schemas can develop or change without reinforcement, because they might be useful at some future time.

Learning by observation offers some demonstrations of this. Bandura (1977b) proposed that reinforcement is more important in getting an organism to display a behaviour than in its initial learning. In a famous study on the learning of aggression (Bandura et al. 1963), children were shown films of adults behaving in unusually aggressive ways towards toys. When the children were put into a room with these same toys, there was no tendency for them to act out aggressive behaviour, unless the children were angered. Only then did they imitate, in detail, the specific acts of aggression that they had seen modelled. Observation of the behaviour had added the new behaviour to their repertoire of aggressive behaviour, so that it was there when needed. It appears that a lot of aggressive behaviour is learnt in this fashion.

It seems paradoxical that people who are abused as children are more likely than other people to grow up to be child abusers. It is expected that they should know how bad child abuse is, and that they would avoid it. It appears that they have learnt—by observing the people that abused them—a strategy for behaving towards children, and when they in turn experience anger and frustration towards their own children, they may act out this latent learning.

Certain characteristics of an observed behaviour may make it more likely to be learnt by observation. Seeing someone else being reinforced for a behaviour is likely to make it appear to be worth learning (this is known as vicarious reinforcement). Behaviours may be acquired if they are novel enough to be interesting in themselves. Children in particular like to learn things that produce spectacular effects. For example, learning dirty words is interesting because adults respond to them in interesting ways.

A major way in which we learn by observation is through the use of language. Although we may never have seen a computer before, by reading the instructions we can obtain information about the correct behaviour; that is, what we have to do in order to make the computer work. Can you imagine the wear and tear on patients if health professionals had to learn about their professions solely through conditioning of randomly occurring behaviours?

PAUSE **&** REFLECT

How would theories of learning explain why people continue to carry out risky health behaviours? Try to explain why someone would drive when they have had too much to drink.

LEARNING TO BE SICK

The earlier description of how one can acquire a phobia illustrates one way in which someone can learn to be sick. There is a variety of others. When temporary tissue damage has occurred, such as when you sprain your ankle, you will very quickly learn what causes pain and avoid doing those things, which is useful because it gives the damaged tissue time to recover. However, it is possible to over-learn avoidance. Consider the case of a young person who has been in an accident and received significant back injuries. During the time that these injuries are healing, the person may develop powerful avoidance learning. Sitting up may cause extreme pain, so the person learns to lie still. Eventually, a point may be reached where the muscles have begun to atrophy through disuse. The person may have learnt avoidance so well that they have great difficulty in bringing themselves to move normally, or they may move awkwardly, thereby increasing the likelihood of re-injury. This can occur even where the person has not become phobic about movement through their experiences of pain, but just because habits of restricted movement have been learnt.

Sometimes being ill carries with it **secondary gains**. If your family and friends have learnt that you are likely to injure yourself if you lift heavy weights, they will tend to move things for you or avoid asking you to help with strenuous activities. The pain patient above, for example, may be excused from doing a variety of things they would otherwise have been asked to do (a right of the sick role). Complaints of pain tend to result in increased caring behaviours from others. The bringing of pain relievers, expressions of sympathy, praise for one's courage and even pillow plumping can all follow from complaining of pain and reinforce the complaining behaviour.

Secondary gain: the gain or advantage an individual gets as a result of being ill.

Treatment of chronic pain usually involves setting up routines for treatment by staff and families that do not reinforce complaining, but reinforce testing the limits of movement. Medication, because it relieves or prevents the onset of pain, is also a reinforcer in chronic pain, and patients often become conditioned to certain dosages and times of medication, even where pain is not present. This is another kind of avoidance learning: the medication prevents the pain occurring, so if medication is missed its absence becomes anxiety-provoking. Ultimately, the patient is taking the medication as much for anxiety relief as pain relief. The kinds of learning just described for pain can occur with almost any other symptom, including nausea, itching and tiredness.

CROSS-REFERENCE
Pain is such an important part of health and behaviour that all of Chapter 11 has been devoted to it.

A more severe kind of learning to be sick can occur when unpleasant events that an individual would like to avoid cannot be avoided. Early studies of escape by animals from electric shock sometimes showed that when shock cannot be avoided or escaped (or when the animal is for some reason unable to find out how to avoid or escape) a pattern called 'learnt helplessness' frequently occurs (Seligman & Maier 1967). In this pattern, distress increases to a point where behaviour is impaired. Learning is retarded, and the animal may quit trying to learn. The stimuli that signal the beginning of shock result in giving-up behaviour such as freezing, whining, shivering or apathy. Researchers found some disturbing similarities between the ways in which the animals behaved and the ways in which some people behave. A wife who is regularly beaten by her husband may come to simply accept the beating without making any attempt to escape. As a result of experience, she has learnt a helpless pattern of behaviour. Even where avoidance or escape appear to an observer to be easy, they are not attempted. In other cases, the helplessness may be more subtle.

The key elements in this kind of learning are helplessness and hopelessness: the organism gives up on behaviour and sometimes shows a pattern of withdrawal from the outside world. It has been suggested that in situations where action is hopeless, this withdrawal protects the organism by conserving resources. It has been observed in children who have been severely abused or neglected, and in prisoners of war. The similarities to the psychiatric disorder of depression are strong enough that **learnt helplessness** is considered to be one of the pathways leading to depression.

Learnt helplessness: distress to a point where behaviour is impaired or the individual gives up in the face of punishment that cannot be controlled.

CASE STUDY

JAMES (CONT.)

Learning without reinforcement could have played a part in James's smoking. He observed his father, some of his friends and characters in films (and, before it was banned, on television) smoking and learnt it as a possible behaviour. He would have learnt a great deal about where and when to smoke, how to hold a cigarette, how to light up and how to blow out the smoke. James might have also learnt through vicarious reinforcement by hearing people say things such as 'That tastes good' or 'I needed that'. These are just some of the reasons why tobacco companies pour a great deal of money into films to have the principal characters smoke—particularly if those characters are attractive, strong or sexy. They are trying to increase learning and memory effects with regard to cigarettes. This also explains why it is so important to decrease these processes by banning smoking from popular entertainment.

James will have stored memories about how cigarettes and smokers look and behave from his observation of others. He will have semantic memories (for example, what smoking-related terms such as 'Have you got a light?' mean), procedural memories (such as how to light a cigarette on a windy day or using a match) and his own episodic memories about smoking (such as how it feels, times when he has tried to quit or information that he has received from other people).

1   How does memory affect James's behaviour?
2   How do all these memory processes fit together?

CROSS-REFERENCE
Depression is discussed in Chapter 10.

Memory: processes (including sensory, short-term and long-term memory) by which experience is retained within the organism.

MEMORY

This section considers how experience is retained once learning has taken place. As with learning, **memory** has a significant impact on how people behave. What we remember about our experiences in terms of being well and being ill are very important in determining how we will react, what we expect to happen and how we will respond to attempts to modify our health.

How is it that an elderly patient suffering from dementia—a global deterioration of intellectual functioning resulting from damage to brain tissue—may be able to recall every detail of their childhood home but not remember the name of the nurse who takes care of them or what they did five minutes ago? Why does your friend remember a story about you that you are certain never actually occurred? Memory is amazing in its ability to hold millions of bits of information, and the ease with which information may be lost or altered. No computer memory can match the flexibility or usefulness of the human memory—or its inaccuracy.

Memory consists of three related processes: sensory memory, short-term memory and long-term memory (see Figure 6.1). Each operates in a different way and serves different functions, but all three have some things in common. Some authors have suggested that there is also a medium-term memory, which we use for things that are likely to be needed in the future but not very far into the future. The need for a process different from long-term memory to explain this is not clear, and there does not seem to be a good theory of how the two types of memory would differ. The discussion that follows looks at the three best established types.

Figure 6.1   Types of memory

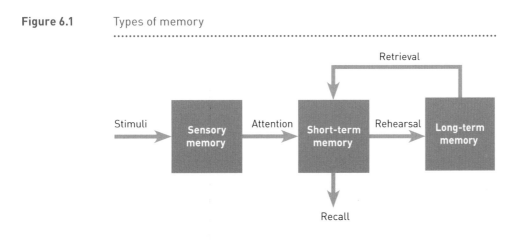

SENSORY MEMORY

Look at the room around you for a moment, then close your eyes and try to remember every detail you can about the wall to your left. You will probably be surprised at how much detail you can recall. However, if you now try to remember the detail of the right hand wall, most of what you remembered about the left will have gone. In the same way, if you hear a bell ring or feel something touch your skin, there will be a momentary lingering—a few seconds of that sensation. For that time the impression will be quite detailed, but it will not be possible to hold on to it for long, particularly if something else happens using the same sense: another sound or touch. It appears that we have a separate sensory store for each of the five senses. This sensory memory seems to serve the function of allowing us time to search for information we need while allowing us to get rid of the detail that we do not. If we had to keep all of the detail that we sense from moment to moment, it would clearly overload the storage capacity of the mind. This is because we have a limited storage capacity within the receptor system (including parts of the nervous system and the sense organs), which is constantly being written over by new information. Once we identify information that is needed, we can then focus our conscious attention on it.

PAUSE & REFLECT

How good is your memory for pain? Can you really remember the sensory memory or only the long-term memories about the experience? What might be the result if you had a really good memory for the sensory experience of pain?

SHORT-TERM MEMORY

The information that we focus on then moves into short-term memory. This is our working memory, and it decays after a short time (Baddeley 1994). When you look up a phone number, for example, it comes into your awareness and stays as long as you actively think about it; that is, long enough to dial the number. If something distracts you, you will probably need to go back to the directory again. Repetition enables you to extend the time over which you keep something in short-term memory, but if you do not repeat the information it will fade in about half a minute. The capacity of short-term memory appears to be surprisingly constant between people. Regardless of individual characteristics such as sex, age or intelligence, we all seem to be able to hold about seven (plus or minus two) separate pieces of information at a time (Miller 1956).

This makes it hard to understand how we manage a task such as reading, in which we need to retain whole sentences made up of lots of letters. We do this by gathering information into larger units, a process called 'chunking'. Instead of remembering individual letters, we remember whole words. Since the rules of language are fairly regular, we can omit remembering words such as 'the' or 'of' and fill them in later. In conversation or reading, and particularly in sending text messages, we can chunk at the level of ideas as well. If something holds our attention, we read at a high rate, balancing 7 ± 2 ideas in short-term memory at a time. If we are less interested, or the information is unfamiliar or difficult, we may have to read seven words at a time, making progress much slower.

Although the physiological basis of short-term memory is not absolutely clear, it is generally believed that impulses circulate around complex loops of neurons. If this circulation of impulses is interrupted by input that interferes with it, or an injury such as a blow to the head, the information is lost. Without short-term operating memory, it would be very difficult to carry on our normal activities. For example, we use short-term memory to store information about goals while we carry out actions, to store the topic of a sentence while we get from the beginning to the end of it, and to store information about the procedure that needs to be carried out while we carry it out.

LONG-TERM MEMORY

The third storage level is long-term memory: our library of reference material. It can hold massive amounts of information indefinitely. In general, information is stored into long-term memory by rehearsal, but important things may be recorded on one trial, which probably results from the fact that important things are related to already present memories and are therefore rehearsed without particular awareness of the fact. Long-term memory capacity is amazing. The process that allows us to remember huge amounts of information indefinitely is structural change in the neurons in the brain. As groups of neurons are affected by information, the interconnections between them are modified. Some connections are strengthened, involving actual physical growth, while others are weakened. Eventually, the changes become relatively stable and we have a long-term memory.

It is useful to classify the kinds of things that we put into long-term memory (Rathus 1997). We remember how things are done, such as how to tie a shoe or use a telephone. These procedural memories become so well established that we can carry out the procedures automatically, without remembering the individual steps in the process. Another kind of memory is for the meanings of things: semantic memories. We hold memory of the words in our language, symbols and other codes that we use regularly, so that we can use them as soon as they are needed. We only have to think about retrieving meanings when we find an item that we do not recognise, or where the meaning does not come easily. Episodic memories are our individual memories about the experiences we have had in our lives: our record of where we have been, what we have done, who we have met and even who we are.

THE ORGANISATION OF MEMORY

The concept of neuroplasticity offers some useful suggestions about how memory may be stored. We know that the brain is producing new neurons all the time, although only in small numbers. It appears that these new neurons are produced in central areas of the brain (the midbrain) and migrate into the cortex. There they may help to form new memories by linking up with other neurons. Although new neurons might be handy to have when we are learning new things, they do not appear to be necessary, and may not even be particularly helpful in some cases. As we rehearse information in order to move it into long-term storage, we will tend to cause the retrieval of existing related memories, which suggests that new information does not create entirely new circuits. Instead, it produces loops of neurons that interconnect with existing ones. The new is added to the old and is coded in related ways. This will not only make the new information easier to retrieve the next time it is needed, but it may also affect the retrieval of the old. As the old loops are fired by the related information, they may become more firmly implanted. In this way, having similar experiences brings order to the memory traces and they become stronger and easier to retrieve. Most of us have the experience of recognising a face that we have seen before, but being unable to retrieve any memory of where or in what context. At this stage, the face is coded as a face only. Repeated experience with the person connects more and more information to the memory of the face, until even seeing a similar face may call up memories that are linked to the original face.

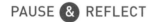

PAUSE **&** REFLECT

How does the organisation of memory help to explain the loss of recent memories but retention of old memories by a patient with brain damage?

MEASURING MEMORY

Remembering consists of more than just recalling total pieces of information and there are several ways that memory can be measured. While it is true that we often test for memory by asking people to recall information (students, for example), there are other more subtle forms of measurement. Even when information cannot be recalled on demand, an individual may still be able to recognise it. Recognition forms the basis of multiple-choice questions. The individual is not asked to reconstruct the memory, but only to recognise what they have seen before. Information may still be retained even when we cannot be sure that we recognise it. An even more subtle measure of memory is how long it takes someone to relearn material to which they have previously been exposed. If, for example, you learnt a poem last year in three hours and cannot now recall or even recognise it, you could relearn it in less than three hours.

FORGETTING

Since long-term memory involves physical change in the arrangement and operation of neurons, it may seem surprising that memory is not more perfect than it is. We do forget, and often find it difficult to recall things as basic as the name of a friend or our own telephone number. How well we remember depends on how efficiently information has been coded for storage and retrieval.

No matter how we search for evidence of remembering, it is clear that some information is lost, even things that we once knew very well. Poems, lists of kings or mathematical formulae that once got us through examinations will prove to be irretrievable for most people; even the face of our first great love can vanish. Psychologists have suggested three basic theories of forgetting. The oldest is decay theory, which suggests that memory traces simply fade away over time—which, for sensory memory and short-term memory, seems to be the case. Problems occur with decay theory when you try to extend it to long-term memory. Why is it that some memories persist, others fade gradually, and some seem to disappear all at once? Why are procedural memories—such as how to ride a bicycle—resistant to fading even over a period of many years? What is it that decays? Is it neurons?

The second proposed cause of forgetting is interference: memories interfere with one another. Earlier events may interfere with the remembering of later events, but the opposite can happen as well.

The third proposal, known as motivated forgetting, suggests that we forget because we want to. Most readers will be familiar with the concept of repression, which suggests that we repress memories that make us feel anxious or uncomfortable. Although this theory suggests that we still keep the memory in our unconscious but just do not retrieve it, this proposal suggests that we may also choose not to store something in our memory at all.

Many people are highly impressed with the ability that they (or others) have to recall extremely detailed episodic memories from the past, often during sleep or under the influence of hypnosis. Similarly, a surgeon named Penfield (1969) reported that, during surgery for epilepsy, stimulation of certain brain areas would produce episodic memories. This kind of report suggests that everything we experience is stored away intact and that we may be able to unlock absolute truths about the past by reaching this memory. It is not uncommon to find that these complete and detailed memories are contradicted by the memories of other people, or by objective information (Loftus & Loftus 1980). What appears to be happening is that we flesh out our memories by adding plausible detail—a process called **confabulation**—without being aware that we are doing so. We may combine several similar events into one. If we are asked to remember our sixth birthday party, say, we may retrieve a jumble of memories from a number of childhood birthday parties and fit them together to make one coherent scene. In the most extreme cases, some people claim to remember past lives, but this is clearly a mixture of details remembered from their current lives, memories of history books and the media, and

Confabulation: the addition of plausible detail to a memory to make it seem more complete; this process takes place without the individual being aware of it.

other material fitted together into plausible confabulations. Keep in mind that there are likely to be reasons for it occurring—and we are not generally aware or those reasons, or even that we are confabulating.

Although much can be done to improve the accuracy of memory, it will always remain fragile. When the basic structures involved in memory fail to function properly, problems inevitably arise. One of the symptoms of dementia is that the process of moving information from short-term to long-term storage becomes faulty. Patients have no trouble remembering the distant past, but the recent past becomes murky. Because this is an unpleasant experience, confabulation may be called on to fill the gaps.

MEMORY AND HEALTH

Much about our personal experience of health is dependent on memory. We have memories about our personal experiences of health and illness. We also have information from outside sources, such as what we have read, heard from others and seen, and many cases that we have observed or been told about. This information influences our understanding of what health, illness and disease are, our reactions to them, and the behaviours that we carry out.

DEMENTIA

Dementia is the loss of cognitive or intellectual functions. It has received an enormous amount of attention in recent years because of its increasing prevalence in the population. Much of this increasing prevalence has to do with the ageing of the population. Better health care can maintain life longer, but longer life can result in a longer time for deterioration in body structures to occur. Although Alzheimer's disease probably receives the vast majority of attention in the media, dementia results from a number of conditions. It is always the result of damage to, or death of, nerve cells in the brain, and it is this that leads to its effects. Once the damage has occurred, it cannot be repaired, so the focus of treatment is to prevent more damage from occurring.

One of the first and most obvious functions to be affected is memory. Not surprisingly, it is the newest and least well-established memories that tend to be affected first, which explains why a childhood memory may remain while the sufferer forgets their doctor's name. Even if at some time in the future biomedical sciences could find a way to regenerate the damaged or dead nerve cells, this would only be able restore function: the memories stored in the original cells would still be gone.

There are something like fifty known causes of dementia, including neurological disease (Alzheimer's and Parkinson's disease are examples), vascular disease (such as multi-infarct dementia, involving death of localised groups of cells due to cutting off of their blood supply) and infections (such as HIV). When the deterioration is progressive, other important mental functions—such as problem solving, decision making, judgment and understanding— are affected. This can result in the loss of all of a person's individual qualities. Such loss is accompanied by personality change.

Because of the loss of function, the sufferer becomes less able to care for themselves. This means the burden of care on other people increases, which means in turn that carers' health may be affected.

CASE STUDY

MARGOT CALWELL AND DRIVING SAFELY

Margot Calwell is a 17-year-old high school student who has just applied for her learner's permit, as she wants to be able to drive a car as soon as she turns 18. Since young people have faster reflexes than older people, she wonders why she needs to keep a record for her driving practice, and why she has to have so many hours of practice before she gets her licence. Her existing knowledge—gained from watching adults drive—suggests to Margot that driving is easy. However, learning how to drive involves developing new manual skills such as steering, braking and watching out for other cars that have not been obvious to her before. In addition, these skills must be integrated with existing skills such as balance and visual scanning that she has already learnt from walking or riding a bicycle or skateboard. Gradually, it becomes clear to her that practice is going to be necessary for these changes in behaviour to happen. Adult drivers may have thousands (and up to hundreds of thousands) of hours of driving experience, under a large variety of conditions. As a result, they will have learnt not just basic skills but also a range of coping strategies for different conditions. Through practice, these become so well learnt that they become automatic. One reason why older women have fewer accidents than other groups of drivers is that they often have coping strategies (such as driving more cautiously, and slowing down or stopping when in doubt) that result in them being in fewer situations that require fast decisions or speedy reaction time.

However, driving seems to come very easily to Margot, and after ten hours of driving around an empty car park on Sunday afternoons, Margot feels that she is competent to drive anywhere and at any time. Margot is a frequent user of her mobile phone, and can read and send texts quickly and confidently almost anywhere. She finds is difficult to ignore her phone, as she feels that she might miss out on something. Having finally persuaded her mother to let her drive the car home from the car park after practising, Margot becomes distracted when her phone rings, and runs into a parked car. Although the damage to both cars is minor, Margot experiences a lot of distress, and subsequently finds it hard to even think about driving without experiencing anxiety. Her parents think she is being 'a bit phobic' about this.

Finally, after getting used to riding with other people, and after a great deal of persuasion by all of her family members, Margot again begins to take lessons. She no longer objects to the long hours of practice, and gradually becomes confident enough to drive in different conditions: at night, during rainy weather, in heavy traffic and at higher speeds on country highways. With her parents' agreement, she takes a 'defensive driving' course. She finally passes her driving test and receives her licence, although she is disappointed to learn that because of her age and her accident, she will have to pay much higher insurance premiums than her older sister (who is 25), and that most rental car companies won't even let her drive one of their cars.

1   How would an understanding of how people learn and remember skills help to understand Margot's story?

2   How could one small accident result in the development of a phobia about driving cars?

3   Would having an accident and subsequent anxiety cause a permanent change in Margot's driving behaviour?

4   What factors could influence her level of risk once she is a fully licensed driver?

Points to consider

Both the activities of driving and texting involve attention, information processing, decision making and physical movement behaviours. As large areas of the brain and memory are involved, the same functions may be called upon by both activities. Anything that interferes with the behaviours involved in safe driving will increase the likelihood of accidents occurring. It is estimated that the risk of using mobile phones while driving is similar to the risk of driving under the influence of alcohol or drugs. It slows reaction times, interferes with motor skills, distracts attention and prevents to recall of important memories for coping with driving—just as the use of substances does.

Insurance companies operate on the basis of probabilities. They need to take actions that will reduce their risk of increased costs resulting from accidents. It is likely that slightly older drivers will have over-learnt coping skills behind the wheel, and will therefore have fewer accidents, and less serious ones. Also, very poor or substance-abusing drivers will be the most likely to have accidents, and these companies will have identified these individuals within the first few years of driving, and subsequently refuse to deal with them.

CHAPTER SUMMARY

- In developed countries in recent decades, behaviour and lifestyle have replaced infections as the main sources of illness and death.
- Modification of behaviour can prevent much illness and help to promote health.
- Risky behaviours—including smoking, alcohol abuse, illegal or prescription drug abuse, obesity and dangerous activities—constitute areas in which behaviour change is particularly important.
- Health behaviours increase levels of health, while risk-reduction behaviours are aimed at reducing the health impacts of risky behaviours.
- The study of learning (that is, the change in the organism as a result of one's experience with the environment) and memory (the processes by which experience is retained with the organism) provide a basis for understanding behaviour change.
- Simple models of learning, such as classical and operant conditioning, indicate that stimuli that lead to behaviour and consequences that follow it are critical to stability and change in behaviour.
- Memory processes provide us with the information that we use to understand health and illness. Dementia is a significant health problem in which memory is affected.

SELF TEST

1   The major causes of death in developed countries in recent times are:

   a   infections such as HIV/AIDS, hepatitis and pneumonia
   b   long-term effects of genetic disorders
   c   accidents, injuries and consequences of war
   d   none of the above.

2 Overuse of alcohol is risky to health because:
  a it causes tissue damage
  b it leads to behaviour that can be risky
  c it interferes with coordination and thinking
  d all of the above.

3 Marian has developed a phobia about doctors. Assuming that this is classically
  conditioned, doctors are:
  a the unconditioned stimulus
  b the unconditioned response
  c the conditioned stimulus
  d the conditioned response.

4 Mr Orson takes his 6-year-old son to see Dr Lee because the boy wets his bed at night.
  Dr Lee suggests a treatment that combines punishment (an alarm that sounds when
  the bed is wet) with positive reinforcement (praise) because:
  a the combination increases the amount of avoidance learning
  b the undesirable behaviours are more likely to be discouraged
  c the desirable behaviours are made more apparent
  d positive reinforcement alone is not very effective.

5 Dai received a sporting injury and began to take medication for his pain. Now, his
  doctor tells Dai that he has recovered and is at risk of becoming addicted to his pain
  medication, but Dai becomes anxious when he thinks about giving it up. It is most likely
  that:
  a the pain will be too much for Dai to bear without medication
  b the medication has become a learnt reinforcement
  c Dai's need for the medication has extinguished without him being aware of it
  d the pain medication is a dangerous narcotic.

FURTHER READING

Doidge, N. (2008) *The brain that changes itself: stories of personal triumph from the frontiers of brain science.* Melbourne: Scribe.

Hammersley, R. (2010) Alcohol and drug use (chap. 6). In D. French, K. Vedhara, A.A. Kaptein & J. Weinman (eds) *Health Psychology* (2nd edn). Chichester: BPS Blackwell.

Hassed, C. (2008) *The essence of health: the seven pillars of wellbeing.* Sydney, Random House.

Various authors (2011) *Index of Learning Theories and Models.* Knowledge Base and Webliography, accessed at www.learning-theories.com.

USEFUL WEBSITES

Healthy Behaviors: Addressing Chronic Illness at its Roots (Grantmakers in Health):
www.gih.org/usr_doc/Healthy_Behaviors_Issue_Brief.pdf

Learned Helplessness (Emotional Competency):
www.emotionalcompetency.com/helpless.htm

Recreational Drugs and Their Effects (Australian Department of Health and Aging):
www.drugs.health.gov.au/internet/drugs/publishing.nsf/content/home-1

Teens are Hardwired for Risky Behavior (WebMD):
www.webmd.com/parenting/news/20070413/teens-are-hardwired-for-risky-behavior

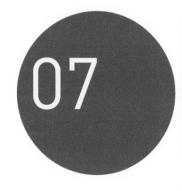

THINKING ABOUT HEALTH BEHAVIOUR: COGNITION AND HEALTH

CHAPTER OBJECTIVES

By the end of your study of this chapter, you should be able to:

- understand the common ways in which individuals make decisions and how this influences decisions about health and illness, and the clinical decision making of health professionals
- describe and compare various models of health beliefs and action regarding health, including why this behaviour may not appear to be in the best interests of the individual
- understand the role of attitudes and expectations in regulating behaviour
- describe placebo effects and how they relate to expectations
- discuss the issues raised by the use of placebo effects in research and treatment of patients.

KEYWORDS

attitudes
agent
algorithm
automatisation
balance theory
cognition
compliance
endorphins
expectancy–value theory

expectations
heuristics
perception explanations
placebo effects
stereotyping
validation
wonder drug effect

INTRODUCTION

In Chapter 4, we looked at the decisions that someone makes when they experience symptoms and about thoughts that people may have about their health. It is time to take a more detailed look at thinking and problem solving in health and illness.

Cognition is a useful psychological term that refers to all of the mental processes that we use. In everyday language this includes reasoning, judging, mulling, problem-solving, deciding, comparing and all of the other ways we have of dealing with information. If we are to look at the ways in which people deal with health and illness, we need to look at the general processes underlying conscious (and possibly unconscious) thinking and decision making.

One way of looking at these processes is to say that they involve the transformation of information that may come from memory, sensory input from the environment, or sensory input from within body. This information is then dealt with in some fashion; for example, by deciding that it is unimportant and can be ignored, by relating it to other information, by comparing it to memories, or by deciding that it is worth holding on to against some future need. These transformations may take place in the forefront of our attention or they may just go on in the background without our paying too much attention to them. Some of the processing is relatively automatic, as when a smell produces a memory without our thinking about why it smells familiar. At other times the transformation requires a lot of effort, as when we are trying to learn a new set of concepts.

Cognition: a general concept embracing all types of knowing, judging, thinking, reasoning and so on.

DAVID AND MARTA BAUM AND IMMUNISATION

CASE STUDY

The aim of this case is to examine the ways in which decisions about health are made.

David and Marta Baum have been told by their doctor, Dr Teresa Ngou, that their daughter Alexis should be immunised against rubella (German measles). They have been told that there is a small risk that Alexis could actually get rubella as a result of the immunisation. If she isn't immunised, however, she could get a much worse case later in life. If she were pregnant at the time, her baby might be born deaf and/or blind. David and Marta would like to make the best decision possible.

They have talked about immunisation within their family, and have some friends who are very strongly opposed to immunisation. They have seen magazine articles about immunisation, and even searched for relevant information on the internet. Some of the information seems contradictory. All in all, it is pretty confusing.

1   What factors would affect David and Marta's decision about immunisation?
2   How could they go about improving the quality of their decision?

RATIONAL DECISION MAKING

Cognition often involves decision making: choosing a preferred option or course of action from among several alternatives. We have to make many of these decisions every day, from major ones such as whether to get married or choose a particular career, to minor ones such as which brand of breakfast cereal to eat, or whether to take the first available parking spot or hope for another one closer to our destination. Decisions often have to be made on the basis of incomplete or uncertain information. How do we decide to take this parking space when we cannot know for sure whether there will be a closer one? Decisions often have to be made in the face of conflicting information; for example, your mother wants you to be a doctor, but your father wants you to be an athlete. Sometimes there is conflict regarding one's own preferences; for example, whether to pursue a potentially huge but very uncertain income as a rock star, or the certainty of an accountant's income. These same issues arise with regard to health-related decisions.

It would be nice to believe that we are rational about our decisions, weighing up the costs and gains and picking the most sensible alternative every time. **Expectancy–value theory** is the name given to one approach to understanding decision making. It suggests that it should be possible to predict our choices by mathematical modelling, based on our attitudes about alternative choices.

Expectancy–value theory: a model that suggests that rational choices between alternatives are based on the perceived probability of occurrence of each option and its value to the individual.

PAUSE & REFLECT

Do you have a health behaviour that seems to be irrational? What about your friends? Can you use expectancy–value theory to explain why that behaviour continues?

Expectancy–value theory assumes that behaviour results from conscious choices among alternatives whose purpose is to maximise gain and minimise loss. 'Expectancy' refers to the strength of the person's belief that an outcome is obtainable. This expectancy has probabilities ranging from 0 (it is impossible) to 1.0 (it is certain). The term 'value' describes the value of the outcome to that individual. To the extent that our decision making is rational and based on the best evidence that we have available, we should be trying to select the alternative that produces the highest combination of expectancy and value. An individual who has low expectancy that smoking is harmful and values smoking highly, for example, may rationally decide to continue smoking. In their case, they gain more from smoking than the health cost they ascribe to it.

Expectancy–value theory can written as a formula:

$$\text{Behaviour} = \text{Expectancy} \times \text{Value}$$

Expectancy–value theory helps to predict many decisions, but works best when the information we have is relatively complete. If we have to choose, say, between buying one car and another, we usually can find out exactly how obtainable each car is and the cost in dollars if the cars are similarly equipped. Similarly, gains in comfort and prestige will be fairly clear. But even in this case, we often waver and struggle to decide, and may be swayed by qualities that we would have trouble defining even to ourselves. It is difficult for expectancy–value theory to explain why people bet on lotteries, for example, since any analysis would show that each bet is likely to be a loss, and that over time the regular gambler is very unlikely to gain any benefit.

Algorithm: a mechanical routine or simple set of rules that can be used to solve all problems of a particular kind.

When we do have complete information we can use **algorithms** to reach decisions. An algorithm is a mechanical routine or simple set of rules that can be used to solve all problems of a particular kind. Mathematical processes such as addition, subtraction, multiplication and division are algorithms. As long as you do not make a mistake while carrying them out, you will get the right answer. Many games—noughts and crosses and checkers, for instance—are simple enough that you can use algorithms and only lose if you make a mistake. The same is true of balancing your bank account.

If, as is often the case, we do not have enough information to enable us to use algorithms, then we run out of rules that can be guaranteed to provide a right answer. Chess, for example, has far too many possible moves for a player to be certain that they have considered them all. Daily choices tend to involve a lot of complex information that is relevant to the decision and a lot of extraneous noise that is not. The choice of what to eat for breakfast would take all day if we were to consider each possible ingredient in the light of rules about nutritional value, possible risk and taste preferences—our own and those of any other people who might be sharing breakfast with us. By the time we finally came to a decision, we would probably have starved to death. It is clear that much of our decision making is less than completely rational.

HEURISTICS

Decision making is often complex and is affected by many variables, including age, gender, experience, the influence of other people, and the beliefs that a person holds. Information about expectancy and value are often very incomplete and fuzzy, yet decisions still have to made—often urgently. The result is that individuals use other, less rigorously rational ways of making decisions. A large group of these are called **heuristics**, with simple ones often referred to as 'rules of thumb'. Examples include, 'Keep your head down and your eye on the ball' in golf, or 'Never talk to strangers'. While these rules of thumb are often based on experience—our own or others'—and can be helpful, they can often lead to irrational decision making.

> **Heuristics:** problem-solving strategies that are based on general rules that usually or often work.

One type of heuristic is means–end analysis. After deciding where you would like to end up, you choose actions that appear to get you closer to that end. If your end with regard to breakfast is to eat in time to get to work, you may select any combination of things that you encounter in the environment that can be eaten safely; all of them will get you fed. Imagine you are a novice chess player, and you have been told that chess players try to control the centre of the board because it greatly increases their chances of winning. If you were to play your first game of chess, you may well adopt strategy in the absence of any other heuristics you could use. However, while it might help you to lose more slowly, it would be unlikely to help you win against the expertise of seasoned players.

Another type of heuristic is reasoning by analogy. It is based on trying to use decision-making rules that have worked in similar situations. If you have tried standing between an opponent and their goal in one sport and it has worked, you might try this in another sport that has opponents and goals. This rule could be taken from basketball and successfully applied in football, but it is not an analogy that one would want to apply in golf.

A lot of problem-solving heuristics are aimed at simplifying the problem. The term 'simplification' is used in mathematics to describe a number of procedures that have been found to improve the ability to see a possible solution. Grouping similar terms is an example. Many non-mathematical problems can be broken down into smaller parts. In subgoal analysis, the aim is to break the final goal into a number of smaller problems with goals that get you part of the way to a solution, and then attempt to find solutions to each of the smaller problems.

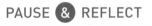

PAUSE & REFLECT

What are some of the heuristics that you use when you are taking notes in class? How do you simplify things so your notes are most useful for studying later?

We frequently use heuristics when making decisions about health. If you are suffering as a result of a cold virus, there is little you can do about the virus except let your immune system develop a defence. In the meantime, taking paracetamol for the fever and pain will get you closer to the goal of not suffering. This is known as a means–end decision.

Complying with the instructions of a health professional is often associated with getting better. By extension, it is probably going to be a good idea to comply with the instructions of the next health professional you consult. Health professionals often use subgoal analysis to decide how to treat the health problems of a particular patient.

Heuristics have two advantages over algorithms: they will work with incomplete information, and they are fast. They have the disadvantage that they can be (and frequently are) wrong. The next section considers some heuristics relevant to health decisions and some of their shortcomings.

CASE STUDY

DAVID AND MARTA (CONT.)

David and Marta might try to make the most rational decision they could by using expectancy-value theory. This would involve comparing the degree and probability of risk of having Alexis immunised against not having her immunised, and comparing the two. In this case, they find that the risks are pretty much guesswork, even when their doctor can tell them something about the probabilities. Since they aren't comfortable that they know enough to make a 'scientific' decision, they think about other things that could help their decision.

There are a number of heuristics that David and Marta could use. They could use the analogy mentioned above: that it is in general a good idea to do what the doctor says. People often reason by analogy with individual cases that they have known about. So David and Marta talk to a neighbour, who tells them about a cousin of his who died as a result of complications arising from immunisation against polio. This information worries David and Marta, as it suggests that Alexis might die.

1   What problems are raised by making decisions based on stories you hear about a single case or anecdote?
2   What are some of the advantages and disadvantages of making health-related decisions by using heuristics such as analogy?

HEALTH HEURISTICS

REPRESENTATIVENESS

People make decisions because they believe that a particular event is representative of a category of event. Consider a couple who had three sons. Although they had always wanted a daughter, they decided not to have any more children because they thought the next child was bound to be a boy. Was this a correct conclusion? Not really. In the absence of a reproductive problem, which had been eliminated in this case, each conception has approximately the same chance of producing a girl as a boy. The sequence of chances that had produced boys three times in a row for this couple was irrelevant to the sex of their next child. To take another example, consider a medical doctor who dismissed his mother's complaints of pain in her hip as not serious because she suffered from arthritis and frequently had pain in her hips. She was subsequently found to have broken her hip as a result of a fall, and he felt very guilty that he had biased his judgment of her pain on this occasion by viewing it as representative of her typical kind of pain.

AVAILABILITY

Because decisions are based on the information that we can call to mind or find in other ways, they will be influenced by the availability of the information—how easy it is to remember or to find. If our cultural background is Chinese or many of our friends are Chinese, we have a high likelihood of encountering individuals who have taken Chinese herbal medicines and become well. If few of our friends are Chinese, we may know very few who have done so. Our judgment as to whether we should try Chinese herbal medicines will be affected by this information, but it should not be. Who we know does not influence the effectiveness of the medicines in any way. The sample we have knowledge of is a biased sample, in a statistical sense. If our cultural background is Chinese or we have many Chinese friends, we will find available examples easily. If we do not, examples will not be available.

Nisbett and Ross (1980) showed that vivid information is given more importance in our decision making than less vivid information, apparently because it is more easily available. Information is likely to attract and hold our attention to the extent that it is emotionally interesting, concrete, image-provoking and/or recent, nearby or involves someone we know. This can explain why media stories about miraculous new treatments attract so much attention and can lead to people trying something that does not have a good evidence base. Wonder drug stories are certainly vivid.

PAUSE & REFLECT

Think of a recent health-related story that has made a great impact on you. What was it about that story that made it so effective?

CLINICAL DECISION MAKING

It may appear that the main difference between experts and others is that the expert has more knowledge. While the decision making of health professionals about patients involves the same processes as those described above, expert health professionals' decision making also differs from less expert individuals in a number of ways.

Some algorithms are used. The process of making a differential diagnosis involves listing the diagnoses that a reasonable professional could make based on the observed symptoms and signs. Results of the history obtained from the patient and tests that have been performed, along with any other data that can be found, are used to eliminate some of the diagnoses from the list, until the most probable one is identified. Other diagnoses of lower probability may not have been fully excluded; the competent professional keeps these in mind until they can be excluded.

Biomedical theories about how particular causes produce particular symptoms and signs produce models of operation for health professionals. These theories may change as more knowledge is obtained, but to the extent that they represent how things really operate, they are algorithms. But they may well be incomplete or only partially accurate, in which case they resemble heuristics more than they do algorithms.

Health professionals use a variety of heuristics that may have been learnt from others or derived from the professionals' own experience. These medical rules of thumb can be as simple as testing all adult patients for high blood pressure. Means–end analysis is frequently used to try to decide how to make a patient feel better as well as treating the cause of their disease. In the absence of a specific diagnosis of a disease—which is very common in practice—subgoal analysis may focus on relieving symptoms, one at a time, until the problem goes away or the diagnosis becomes clearer. Simplification strategies could include identifying what the most important symptom is for the patient and concentrating on that first, or grouping problems that have similar treatments.

Pattern recognition is an important decision-making process. As a result of training or experience, health professionals develop an ability to recognise combinations of elements that may signal the presence of a meaningful pattern, which could include information from an observation of the patient's appearance and behaviour that leads to a feeling that the problem is likely to be a specific one. This can lead to the professional making correct choices about what questions to ask, how to ask them, or how to respond to the patient—questions that speed up or smooth the process of diagnosis and treatment.

Automatisation: the carrying out of patterns of behaviour or thinking that are so well learnt that they require no apparent thought.

Automatisation refers to patterns of behaviour or thinking that are so well learnt that they require no apparent thought. Hand washing becomes automatised for many health professionals, as does the care of equipment and touching of patients. Taking histories may also become automatic. A problem for students in the health professions is that their clinical teachers may forget that a decision-making process that is automatised for them will need careful step-by-step explanation for students. This is as true for diagnostic heuristics as it is for the proper way to give an injection. Automatisation is not restricted to the behaviour of health professionals, however. It is common through all aspects of our lives, from the way in which we hold our cutlery or chopsticks while we eat, to the way we type when we are writing an essay.

HEALTH BELIEFS

The cognitions that an individual has regarding health are a major influence on health behaviour. An important part of these cognitions is **attitudes**. Attitudes consist of the thoughts, feelings and readiness to act that we have about any object, person or event. Our attitude to peanut butter, for example, may include knowledge about its nutritional value, feelings about its taste and stickiness, and readiness to eat peanut butter if it is offered, or to go out and buy some if there is none available in the house.

Attitudes: the thoughts, feelings and readiness to act that an individual has about any object, person or event.

To take an example from a health-related area, attitudes to exercise would include not only knowledge of what it is and what effects it can have on cardiovascular fitness, but also how exercising makes the individual feel and whether that individual is prepared to go out and exercise in the face of competing time and energy demands. Health psychologists—along with advertisers, politicians and many others—have an interest in understanding how we make decisions about health. One primary focus in the study of health behaviour has been on the interaction between attitudes—our thoughts, feelings and behavioural intentions—and their relationship to actual behaviour.

CROSS-REFERENCE
The sick role is discussed in Chapter 4.

CROSS-REFERENCE
The influence of culture, social class and family are discussed in Chapter 14.

By understanding people's attitudes, researchers can use them in promoting health. Using a vivid emotional story, for example, may be more helpful in persuading people to adopt certain health behaviours than using statistics to convey similar information. A very important influence on health decision making is being part of a group. Groups share knowledge, attitudes and biases. They also confer the rights and obligations of the sick role.

Because of differences in health beliefs between cultures, it is important that health professionals have at least a general knowledge of what those health beliefs are. For example, Vickery and Westerman (2004) found that many Aboriginal people in Western Australia did not think of depression as a disease that could be treated. Similar issues arise with First Peoples in other countries, and with immigrants and refugees.

The general principles of decision making discussed above are all relevant to health decision making, but a number of theories have been proposed that are specifically aimed at predicting important choices about health. The persistence of unhealthy behaviour—which should be very unlikely if decision making is rational—indicates the importance of understanding the process. There are quite a number of theories about health behaviour, which is in itself a problem (Noar & Zimmerman 2005; Weinstein 2007) because it can lead to confusion and even be misleading. This issue is discussed after a brief presentation of some sample theories.

THEORIES ABOUT HEALTH BELIEFS

The health belief model (HBM), depicted in Figure 7.1, was developed by people who were interested in patient compliance with recommended health behaviours (Taylor 2006; Rosenstock 1974). There is a degree of resemblance between the HBM and expectancy–value theory. The degree of perceived threat (value) to individuals is made up of their general views about the importance of health, their personal vulnerability to a particular threat, and the severity of that threat if it were to occur. The individual's perception of the benefits that would come from a particular health behaviour and the barriers to that health behaviour are important in determining whether they will believe that the health behaviour is possible and likely to be effective in averting the threat (expectancy). This model predicts some behaviour quite well, but does not seem to account for all of the cognitive factors involved in health behaviour (Taylor 2006; Allen 1998). Noar and Zimmerman (2005) suggest that the HBM might be most useful when the health threat presented by a particular behaviour is obvious to the individual.

Figure 7.1   Health belief model

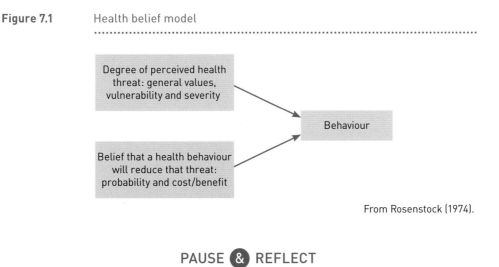

From Rosenstock (1974).

PAUSE **&** REFLECT

Where have your own attitudes towards smoking come from? Have media campaigns played a significant part? What about your parents?

The HBM did not take into account the social influence of others (approval or disapproval of the behaviour) in the decision-making process (Fishbein & Ajzen 1975). In many cases, people's decisions about health behaviour are influenced by what they hear from others, what is presented in the media, and what the general opinions of health professionals are. The theory of reasoned action (Fishbein & Ajzen 1975; see Figure 7.2) tried to predict motivations for health behaviours, including social influence. Norms (the person's perception of what others believe should be done) and attitudes (the person's perception of the consequences of a behaviour) were seen to impact on the individual's intentions to behave. It was predicted that intentions would accurately predict actual behaviour.

Figure 7.2   The theory of reasoned action

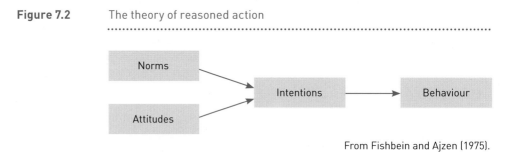

From Fishbein and Ajzen (1975).

This model of decision making about health has enabled people to predict health behaviours in a variety of settings, but begins to have trouble when people either do not control the behaviour in question or at least believe that they do not control it. This modification leads to the theory of planned behaviour (Ajzen & Madden 1986; see Figure 7.3).

Figure 7.3   The theory of planned behaviour

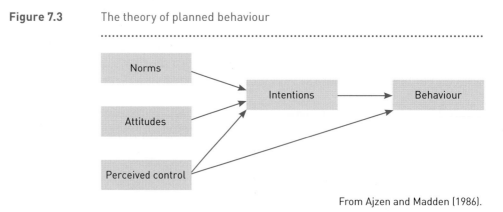

From Ajzen and Madden (1986).

Neither of these models appears to take much account of the past behaviour or habits of the individual on present behaviour. Noar and Zimmerman (2005) suggest that they may be most useful when the connection between intention and behaviour is strong and clear to the individual.

Clearly, the influence of our thought processes on our behaviour is complex. We cannot expect all health behaviour to be rational.

TOO MANY THEORIES?

There are thousands of studies that have looked at whether theories of health behaviour really explain health behaviour (Weinstein 2007). The typical conclusion is that a particular set of cognitions occurs in those individuals whose behaviour changes, and does not occur in those whose behaviour does not change. This is usually demonstrated by correlations between cognitions and behaviours at the end of the process, which, unfortunately, doesn't enable us to be certain that it was the existence of the cognitions in the first place that led to the behaviour. There could have been common factors that produced both, or it could be the behaviour that led to the cognitions (Bandura 1998).

Noar and Zimmerman (2005) suggest that the result of this mass of research is not really advancing our knowledge about what regulates behaviour, and that we need a different approach if we are to move forward. They recommend comparing different theories within the same study to see if we can determine whether there are particular cognitions that are more important than others. These studies would still need to be carried out with many different behaviours because any single theory may predict better in one situation than another. They would also need to begin before the behaviour change attempt started, so that the order of events could be studied all the way through the process. There is also a problem with the multiplication of concepts used in various studies. Weinstein (1984) suggested that we need to consider unrealistic optimism as a factor, and Rogers (1985) suggested including fear in the health belief model. This increase in the number of concepts can result in confusion and a lack of comparability between studies. Ogden (2007) describes the addition of ethical/moral norms, anticipated regret, self-identity, ambivalence, emotion, personality and self-prediction to various models—adding further to these conceptual issues.

Another problem with the large number of theories is that just because they use different terms, they don't necessarily differ from one another (Weinstein 2007). A lot of the concepts used are very similar to one another. The most obvious case is the theory of planned behaviour, which was developed out of the theory of reasoned action by the addition of the concept of perceived control. How different is that from the importance of cognitions in the health belief model regarding whether a healthy behaviour is possible and likely to be effective in averting a threat to health? Ogden (2003) has advanced the view that while each of these theories may help predict some behaviours some of the time, they may lead to circular reasoning; that is, the conclusions drawn from them may be 'true by definition rather than by observation' (p. 424). There are common elements in these theories that are almost certainly of importance. One of these is knowledge about a link between a particular behaviour and some aspect of health. If the person is not aware that a behaviour is unhealthy, they will not be motivated to change that behaviour. A second common element is the perceptions that a person has about their control over the behaviour. The person who doesn't believe that the behaviour is controllable, or who believes that they can't control it for some reason, is unlikely to make the effort. These beliefs about control may relate to barriers (for example, they may not be able to afford professional help) or personal capabilities (they may have an external locus of control and believe that powerful others control their outcomes).

One way of simplifying these models is to look at how a variety of factors may act through a more general factor. The integrative model of behavioural prediction (IM; Fishbein 2008) focuses on how a number of the factors described above impact on motivation. In the IM, intention to behave in a particular way, along with relevant behavioural skills and environmental factors that allow or constrain the behaviour, are seen as exerting direct influence on behaviour. Understanding these three elements can lead to predictions about both individual behaviour change and the effectiveness of broader inventions aimed at groups or populations. (See Chapter 16 for more about health promotion.)

Most of the factors discussed in the previous paragraphs exert influence by changing the individual's intention to behave. For example, beliefs that a behaviour will affect health or emotions such as fear both act on our intentions to behave. If we have the necessary skills to carry out the behaviour, and nothing in the environment prevents it (or if something promotes it), we will have a higher likelihood of carrying out the behaviour. While is it more general than most models, the IM still does not necessarily answer all of the objections given above. One general theory of behaviour (not just health behaviour) that takes these aspects into account is social cognitive theory (Bandura 1986).

SOCIAL COGNITIVE THEORY

Agent: the person who has control over the stimuli and/or reinforcements for change.

As applied to health behaviour, the emphasis of social cognitive theory is on the individual as the **agent** of change. The central links between the person and the outcome are efficacy beliefs and outcome expectations (Bandura 1998). Efficacy beliefs can come about through four main influences. The most effective of these influences are mastery experiences. When the individual attempts to exert control and is successful, these mastery experiences increase the individual's sense of self-efficacy; conversely, failure undermines self-efficacy. The second influence comes from vicarious experiences, in which the individual observes what happens to others (role models) when they exert control and succeed or fail. The third influence is social persuasion, which involves direct or indirect attempts to convey to individuals that they can influence their outcomes through their own efforts and that change is possible. Within all of these situations, it is important not to overlook the influence of the somatic and emotional states of the individual, which may have nothing to do with the actual demands they face. Tiredness can lead to a lowered sense of control, for example, even if it has resulted from illness rather than from efforts to exert control. Depression arises in biochemical processes within the brain, but has profound effects on cognitions. The depressed individual feels helpless to influence events or their own feelings, and the hopelessness that accompanies depression saps motivation to behave at all.

CROSS-REFERENCE
The relationship between self-efficacy and reinforcement is discussed in Chapter 5.

CROSS-REFERENCE
Expectations are discussed in more detail later in the chapter, with particular reference to placebo effects.

Outcome expectations refers to cognitions that the individual has about what will follow a particular behaviour. This is related to expectancy in expectancy–value theory and elements of most health beliefs models. Bandura (1998) states that these expectations include beliefs about how the behaviour will make the individual feel (physical), what kinds of reactions the behaviour will produce in other people who observe it (social) and how the individual will view themselves following the behaviour (self-evaluative). This latter aspect is, in Bandura's view, often overlooked in theories about health behaviour.

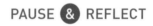

PAUSE & REFLECT

Write down a list of your outcome expectations regarding exercise. How many are physical, social and self-evaluative?

One of the differences between social cognitive theory and many of the others described above is that it is more general; that is, it is intended to describe a broader range of behaviour than just health behaviour. As a result, it can be helpful in integrating theories of health behaviour and in designing ways to compare them. There are, of course, other theories of this more general sort, such as self-determination theory (Ryan & Deci 2000). Attempts to compare theories are not common, however, and there appears to be a great deal of overlap between them. Cognitive theories are useful in explaining a variety of behaviours that are important to health; compliance with healthy behaviour or treatment is one of the most important of these.

THE STEPS LEADING TO HEALTH BEHAVIOUR CHANGE

Prochaska and DiClemente (1984) looked at the steps that people tend to go through when moving towards a change in health-related behaviour. Their model is called the transtheoretical model as it enables other theories to be brought together to map the process of change. It can be used to guide thinking about what kinds of intervention are most likely to help people to move in the direction of change. It also serves as a useful model of decision making. It is often described as a spiral model, because individuals frequently drop back from a higher stage to a lower one as motivation wavers, as accidents interfere with change, or if relapses occur.

CROSS-REFERENCE

You should be able to see similarities between this model and the model of illness behaviour as a process discussed in Chapter 4.

1   The *precontemplation stage* refers to the time before behaviour change is considered. The individual either does not realise they have a problem or has no thoughts that the problem can be changed. Interventions at this stage need to be aimed at bringing about awareness of the problem.

PAUSE & REFLECT

What strategy might you use to encourage change in a patient who has no intention of altering their risky behaviour? How could you introduce the idea of change (without confrontation) with, for example, a cyclist who won't wear a helmet?

2   The *contemplation stage* begins when the individual recognises that something is wrong and needs to be changed. This does not mean that a decision has been made to do something or that they have a plan for doing something. Interventions at this stage should focus on the probability that change is possible and that it would have a significant effect on the individual's risk of ill health.

3   The *preparation stage* refers to the time during which the individual is thinking about how to go about changing a behaviour. They may be evaluating strategies they have heard about, talking to others who have made the change, and developing the commitment to try. Interventions at this stage aim at motivating and educating about change rather than just about the problem itself.

4   The *action stage* is when the individual has begun to modify the behaviour. This does not mean that the change has taken place, or that it is certain to occur, only that the change attempt has begun. At this stage, it is best if interventions focus on encouragement and motivation.

5   Once the behaviour is changed, the individual is in the *maintenance stage*. The importance of this stage is often overlooked in the enthusiasm over the fact that a change has occurred. Maintenance is critical: many well-planned change programs fall apart because the individual has no strategies for keeping the change going and dealing with relapses. Interventions here can look at the benefits gained from the change and what would be lost if the individual returned to the earlier behaviour. Specific relapse management strategies

(which are discussed in Chapter 8) and coping strategies to deal with temptation may be helpful.

Not all experts find this model useful. Bandura (1998) suggests that the boundaries between the stages of the transtheoretical model are fuzzy: matters of degree rather than true boundaries. How long, for example, does one stay in the action stage before they are in the maintenance stage? One month? Six? Another criticism of the stages of change is that the most effective intervention for a particular individual may include several elements that are linked to different stages. In fact, a general criticism of all stage theories is that they don't allow for individual variation.

CASE STUDY

DAVID AND MARTA (CONT.)

Dr Ngou maintains that it would be a good idea to have Alexis immunised against rubella. David and Marta decide to accept whatever she recommends, because to them she is the expert where matters pertaining to health are concerned (a heuristic).

Although David and Marta seem to be willing to accept her word in this specific case, Alexis will need other immunisations in the future and Dr Ngou would like to persuade them that immunisation in general is a good idea. She would like to change their attitudes and, more importantly, their behaviour for the future.

Dr Ngou decides that, as far as immunisation behaviour is concerned, David and Marta are in the contemplation stage because they are thinking about it. She knows then that she should try to increase their knowledge about the effectiveness of immunisation in preventing disease, and the importance of that prevention for Alexis's health and well-being. By talking to David and Marta about immunisation, Dr Ngou is providing them with norms, with the aim of modifying their intentions to immunise, which will encourage them to behave in a way that Dr Ngou believes is in Alexis's best interests.

Alexis is given her immunisation. Because her school friends have told her so, she expects that she will feel awful after the immunisation. If Alexis expects to feel bad after her immunisation, there is a high probability that she will (this is a variety of placebo effect). If her school friends have described a particular kind of feeling that follows immunisations, this is the kind that Alexis is likely to experience. If the doctor anticipates this, however, she can head off the side effects by using reassurance, persuasion and expectations.

1 How would giving David and Marta norms about having Alexis immunised for rubella be likely to affect their decisions about being immunised themselves?
2 Could Alexis's expectations about immunisation actually make it more likely that she will feel better?
3 Could an injection produce placebo effects?

COMPLIANCE

Given that we like to think of ourselves as rational beings, it is instructive to note that non-compliance with advice and instructions from health professionals is considered to be a serious and common problem. A majority of patients do not, for example, take medication in the doses or time patterns that doctors recommend. Sometimes this is because the patient did not understand the instructions, but usually it is because the patient was not motivated to follow instructions that they did understand. Shelton (1994: 15) lists the following as factors that reduce **compliance**: low levels of experienced distress, denial of the illness, poor communications, complexity of the treatment program, embarrassment about the treatment, side effects, and gains from remaining ill. Factors that encourage compliance include good communication, simple programs, clear instructions, positive reinforcement of compliance and, of course, any decrease in distress that comes with following the treatment program.

It is clear from this that compliance will be particularly low when the individual's diagnosis is not accompanied by a sense of being ill, such as treatment for high blood pressure, treatment for asthma aimed at preventing rather than relieving attacks, or antibiotic treatment where the individual should take all of the course of tablets regardless of whether the symptoms have gone away. Compliance will also be low if the side effects of treatment are unpleasant or embarrassing, such as when drugs cause stomach upset, headache or drowsiness.

There is much that can be done by both the health professional and health education to improve compliance. It is perhaps surprising that little is being done when the problem is so significant. The reason may well be found in the assumption that we are all more rational in our thinking and decision making about health than in other areas of life—because of the benefits to be gained and risks of not complying—but the study of health beliefs tends to indicate that this is not necessarily the case.

Compliance: obeying another's instruction, or acting as they would like; it does not necessarily mean agreeing with the reasons behind the instructions.

EXPECTATIONS AND HEALING

As these health beliefs models indicate, a wide variety of expectations may influence our behaviour: the beliefs of important others, our past experiences and our expectations about how the world works. These expectations play a very large role in regulating our thoughts, emotions and behaviours.

EXPECTATIONS

Expectations refer to the cognitions that individuals have about what is likely to happen in a given situation. When we flip a light switch, we expect to get light, not water. When we say to someone, 'How are you?' we expect to get a ritual response such as 'I'm fine', not details of digestion and respiration. Expectations allow us to simplify our interactions with the world so that they are predictable. (Recall that beliefs are expectations about the workings of the world, while health beliefs are expectations about the workings of health.)

Not surprisingly, we like to have our expectations confirmed. When we expect to do well in an examination, and we do well, we are pleased. If we do not do well, we are disappointed. When we do not expect to do well and do not, it gives us some satisfaction to prove ourselves right. Punishment can be satisfying if it confirms our expectations. It means that the world is a predictable place and that we can organise ourselves to meet it. A stable life is predictable. Research on life stress—the effect on someone's health of the events that occur to them—has shown that change is always stressful, whether it is positive change such as a promotion, or negative change such as loss of a job. In either case, change decreases our certainty about how to behave and what to expect.

Expectations: the cognitions that individuals have about what is likely to happen in a given situation.

CROSS-REFERENCE
Life events and stress are discussed in Chapter 12.

Balance theory: an approach that suggests consistency is the organising principle of our cognitions.

Balance theory (Heider 1967) suggests that consistency is the organising principle of our cognitions. Thus, if our cognitions are consistent with one another, we are in a state of balance—a satisfactory state. For example, you might want all of your friends to like one another. If your two best friends hate one another, it creates a state of imbalance within you, and you will work to produce a more balanced state. You might drop one friend, deciding that the other friend is right and the dropped one is really not so nice after all. You might work to change both your friends' minds by getting them to like one another. If all else fails, you may deny the imbalance by convincing yourself (inaccurately) that they really do like one another but just cannot manage to be in the same place at the same time because of chance factors. Consistency is also important to the way in which we form expectations about people.

PAUSE & REFLECT

Try to remember a time when your cognitions were unbalanced: when you felt stressed because things didn't seem to make sense. What happened? Did you choose to change some of your thinking to make yourself more comfortable?

The importance of the individual's expectations of a medical treatment to its outcome was demonstrated in a study done by Dix (1985), who looked at the expectations of patients with long-term pain resulting from osteoarthritis of the knee. All patients took part in three treatment conditions over a three-month period. At the end of this period, the subjects who reported the most improvement were those who had moderate expectations at the beginning. By comparison, those who had either low or high expectations showed little improvement. Those with low expectations got what they expected—not much. Those whose expectations were too high could not have been satisfied by any treatment and were disappointed. Moderate and realistic expectations seem to be crucial to the achievement of improvement, whatever the treatment.

PLACEBO EFFECTS

Historically, a placebo (from the Latin for 'I will please') was thought of as a sugar pill: a substance of no worth given to humour a difficult patient. A clear distinction has existed in people's minds between treatments (which work) and placebos (which do not). From time to time, every health professional will encounter patients who have been cured by a faith healer, a magic device or a sugar pill. The patient will not be lying or crazy. The health professional will find that clear clinical signs of an infection, an emotional symptom or even a tumour that was present before have now disappeared. Such incidents cannot be dismissed as simple coincidences. They demonstrate the strength of **placebo effects**.

Placebo effects: the non-specific effects that any treatment produces.

The very best treatments do not always work and so-called placebos often do (Shapiro & Morris 1978). Recognition of this fact has led to a change in the way treatments are understood, especially in the way in which treatments are evaluated. Any treatment has some specific effects: diuretics, for example, are drugs that cause cells to lose water, while morphine is a drug that binds to receptors on cells that respond to pain. At the same time, every treatment will produce some non-specific effects; that is, ones for which no direct consequence of the treatment seems responsible. Placebo effects refer to these non-specific (or non-pharmacological or non-surgical) effects that a treatment produces.

A placebo effect is generally defined by the proportion of subjects who respond to a (supposedly) inert treatment in a randomised control trial, preferably double-blind: a trial in which neither the researcher nor the recipient knows whether a real treatment or a placebo is being administered. A randomised control trial is one in which patients are assigned at random to receive either the experimental treatment or a placebo. Beecher (reported in Balis 1978) studied the effects of morphine on post-surgical pain. Patients who had undergone abdominal surgery, which is extremely painful, were given injections of either morphine or sterile saline. Saline is considered a placebo in this case because there is no particular reason for assuming that it will have any effect on pain. It was estimated that about half of the effect of morphine could be attributed to its placebo effects. It is worth remembering in this case that the patients given morphine knew that there was a 50:50 chance that they were getting saline. As a result, they may have been experiencing a negative placebo effect, which is discussed later in this chapter.

PAUSE & REFLECT

One major difference between treatments prescribed by health professionals and complementary treatments such as herbal remedies is that the former have been tested in randomised control trials and most of the latter haven't. What risks to health of the community might result from this?

Because of the strength of placebo effects, most new treatments now undergo rigorous testing involving double-blind, placebo-controlled trials, which has provided a considerable amount of information about the scope of placebo effects. When tested without a placebo control condition, treatments are very much more likely to be judged to be effective. Unfortunately, many so-called 'alternative' or 'natural' treatments have never been tested against placebos. This means that they may seem at first glance to be more effective and less prone to side effects than 'medical' treatments. When properly tested, many of these untested alternative treatments turn out to be ineffective, to interfere with other treatments, or even to have dangerous side effects. Without such testing, however, any effects that these treatments may appear to have may simply be placebo effects.

Placebo effects are reported by between 30 and 50 per cent of subjects in all treatments when controlled studies are done, although some authors report the range to be 0–100 per cent, depending on the conditions (Shapiro & Morris 1978). The proportion of placebo responders tends to vary depending on the treatment, with higher proportions of patients responding to placebos in trials of mood-altering treatments, for example, and lower proportions in trials of pain relievers.

Results produced by placebos can include every effect produced by any treatment (Balis 1978). They have been shown to affect not just symptoms such as pain, headache, coughing, nausea and depression, but also underlying bodily states. They have been reported to be able to produce dilation of airways, reduce blood sugar in people with diabetes, reduce swelling following injury, improve (or impair) immune function, and even slow or reverse tumour growth. Spiro (1986) examined a large number of these reports and concluded that there is better evidence that placebos affect illness than that they affect disease.

This finding includes surgical procedures as well as any other. In the 1950s, one treatment for angina pectoris (chest pain resulting from coronary artery disease) was internal mammary artery ligation, a procedure that involved operating to tie off the internal mammary artery. Many patients reported considerable, although usually temporary, pain relief after the operation. Dimond et al. (1960) reported the results of a placebo-controlled trial using sham surgery, in which some patients (double-blind) received an anaesthetic, had their chests opened and then immediately sewn back up. The results were quite clear: the same proportion of sham-operated patients reported pain relief as for the ligation patients, and some of them reported greater pain relief than most of the ligation patients. The authors of this study summed up their discussion by referring to the powerful psychological effects of surgery. Needless to say, internal mammary artery ligation is no longer performed. Less strict ethical restrictions existed at the time of this research, and because this experiment involved deception of subjects and unnecessary anaesthesia, it would be considered unethical by current standards.

Placebos also produce side effects. If the common side effects of a real treatment are well known, a placebo will often produce them (for example, gastric symptoms with placebo antibiotics). Logically enough, then, the more medicinal a placebo, the more effective it is likely to be. A big pill would work better than a small one, a capsule better than a pill, an injection even better, and a painful injection best of all. Side effects resulting from placebos are so consistent that it is hard to remember that we are discussing the effects of inert substances.

FACTORS AFFECTING OCCURRENCE OF PLACEBO EFFECTS

It has often been assumed that placebo-responders are a particular group—neurotics perhaps, or unintelligent. However, there is little evidence to suggest that placebo-responders can be identified as a particular group. Whether an individual responds to a treatment seems to have more to do with their outcome expectations for that treatment at that time than with any enduring characteristic of the patient (Shapiro & Morris 1978). Scientifically oriented people may be less likely to respond to a spiritually based treatment, but may in turn be more likely to respond to a plausible scientific placebo than might a religious person. In fact, placebo effects vary within a given individual over time, across bodily systems, between types of treatments, and from one treating health professional to another. If there are any characteristics that go to make up a placebo personality, they include a lack of confidence in one's knowledge in a particular area, and persuasibility. Even these characteristics can, in a particular case, be overwhelmed by situational factors.

Different health professionals get differing levels of response from their patients to almost any treatment. Placebo treatments are just another case. Enthusiasm on the part of the health professional for the treatment is important, and probably one of the major factors behind the **wonder drug effect**, which is the observed tendency for a new treatment to work better while it is still new to the market. A better relationship with patients produces bigger placebo responses. It is likely that these things lead to greater trust by patients of the health professional and, as a result, better expectations for outcome.

The situation in which treatment takes place has all the elements of **stereotyping**. Health professionals often wear uniforms and have professional manners. Walls and desks are covered with the symbols and tools of the trade, and interaction tends to proceed in a stereotypical way. The setting and interaction themselves can have healing effects, some of which may result from conditioning. As you gain experience with attending health professionals, you experience repetition of the pattern: 'See a health professional—get better.' Since the natural history of most disorders is to get better, this repetition of stimulus and response will tend to occur whatever the health professional does. The person may become conditioned to get better. Certainly,

Wonder drug effect: the observed tendency for a new treatment to work better while it is still new to the market.

Stereotyping: making the assumption that a member of a category of people will share all of the characteristics attributed to that category.

patients' anxiety levels drop considerably when they have seen a health professional (in most cases) because they have a clearer idea of what to expect, including that they will get better.

One important element of the doctor stereotype is that the consultation usually ends with a prescription. If the patient does not get the prescription—whether or not they need one—they may be unhappy. This, in turn, puts pressure on the doctor to give something, even where nothing is likely to help the patient, just to humour the patient and take advantage of any placebo effects that might occur. This shot-in-the-dark approach is often justified on the basis that it does little harm. Unfortunately, many of the substances given in this way, such as antibiotics, do have considerable potential to do harm. In addition, going along with the situation stereotype tends to lead patients to trust medication rather than their own resources. More and more doctors are now coming to recognise that patients can accept reassurance and behavioural interventions just as readily and still show the same kind of conditioned healing with many fewer side effects. The Australian government is currently encouraging doctors to give behavioural prescriptions, written on a standard prescription form, to take advantage of this stereotype.

CROSS-REFERENCE
Stereotypes are biases in person perception, as discussed in Chapter 4.

PAUSE 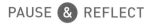 REFLECT

Imagine that you are being treated by a health professional for some health problem. What are the stereotypes present in your image?

PSYCHOLOGICAL EXPLANATIONS OF PLACEBO EFFECTS

A number of psychological explanations have been offered for placebo responses. Most of these have been mentioned already in relation to expectations, but you may find that a review will help you to organise them in your mind. All of them are true in some degree, which is why they have continually been referred to in the plural—placebo effects. There are many of them: as many as there are explanations, conditions, treatments and patients.

Conditioning was discussed above. Prior experience with treatments in general leads to conditioned healing. It does not give a precise explanation for the mechanism by which change takes place. The other explanations given below may provide that mechanism.

Perception explanations suggest that placebos actually affect the perception of the symptom rather than the symptom itself. If you have pain and take a sugar pill, the pain is still the same as it was, but it seems to be less severe. There is a large body of work that supports this explanation, and it is undeniable that placebos have a major influence on our perceptions. It is not the whole explanation, however, since placebos have been shown to affect underlying conditions as well. It is difficult to see how altered perception could lower blood pressure, for example, or increase someone's resistance to infection.

Validation (also known as Hawthorne effects) is based on the idea that patients will assume that a health professional will not give them a diagnosis or a treatment unless they have valid reasons for seeking them. In the 1930s, Western Electric factories were used for a series of studies—subsequently known as the Hawthorne studies—conducted to improve the output of workers. The result was that almost anything the researchers did, even if it produced a deterioration in working conditions, resulted in improved output. It seems that the fact that someone cared enough about the workers to try to encourage them to produce more work by changing their situation made them feel appreciated. It implied that they mattered, that

Perception explanations: the idea that placebos actually affect the perception of the symptom rather than the symptom itself.

Validation: the idea that patients will assume that a health professional will not give them a diagnosis or a treatment unless they have valid reasons for seeking them (also known as Hawthorne effects).

the complaints they had been making for years were being heard, and that solutions to their problems were being sought. In many cases, patients may not have been sure of—or not been able to persuade people around them of—their right to the sick role. When a health professional gives a patient any treatment, they have done several other things: they have validated the illness by saying, 'Yes, you really are ill', indicated that the illness is significant enough to merit treatment, and that the effort of providing that treatment is worthwhile, all of which can give the individual hope that improvement in their condition is achievable. As well as improving their mood, this validation can mobilise the resources of the patient to their own benefit (Frank 1973) and also mobilise others to help them. Subsequent effects might be produced by the hope and the mobilisation of resources. The role of such validation effects in placebo should not be overlooked.

CROSS-REFERENCE
Persuasion is discussed as one of the influences on self-efficacy beliefs within the social cognitive theory earlier in this chapter.

Theories of placebo effects often are based on suggestion, either by the health professional or patient, which leads to the individual being persuaded that they are getting better. This leads to actual improvement. Suggestion may arise from direct attempts to influence the patient, the nature of the treatment relationship (sometimes called 'transference') or role demands (Shapiro & Morris 1978), or possibly even the use of hypnotism. Persuasion certainly occurs in healing, but the question remains: If we have that much control over our bodily processes, why are we unable to learn to use it without the intervention of some inert treatment?

People try to get their responses to treatments to add up, to make sense, which leads them to expect change, then to evaluate the results that appear to come from the treatment, and then to re-evaluate their thinking about their illness and the treatment. The study by Dix (1985) cited earlier would indicate that such mental arithmetic occurs for patients who expect too little or too much from their treatment.

Storms and Nisbett (1970) suggested that a reason why some people get little benefit from sleeping pills is a negative placebo effect based on mental arithmetic. These individuals take a pill, go to bed and begin to think: 'I have taken the pill, so I should sleep. But I am not sleeping, therefore I must be worse than I thought.' Then they lie there and worry about the significance of the sleeping pill not working. The researchers suggested that, if this occurs, giving people an arousal placebo might work better than a relaxation placebo. Subjects could then attribute feeling awake to the effects of the pill, which would lead them to stop worrying about their state of alertness and go to sleep. The subjects that received the arousal pill went to sleep sooner and reported better sleep than the subjects given the relaxation pill. While mental arithmetic probably serves to modify increasing or decreasing placebo effects, and may be very useful in explaining side effects of placebos, it is too narrow an explanation to cover very much.

All of the above explanations, and others as well, ultimately result in a reduction in uncertainty about the future for the patient. This can decrease anxiety, improve compliance and alter risky behaviours.

PHYSIOLOGICAL EXPLANATIONS

Endorphins:
endogenous substances that are considered to be the body's own pain relievers, binding to the same receptor sites on neurons as morphine.

In addition to—or resulting from—these psychological factors, placebos also produce biochemical and physiological changes that can help explain the phenomena observed. A few of these explanations are given here.

The body produces a number of substances that can change physical states or affect ongoing physical processes. Examples include **endorphins**, which are considered to be the body's own pain relievers and bind to the same sites as morphine. Circulating levels of endorphins are known to be increased in exercise, (sometimes) in yoga, and in chronic pain. Levine, Gordon and Fields (1978) suggested that endorphins may help to account for placebo pain relief (analgesia). They analysed blood from pain sufferers who had been given a placebo treatment for pain following the extraction of wisdom teeth and found more increased levels of circulating endorphins in placebo responders than in non-responders. In addition, when subjects were given a blocking dose of a drug (an endorphin antagonist called Naloxone), placebo effects were significantly reduced. Although other researchers have failed to replicate the results quite as clearly, this research suggests an interesting model for the physiological process underlying placebo pain relief. However, it only relates to pain relief, and while it explains the 'how', it does not offer much help on the 'why' of placebo responding in that area.

It has been noted that immune function can be affected by a variety of events at the cognitive level. Stress, anxiety and depression have all been linked to poorer immune function. Also, treatments aimed at reducing stress—such as relaxation, hypnosis, meditation and mental imaging—have all been linked to improved immune function. It is not surprising, therefore, to find that placebos may have a considerable effect on immune functioning, which may help to explain how things as varied as AIDS, colds and cancer may be affected by placebos. It is also closely related to the next explanation.

CROSS-REFERENCE
Psychoneuroimmunology is discussed in Chapter 10.

Placebos may cause a reduction in damping effects caused by stress. Stress has a mobilising effect on the organism. Partly as a result of this, some systems of the body are put into an emergency mode, which may actually be detrimental to the body over the long term. The immune system is one that seems to be changed considerably by stress. The body begins to patrol aggressively for intruders. The cardiovascular system also responds by raising the output of the heart and, coincidentally, blood pressure. On the recuperative side—that is, healing functions and the replacement of resources—things seem to be damped down or put aside until the organism has the leisure to spare from the emergency. If the organism is continually stressed, this damping down may interfere with long-term healing. What placebo effects may do is decrease this damping down by redefining the situation as no longer an emergency.

THERAPEUTIC USES OF PLACEBO EFFECTS

The health professional also functions as a placebo. The non-specific effects of the professional's behaviour on the patient's health result from the same causes as the non-specific effects of drugs. The professional's value—in validating the patient's illness, providing stimuli that have been conditioned to healing, and just being present—can add to the real effect of every treatment that they provide. This additional effect can be encouraged by the professional by providing patients with positive, but also moderate and realistic, expectations for the outcome of the treatment, as well as by validating the patient's sense that something is wrong and needs attention, and by mobilising the patient's own resources, including physiological ones, in healing.

Significant ethical issues are raised when using inert substances in an attempt to humour the patient, particularly if the patient is considered by the professional to be a hypochondriac or neurotic. It is under these conditions that placebos are most likely to do harm, first through mental arithmetic leading the patient to believe that they are sicker than they believed before, and second by encouraging a dependence on pills for what are really problems of communication between doctor and patient.

CASE STUDY

MICHAEL OBUNO AND FLOSSING

Michael Obuno is a 30-year-old accountant. He is married, with two children aged 4 and 2. During a routine check-up with his dentist, he is told that he is developing a lot of plaque in between his teeth, and needs to use dental floss after every meal—or at least before going to bed every night—if he is to avoid having increasing problems with decay. Michael has never used floss before. Flossing is a risk-reduction behaviour that he hasn't given any particular thought to, but now Michael's dentist has indicated that it is an important one. This makes Michael think about flossing for the first time. However, no one in his family uses dental floss, so there is none in the house. However, he doesn't want to have decay or gum disease.

Up to now, he has gained most of his ideas about flossing from second-hand sources. For example, one of his friends has told him that they have tried flossing and it caused a lot of bleeding from the gums. Michael feels very queasy when he sees blood, so this makes him feel anxious about the idea of having 'a lot' of blood in his mouth. However, he now has to integrate new information, from a health professional that he trusts, into his existing beliefs. Michael already has a number of good health habits, such as doing regular exercise, and so he believes that healthy behaviour is important. He also has a strong belief that he can do new things if he wants to. He asks another friend who flosses regularly about the bleeding problem and is told that the bleeding stops quickly once regular flossing takes place. While in the supermarket, Michael sees floss on special, so buys some to try out.

After using dental floss for the first time, he discovers that it is mint-flavoured, and he likes the taste and that his mouth feels fresher. A colleague tells Michael that she used to avoid him because of his bad breath, but has noticed that this is now gone. He also finds that the bleeding is slight, and quickly decreases as he flosses regularly. He finds flossing easy, and quick.

After a few weeks, flossing has become part of Michael's regular teeth-cleaning routine, so that he no longer has to even think about doing it. If he forgets, he finds that he becomes aware of an unpleasant taste in his mouth, and this reminds him about flossing. He even suggests to the other members of his family that they should start flossing. His parents have had a lot of trouble with dental disease during their lives—both tooth decay and gum problems—and Michael doesn't want his own children to have to put up with these problems in the future.

1 How much influence do simple environmental effects—such as the lack of dental floss in the house—have over your own health behaviour?

2 What could Michael's dentist have done to improve the likelihood that Michael would begin to floss? How could the knowledge of Michael's stage of change have guided the dentist's behaviour?

3 Flossing is a fairly simple health behaviour with hardly any side effects. How does modifying it differ from modifying a major health behaviour such as compliance with medication for lowering blood pressure?

4 Over time, are there any other changes in behaviour that are likely to be observed as Michael continues to use dental floss?

Points to consider

A number of theories of health behaviour can be seen in this case. Michael has progressed through the stages of change, from pre-contemplation (when he hadn't given much thought to using dental floss as a health behaviour), through contemplation, action and maintenance. He has experienced changes to his cognitions about dental health—some of which have to do with the link between the behaviour of flossing and the outcome of dental health; and some about the likelihood that flossing will produce the desired change in his risk. He has encountered barriers to the behaviour: unavailability of floss, and negative feelings about bleeding. He has sought out information about possible effects of the behaviour, and found some good and bad sources of information. Self-efficacy has played a significant role in his behaviour change and, in return, the behaviour change has probably increased his sense of self-efficacy.

CHAPTER SUMMARY

- Cognition refers to the variety of thinking processes that people use. We would like to believe that our thinking and decision making are rational, but we often ignore objective information, instead making subjective evaluations of the likelihood and value of particular outcomes.
- Instead of using algorithms—mechanical routines that guarantee a correct solution but are slow—we frequently use heuristics: rules of thumb that are fast and can work with incomplete information but may lead to incorrect decisions.
- Health professionals also may use heuristics of various kinds to assist clinical decision making; the same issues arise from this use.
- A number of specific models have been developed to try to explain our thinking and decision making about health. Most of these models are only partially effective in explaining behaviour, but can give some assistance in explaining why that behaviour is often not very rational.
- Compliance with the recommendations of health professionals is often poor and many of the reasons for this have to do with health beliefs.
- An understanding of how expectations affect behaviour can be useful in the study of health and illness.
- Placebo effects provide a good example of the ways in which expectations can produce outcomes that differ from those that an objective observer might expect. Placebo effects may arise from a variety of psychological processes and the ways in which these processes influence the physiology of the body.
- It is important for health professionals to recognise the power of placebo effects and to use them ethically in the treatment of patients.

SELF TEST

1   In the theory of planned behaviour, a person's intentions regarding health behaviour will be the result of interaction between:
    a   behavioural beliefs and outcome evaluations
    b   motivation to comply and social control
    c   control beliefs and perceived power
    d   attitudes and subjective norms.

2   Joan is a pack-a-day smoker. She knows this is bad for her and her family. She wants to quit, and has contacted a government-funded smoking cessation program. Which stage of the change process is Joan most likely to be in?
    a   preparation
    b   precontemplation
    c   contemplation
    d   maintenance

3   Dr Blogg believes that people experience placebo effects because consulting with a health professional gives them the feeling that their illness is genuine and this gives them confidence that something can be done about it. This is most similar to theories of placebo effects based on:
    a   validation or Hawthorne effects
    b   misperception of symptoms
    c   classical conditioning
    d   circulating endorphins.

4   The most general psychological explanation of placebo effects is that:
    a   the individual experiences an increase in circulating endorphins
    b   mental arithmetic leads the individual to incorrect conclusions
    c   the patient's uncertainty about the future is reduced
    d   none of the above: placebo effects are physiological and not psychological.

5   The finding that the placebo effect on insomnia of so-called arousal pills is greater than that of sleeping pills would tend to support a psychological theory based on:
    a   Hawthorne effects
    b   perception of symptoms
    c   mental arithmetic
    d   classical conditioning.

FURTHER READING

Fishbein, M. (2008) A reasoned action approach to health promotion. *Medical Decision Making*, 28, 834–44.

Higgs, J., Jones, M.A., Loftus, F. & Christensen, N. (2008) *Clinical Reasoning in the Health Professions* (3rd edn). Edinburgh: Elsevier.

Maher, P. (1999) A review of 'traditional' Aboriginal health beliefs. *Australian Journal of Rural Health*, 7(4), 229–36.

Noar, S.M. & Zimmerman, R.S. (2005) Health Behavior Theory and cumulative knowledge regarding health behaviors: are we moving in the right direction? *Health Education Research*, 20, 275–90.

USEFUL WEBSITES

A stages of change approach to helping patients change behaviour (AAFP):
www.aafp.org/afp/2000/0301/p1409.html

A tonic for sceptics: Placebos are just as effective as treatments such as homeopathy because they work the same way (*The Guardian*):
www.guardian.co.uk/science/2005/aug/29/badscience.health

Compliance, culture and the health of Indigenous people (Rural and Remote Health):
www.rrh.org.au/publishedarticles/article_print_190.pdf

Placebo effect: a cure in the mind (*Scientific American*):
www.scientificamerican.com/article.cfm?id=placebo-effect-a-cure-in-the-mind

HOW TO CHANGE HEALTH BEHAVIOUR

CHAPTER OBJECTIVES

By the end of your study of this chapter, you should be able to:

- understand the process of behaviour change and the importance to the process of selection of appropriate target behaviours
- define and contrast antecedents and reinforcements of behaviours and the role these play in behaviour change
- understand the principles for selecting an appropriate method for behaviour change
- apply the methods of behaviour change—including stimulus control, behaviour bonds and self-reinforcement—and know how to manage lapses.

KEYWORDS

antecedents

extinction

good behaviour bond

habituation

homeostasis

hypothalamus

incentive

instincts

low-awareness habits

motivation

opponent–process theory

optimal level theory

primary drive

schedule of reinforcement

self-efficacy

stimulus control

MOTIVATION FOR CHANGE

'How many psychologists does it take to change a light bulb?' Answer: 'Only one, but the light bulb really has to want to change.' As this joke indicates, the most important factor in determining whether an individual will modify behaviour is how motivated the individual is to change. Before considering strategies for change, it is necessary to consider the general issue of motivation.

When we are hungry, we eat: a simple case of motivated behaviour that we can easily understand. However, many people in the world would, and do, starve to death rather than eat readily available and perfectly nutritious food. Think of the sacred cows of India, for example. How easy would you find it to eat insects? Many people around the world eat them. It might depend on whether you knew you were doing so (crayfish and crabs, for example, are *Arthropodae*—related to spiders). It might also depend on whether it was your only way of staying alive. People suffering from anorexia nervosa starve themselves in the midst of plenty in order to attain their ideal of body shape. The further we get from the simple case that we started with, the harder we tend to find it to understand what motivates the behaviour.

Most people think about **motivation** in terms of needs that must be met to achieve a state of comfort. When behaviour occurs, we assume that it has done so to achieve some goal. If the behaviour succeeds, the result is satisfaction; if not, frustration. The study of motivation, therefore, is concerned with those factors that arouse, sustain and direct behaviour.

Motivation: factors that arouse, sustain and direct behaviour.

One useful analysis of human motivation (Maslow 1970) suggests that we have a hierarchy of needs that we will be concerned with satisfying. Our most basic needs come first, then we are able to direct energy at higher-level needs (see Figure 8.1). The most basic needs are the fundamental physiological ones: hunger, thirst and avoidance of pain. Only when these are satisfied are we able to worry about the next level, which Maslow described as the safety needs: to feel secure and out of danger. The next level of needs is seen to be social: the need to belong to a group, to be loved and wanted. Esteem needs come next: the need to feel competent, to achieve something, to gain the approval of our fellows. Maslow completes his pyramid of needs with the need for self-actualisation: to be the best that we possibly can be, to fulfil our own unique potential.

Figure 8.1 Maslow's hierarchy of needs

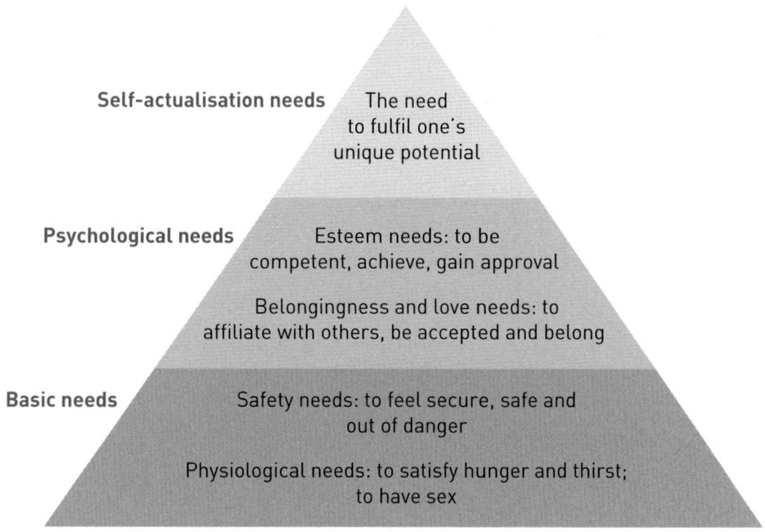

Self-actualisation needs — The need to fulfil one's unique potential

Psychological needs — Esteem needs: to be competent, achieve, gain approval

Belongingness and love needs: to affiliate with others, be accepted and belong

Basic needs — Safety needs: to feel secure, safe and out of danger

Physiological needs: to satisfy hunger and thirst; to have sex

CASE STUDY

DANIELLE ANGELOU AND HAND WASHING

Danielle is a 19-year-old university student who is training to be a radiographer. Although her teachers have discussed the importance of hand hygiene in lectures, and demonstrated the use of alcohol hand washes in laboratories, when she goes on clinical placements to radiography departments, few of the staff—even the senior radiographers—ever clean their hands between patients. Gradually, Danielle stops cleaning her own hands regularly. Danielle's motivation to clean her hands is likely to have been affected by the time and effort required. For example, the dispensers for alcohol hand washes might be located in the corridor instead of the examination rooms. The lack of role models may lead her to feel that hand washing is not necessary, or even effective, as an infection-control strategy. This means that the gains of the behaviour become less obvious. Also, the habit of hand washing has not developed sufficiently to resist extinction. At this point, Danielle's behaviour is unlikely to change—unless there is a change in her motivation.

1   What might stimulate such a change for her?

2   Who should be responsible for making sure that appropriate hand washing takes place in this clinical setting?

While Maslow's theory makes good intuitive sense, a number of objections have been made to it. All of us can think of times when we ignored a basic need to look after a higher one, and examples of people who have sacrificed their own security for the benefit of others are too common to ignore. Clearly, circumstances can lead to a reordering of the hierarchy. Maslow's theory also does not really give a detailed picture of the workings of needs: where they originate, how they push or pull behaviour, and why humans do things that are quite clearly not in their own interests. To begin to understand them, we need to examine genetic, biological and higher mental (cognitive) factors that influence motivation.

GENETIC FACTORS

Instincts: patterns of behaviour that are genetically programmed to occur in response to internal or external events.

Much of animal behaviour seems to be based on **instincts**: patterns that are hard-wired or programmed to occur in response to internal or external events, including events such as the migration of birds, aggression between species, and so on. What holds for animals might hold for humans as well. Early psychologists such as James (1890) believed that social behaviour showed patterns that looked like instinct, while the psychoanalyst Freud (see, for example, Hall 1979) believed that instincts relating to sex and aggression were the basis of much of human behaviour.

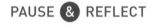

PAUSE **&** REFLECT

How much of your behaviour do you think is based on instincts? Can you give any additional examples to those in the text?

Some patterns of human behaviour appear to be so universal that an instinctual basis seems likely. One example is the protectiveness that almost all adult humans feel for babies. The head size and the shape of a baby's facial features seem to produce an internal state and a readiness to respond protectively in the adult. Stimuli that perform this kind of preparatory function are called 'releasing stimuli'. Releasing stimuli in lower animals may produce mating behaviour (such as the mating dances that many birds go through) or aggression (attacking any bird that approaches too closely to the nest). Some authors have considered which human behaviours appear to be most instinctive. Attention has generally focused on behaviours that ensure the transmission of genes to the next generation. Attachment in mothers and babies helps to ensure the survival of those who share genetic endowment; some authors have suggested that territoriality and dominance in males serve the same purpose. In humans, most behaviours are too variable to have been caused by instinct. There is quite clearly a heavy overlay of learnt behaviour as well.

CROSS-REFERENCE
Attachment is considered in more detail in Chapter 2.

BIOLOGICAL FACTORS

Some drives do quite clearly ensure the survival of the individual and are so based in bodily states that they must have a key biological focus. Physiological needs, in Maslow's terms, give rise to internal states focused on satisfying those needs, states that are commonly referred to as **primary drives** (Hull 1943). In a primary drive, either deprivation (of food or water, for example) or stimulation (pain or sexual arousal, for example) produce a need state in the organism, which in turn gives rise to a drive to satisfy that need. This drive is not just a general state; it also has a direction. This direction in the case of hunger is to find food; in the case of pain it is to move away from the source. Thus, a drive does not just produce behaviour but also produces certain specific behaviours related to the desired goal. The behaviours may succeed in reaching the goal, in which case need is reduced. If not, the drive state continues to produce behaviour aimed at the goal until either the need is reduced or the organism is exhausted (see Figure 8.2).

Primary drive: an unlearnt drive, for which there is an organic or physiological basis.

Figure 8.2   Drive cycle

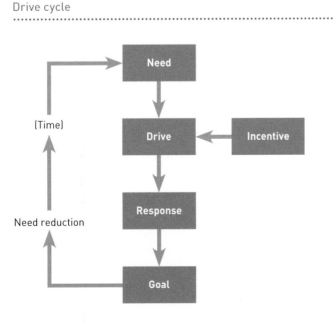

Sometimes, even after we have eaten until we are full, some especially desirable food can tempt us to eat again. This ability of an object to draw out behaviour is called **incentive**. Pain avoidance and sex are essentially incentive-based drives. No one ever died from a lack of pain or a lack of sex, which are needs that are based on the presence of environmental (or, less commonly, internal) stimuli.

Not all of our behaviour is related to the reduction of a handful of biological needs. Why, for example, are we willing to work hard just to receive a few words of praise or a mark on a piece of paper? Most theories that consider drives to be the basis of behaviour have argued that such behaviour is based on learnt drives (or acquired drives) that have been acquired through association with primary drives. Because our experiences of the satisfaction of hunger and thirst during the dependency of infancy are closely tied up with the social relationship between infant and caregiver, we learn to have a need for social contact. This learnt state of need gradually becomes more or less independent of the physiological need that gave rise to it. The occurrence of a state of need leads to a secondary (or learnt) drive, aimed at reducing the internal need state. All sorts of learnt drives have been proposed (Murray 1938; McClelland 1961)—for affiliation, approval, nurture, succour, achievement and dominance, among others. Although few of the proposed lists have satisfied everyone, there seems to be general agreement that learnt drives act very much like physiological drives with both deprivation and incentive effects.

As Figure 8.2 indicates, need reduction theories describe a feedback system, with the arousal of a need producing a change in the system. This change results in a drive to attain a goal in order to return to a state where the need has been reduced. The concept of **homeostasis** (Kimble 1992) has been developed to describe the nature of this process. Like the thermostat on a heater or air-conditioner, there is a regulatory mechanism that responds to deviations from some desired level by producing system activity. Once the desired level is achieved, activity is turned off. In terms of our biological homeostasis, much of this regulation appears to take place in the **hypothalamus**, a small structure in the midbrain that is involved in temperature control, pain and pleasure, and emotional regulation. Electrical stimulation of parts of the hypothalamus produces effects on regulation of behaviour: stimulation of some spots can, for example, produce gorging of food or water in already full animals; others can produce a refusal to eat or drink.

COGNITIVE FACTORS

The fact that motivated behaviour has direction (for example, we tend to hold off eating until we can eat preferred foods) clearly indicates the role of cognition (our thought processes) in motivation. As already mentioned, motivation can be modified by learning, which means that higher mental processes can play a significant role in our understanding of motivation and our responses to it. Much (if not most) of the time, our behaviour appears to be mindful; that is, rational and sensible. We do not usually grab and eat other people's lunches just because we are hungry, or sexually assault everyone who appeals to us. There is a considerable degree of cognitive regulation at work. We balance costs and returns of our behaviour to produce the maximal overall outcome (dependent on the probability and desirability of each outcome). If we behave in too asocial or antisocial a way, other people will regulate our behaviour for us in undesirable ways (for example, imprisonment, rejection or a punch in the nose).

In some cases, cognitive appraisals—judgments that people make about the situations they are in—lead individuals to make regulatory decisions that look pretty irrational in terms of their biological needs. Some people have chosen to be arrested, tortured and even executed rather than

Incentive: an external object or stimulus that draws out behaviour or creates motivation in the absence of a need.

Homeostasis: the tendency of the body to maintain internal constancy, and to try to restore equilibrium when that constancy is disturbed.

Hypothalamus: a small structure in the midbrain that regulates behaviour to maintain homeostasis.

CROSS-REFERENCE
Cognitive factors are discussed in more detail in Chapter 7.

fight in a war, while others may be willing to fight to the death over a minor insult. Although we may need to be recognised, most of us would stop a long way short of self-mutilation to get that recognition. Another way we regulate behaviour is by the postponement of gratification, at which we are far better than most other organisms. Graduation, for example, is hard to predict on the basis of biological needs, yet you will work hard over a number of years to become university graduates.

As discussed in Chapter 7, cognitions about health are critical to our motivation towards behaviour change. The integrative model of behavioural prediction (IM; Fishbein 2008), like other cognitive theories about health, focuses not just on our cognitions about disease and health and what causes them, but also on our beliefs about our own capacities and limitations (behavioural skills), whether or not the costs and gains of a behaviour change come out in favour of going through with it (intentions), and whether or not we believe that factors which we can't control (environmental factors) will be likely to assist us or block us in trying to change.

MOTIVATIONAL INTERVIEWING

One approach to changing behaviour specifically by targeting motivation is called motivational interviewing (MI) (Miller & Rollnick 2002). The basis of this approach is that people are often ambivalent about changing health related behaviours; that is, they have positive and negative motivations. For example, most people who smoke, or are very overweight, know that they should change their behaviour in order to improve their health (positive motivation toward change). However, they don't want to give up their established behaviours, or the comfort that they may get from them, or are concerned about the unpleasant feelings that may arise from trying to change (negative motivation toward change). MI involves counselling people to explore their feelings about behaviour change, with the aim of helping them to resolve the ambivalence and find strong enough motivation for change to bring about action. There is a substantial literature (Rubak et al. 2005) that shows that this approach—whether carried out by psychologists or by general practitioners or other health professionals—can be quite effective in many cases.

As with all approaches to behaviour change, MI is likely to work best when it is seen as just one element of the behaviour change process. Motivation is critical to bringing about change, but is usually insufficient on its own. This is often because the individual simply doesn't know how to go about it, even if they are highly motivated to change. They need to have strategies as well. We focus on how strategies are developed and carried out later in this chapter.

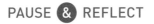

PAUSE & REFLECT

What is it that motivates you to do well at university? Where do think your motivation comes from?

In summary, motivation is an interaction of influences that come from the genetic, biological, cognitive and social levels.

MOTIVATION WITHOUT NEEDS OR DRIVES

What happens when all drives are satisfied? The organism does not just sit there waiting for a need to develop. We actually find a lack of stimulation unpleasant and, if deprived of it, will

Optimal level theory:
the idea that organisms
have a preferred range
of environmental
stimulation, and that
they will work to
maintain themselves in
that range.

seek it out. **Optimal level theory** suggests that we have a preferred range of environmental stimulation. If there is too little stimulation, we seek more; if there is too much, we seek to reduce it, all of which relates fairly clearly to the concepts of homeostasis and the idea that we have certain set points for internal regulation.

Even when we obtain the right amount of stimulation, we tend not to be satisfied for long. As we become accustomed to a given stimulus—a process called **habituation**—it becomes less pleasant to us. It has been shown, for example, that once we have become habituated to a particular stimulus, our preferred level of stimulus is one just slightly different from it. Imagine that you place your hand in a pan of cold water. At first it may be uncomfortable, but after you habituate, you will find that water is more pleasant when it is just a little warmer or colder. Water that would have been pleasantly warm at first may now be too warm. Figure 8.3 represents this in graphic form. Experimenters have shown that animals placed in a boring environment will actually work fairly hard to earn a little stimulation, such as the opportunity to watch the outside world or watch a toy train going around in circles.

Habituation: adapting
to a stimulus so that it
no longer arouses the
same level of response
that it originally
aroused.

Figure 8.3   The pleasantness of an unfamiliar temperature

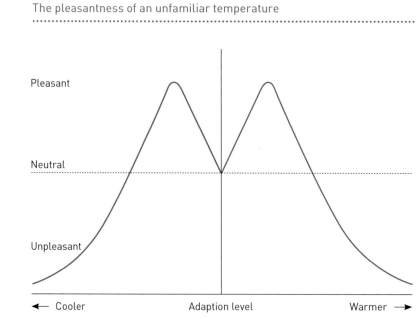

One way of accounting for this kind of phenomenon, and others such as drug addiction, is **opponent–process theory** (Solomon 1980), which proposes that there are always two processes in motivation—the primary process and a secondary and opposite one, set up within the nervous system. This secondary process comes on more slowly than the primary, but also fades more slowly. The purpose of the secondary process is to protect the system from intense stimulation. Thus, in the cold water example, the primary process of discomfort with the cold water is opposed by a secondary process that decreases the discomfort. At this new level of adaptation, a new opposing process diminishes our pleasure in this comfort to the extent that a change is preferred.

Opponent–process
theory: the idea that
there are always two
processes in motivation:
the primary motivation
or process, and a
secondary and opposite
one set up within the
nervous system.

In the case of heroin addiction, the novice drug user experiences a strong primary rush, which, because of a secondary opponent process, reduces to a pleasurable state. When this pleasurable state fades with the drug, the secondary process (fading more slowly) is experienced as unpleasant. With continued use, the secondary process becomes better and better at reducing the rush to protect the nervous system from overload. This requires that more drugs need to be taken to continue to achieve a pleasurable state and also that withdrawal produces a more unpleasant set of sensations.

STRATEGIES FOR BEHAVIOUR CHANGE

It is possible to modify behaviour by using the same principles of perception, learning and memory, and motivation that produced those behaviours in the first place. There are some basic assumptions implied by that statement, however, and it is important to make those assumptions clear in order to understand the ways in which behaviour can be changed.

The first assumption is that we need to be able to see what it is we want to change; that is, it is only observable behaviour that we can work with. We also need to have clear goals for how we wish the behaviour to change: in what ways, how much and within what time frame. Then, we need to assume that maladaptive behaviours are learnt, and therefore can be unlearnt—or replaced by adaptive behaviours. It is not particularly important in most cases to know just how a behaviour was learnt in the first place. It is not possible to go back and change the events that produced that learning. Change has to take place in the present. This does not mean that we can't benefit from looking at past experience. As you will see below, this can help us to pick methods that are appropriate to the behaviour we wish to change. Finally, it is much easier to change a behaviour if we have evidence that the behaviour is actually changing.

There are some basic principles that should be kept in mind in planning how to modify behaviour.

PICK APPROPRIATE BEHAVIOURS

The techniques, based on simple psychological principles, that are described in this chapter are mainly aimed at producing small and gradual changes in behaviour; however, the importance of this kind of small and gradual change should never be underestimated. Behaviour change has several advantages: it is realistic, it is cheap, once change has occurred it tends to be resistant to **extinction** and, unlike many medical interventions, it doesn't have side effects. The federal government has recognised these advantages and encourages health professionals to use behaviour change in the treatment of many health-related behaviours, including support of the development of a series of Lifescripts (Department of Health 2011). 'Script' here is related to 'prescription'—these are behavioural prescriptions. As defined on the website, 'The Lifescripts initiative provides general practice with evidence-based tools and skills to help patients address the main lifestyle risk factors for chronic disease: smoking; poor nutrition; alcohol misuse; physical inactivity; and unhealthy weight.' As you will see from this chapter, behaviour change can actually include far more than this list.

It should be noted that behaviour change will never entirely replace medication, whether that medication is for the treatment of infectious diseases or major depression. Nor will it replace more intensive psychological treatments. People who have major psychological or physical health problems should always work with a qualified health professional to manage their conditions, but behaviour change is often useful or necessary in combination with medical or surgical treatments. Total lifestyle programs such as the Ornish program (Ornish 1990) or Multiple Risk

Extinction: the gradual diminution of a conditioned response when reinforcement is removed.

Factor Intervention Trial Group (MrFit) (1982), which involve medication, diet, exercise, coping skills, relaxation and so on, can greatly decrease the incidence of heart attacks and strokes for those at risk. However, behaviour change cannot, and should not, entirely replace other medical treatments in serious medical conditions.

Individuals can improve their chances of a successful behaviour change by selecting appropriate behaviours, though what they are is not always clear-cut. Help in selecting behaviours that are appropriate for change can be found by using a mnemonic (memory jogging) device. A common one is SAME (Hassed 2000). The S stands for *specific*: the behaviour should be clearly identified, as should the amount of change desired. The A stands for *achievable*: a realistic amount and timescale for change should be selected. The M stands for *measurable*: if we don't pick a way to measure the behaviour (say, how frequently it occurs), we can't really tell that change is occurring. The E stands for *enjoyable*: unless sufficient motivation can be found, the process of behaviour change is unlikely to go ahead. Motivation (enjoyment) can be manipulated.

PAUSE & REFLECT

What health-related behaviours do you think you need to change? Are there others that you would like to change? Are there others that you think you will need to change at some time in the future?

PICK APPROPRIATE METHODS

CROSS-REFERENCE
Stress management is discussed in detail in Chapter 13.

Some methods of behaviour change are appropriate for some behaviours, or for some people, but not for others. It is important to understand the nature of the behaviour targeted for change before selecting methods. Like the selection of appropriate behaviours, this is related to the *specific* part of the SAME model. Some problems will be best handled with the behaviour change approaches discussed in this chapter; others will require stress management approaches.

Just as losing weight is best handled by increased exercise combined with changes in the food eaten (not necessarily dieting), some health behaviours need more than one technique. Given the demonstrated benefits of relaxation and stress management, there is probably no one who would not gain from a bit of technique and practice, but even these will not help with all healthy or risky behaviours. Some guidelines for selecting methods are included in later sections of this chapter and in Chapter 13.

DO NOT EXPECT TOO MUCH

The most common reason for failure of any treatment procedure is unrealistic expectations: the *achievable* part of the SAME model. The truth is that about 70 per cent of smokers trying to quit will fail at first, no matter what method they use. Eventually, though, more than 70 per cent of smokers will succeed in quitting. It is more realistic to aim for a partial change—cutting down, for example—and once that change is achieved to change the target. Success in meeting interim targets will add to feelings of confidence that the ultimate target can be reached as well, which is one of the reasons why it is so important that behaviours be *measurable*.

GIVE METHODS A CHANCE TO WORK

Closely related to expecting too much, methods frequently fail because the individual gives up too soon or fails to stick to the rules. Behaviour change programs need to be able to deal with slow progress, temporary setbacks and small (and even big) lapses without the individual giving up. To maintain a behaviour change, some basic characteristics underlying the behaviour need to change and stay changed. In some cases, this will be for a fixed period of time; in others, forever. Patience is needed, and enough time for success to be achieved. To take the weight-loss example, crash dieting simply does not work.

PEOPLE ARE NOT FAILURES, ALTHOUGH METHODS MAY BE

If behaviour does not change dramatically in a short period of time, it does not mean that the person who tried it is a weak or flawed person. Most habitual behaviours are hard to change. If they were not, unhealthy habits would not exist. Low self-esteem can be a cause of risky behaviours, and if behaviour does not change, self-esteem can be lowered as a result, thereby creating a vicious cycle. There are many ways to prevent this happening, the most important being for each individual to select the right behaviour and method for themselves.

DANIELLE (CONT.)

CASE STUDY

After hearing another teacher speak about the importance of hand hygiene, Danielle decides that she really needs to clean her hands between patients. This is because of the severity of the risks of transmitting diseases from a patient to herself or, even worse, to one of her often very vulnerable patients. Aside from the health issues, there could even be issues with legal liabilities. She sets out to modify her behaviour. Now that she has found the motivation to change her behaviour—which could be considered to be a combination of safety needs (her own health) and belongingness needs (to help her patients)—she needs to identify when she thinks about washing, and when she doesn't. The triggers turn out to be: she washes her hands when she happens to be passing the dispenser and notices it, when a patient seems to her to be an obvious infection risk (for example, with an open or bandaged wound, or a cold) and when someone else washes their hands. The triggers of not washing turn out to be: when she is busy or distracted, when the patient is not obviously an infection risk, and when she doesn't pass the dispenser during the procedure.

Danielle decides that a number of these triggers for behaviour could be changed (stimulus control). A hand-wash dispenser could be placed in a more obvious location, preferably one she has to pass with every patient, or the dispenser could be made more obvious by placing a poster or arrow next to it. These are strategies that she could introduce herself, but she could also encourage the unit to introduce them for everyone's benefit.

She could also practise thinking that every patient is a potential infection risk, or about the potential consequences of infection. She could encourage others around her to use the hand wash more often—even becoming a role model herself for others.

1 What kind of behaviour change process has she gone through with this analysis?
2 What changes could she make in her health cognitions that would increase her motivation to wash her hands?

PAUSE & REFLECT

Think of someone you know who has tried to change a behaviour and failed. How did it make them feel? What effect do you think it had on their future behaviour?

CHANGING BEHAVIOUR BY CHANGING STIMULI

Antecedents: stimuli that precede its occurrence and lead to the behaviour.

In order to change a behaviour, we need to know two things about it. The first of these involves the **antecedents**: the stimuli that precede its occurrence and lead to the behaviour. The second involves the reinforcements: the consequences associated with the behaviour that keep it occurring.

ANTECEDENTS

There are a lot of things that trigger behaviour. Some of these are obvious, such as looking at the clock, seeing that it is time to go to work, and going. Some are a lot less obvious, such as why we looked at the clock in the first place. Sometimes, the best way to explain a behaviour is habit: we do something because we have learnt through experience to do it. We do not give much thought to tying shoelaces, for instance, but when we put on shoes with laces, habit takes over and we tie them. If we had to describe how we tie shoelaces to someone else, it is not unlikely that we would have a lot of trouble. If we wanted to change our method of tying shoelaces, our habits would interfere. We might have to do some unlearning before we could learn a new approach. Many of our habits are so well learnt that we are not especially aware of the behaviour, much less what triggers it, which frequently produces problems when we want to change a behaviour. So step one is to identify the antecedents. This self-monitoring is an important component of successful health behaviour change (van Achterberg et al. 2011). There are several useful tools for doing this.

THINK BACK TO PAST BEHAVIOURS

If an individual would like to eat more fruit, they need to think about times in the past when they have eaten fruit with pleasure and try to decide what preceded eating. Was the fruit given to them? Was it new and interesting? Was it simply handy at the time they were eating something else? Did it look particularly good? Were they especially hungry? These kinds of clues to antecedents for fruit eating will provide hints as to how to increase it.

OBSERVE PRESENT BEHAVIOURS

When does the individual eat fruit? How do they feel before they eat it? When do they think about eating fruit? When do they think about eating fruit without actually eating any, and what stops them at that particular time? There is much research which shows that present behaviour is the best predictor of future behaviour (Ogden 2007; French et al. 2010).

KEEP A FORMAL RECORD

This goes together with points one and two. When eating fruit, or thinking about eating fruit, it is useful to keep a record that can then be analysed for clues about antecedents. Diaries are often used in behaviour change programs, because time can be an important trigger for many behaviours. If we regularly eat fruit at breakfast but never at other times, then the time of day may be an antecedent to fruit eating that the individual can work with.

This kind of monitoring of our own behaviour can be enough to change the behaviour. Thinking about why we do something alters the way we think about that behaviour and this in itself changes the antecedents. People may say that they quit smoking by sheer will power and without a plan, but by will power they really mean that they thought about the stimuli for doing it and for not doing it, and this changed the antecedents of the behaviour. It is often the case that their will power was boosted by thinking about the damage a cigarette would do, or by keeping the mouth busy with something else, such as chewing gum or sucking on a blade of grass or a toothpick instead of smoking. This is the other side of behaviour change—motivation—and methods for changing this are discussed later in the chapter.

STIMULUS CONTROL

The basis of changing behaviour by changing its antecedents is called **stimulus control**. Sometimes this involves eliminating a stimulus that produces the wrong kind of behaviour. Watching television in bed may make it harder to fall asleep, as the bed is then conditioned to (associated with) interesting and exciting events rather than sleeping. We can control the stimulus by using the bed only for sleeping. This means that the stimuli associated with the bed are all clearly connected with sleeping and only with sleeping. (Sex may need to be considered an acceptable behaviour for the bed as well.)

Stimulus control: changing behaviour by changing its antecedents.

Sometimes a stimulus that leads to a behaviour is not eliminated but modified, perhaps by changing its meaning or making it a stimulus for a different and competing behaviour. Instead of sitting in front of the television news on arriving home, an individual might go for a run and listen to the radio news instead. The same stimulus—coming home—becomes the antecedent for a different behaviour.

Other people can serve as stimuli to trigger behaviours. Problem drinkers often find that the hardest thing to control is their friends. If the individual's social life revolves around the pub or friends who drink quite a lot, then it may be necessary to change those elements in order to reduce drinking. Sometimes others can be motivated to change, as when a parent changes the family's food-buying habits and menus to help diet improvement in a child. At other times, certain people or places may need to be avoided. Smokers often go to specific places—special rooms in the house or outdoors—to smoke. Someone who is quitting is well advised to avoid these places because they will be full of smoking cues: smells, sights, cigarette butts and ashtrays, and smokers and their positive comments.

Table 8.1 gives a summary of some of the antecedents for health behaviours, and some techniques (described in the text) that can be used to control them.

Table 8.1　　Summary of stimulus control

ANTECEDENT	STIMULUS CONTROL METHOD
I forget to (exercise, eat fruit etc.)	Provide reminders for the behaviour.
I don't have the time to ...	Schedule a regular time; reorganise program to make time; eliminate wasted time.
I never seem to have the right (food, equipment, material etc.)	Put the equipment in a convenient place; get it ready ahead of time.
(A healthy meal, gym time) is too expensive or too hard to find.	Take your meal with you from home; buy tickets in bulk; join a club.
I'm not aware that I'm ...	Create a signal so that you can't do the behaviour without being aware of it. Organise surveillance; ask others to tell you when you are doing it.

PAUSE **&** REFLECT

How could you use stimulus control methods to improve your study behaviour? Think about where, when and how you study.

INCREASING AND DECREASING BEHAVIOURS

To begin with, it will be useful to break behaviour change down into three groups: behaviours we want to increase (health behaviours), those we want to decrease (risky behaviours) and behaviours that we are not particularly aware of doing (**low-awareness habits**) that we want to increase or decrease. Slightly different techniques are useful with these three types of behaviour change, although there is considerable overlap, as you will see.

Low-awareness habits: habitual behaviours that the individual carries out without being particularly aware that they are doing so, such as nail-biting.

If the goal is to increase a behaviour, such as exercise, the problem is often that there are not enough relevant stimuli for exercise in the ordinary environment. An important step in changing the behaviour is to change the environment so that those stimuli are present. The hopeful exerciser could, for instance, put up posters featuring exercise, place reminder notes around the house or workplace, and keep exercise equipment in an obvious and easily accessible place. Someone who wanted to eat more fibre might keep high-fibre recipes on the refrigerator door, or a list of the fibre content of snack food on the door of the cupboard where that food is kept.

Decreasing behaviours involves reducing either the occurrence of stimuli related to those behaviours or changing the meaning of those stimuli. If an individual stops at a vending machine to buy chocolate every time they go down a particular staircase, simply finding a different path may be enough to stop the behaviour. If they feel the need of a cigarette most often when drinking at the pub, they may need to stay away from the pub, or drink less, while trying to change the behaviour.

Eating and sleeping are heavily habit-dependent, a fact that often surprises people, who tend to think of them as bodily processes that are not consciously controlled. The truth is that a common trigger for eating is the presence of food. (Remember incentives from the section on motivation?) Eating and sleeping often respond very well to stimulus control. For this reason, weight-management programs often ask people to develop different eating routines that might include rules such as never eat standing up; eat only in the dining room with the table set, others present and no television or other distractions; always wash dishes and utensils as soon as eating is finished and put them away out of sight; keep all food in difficult-to-access cupboards so that it is harder to get to; and never have food lying around unless it is part of the diet plan.

In a similar fashion, the first rule for people who have trouble getting to sleep at night is to never nap during the day, no matter how sleepy they become. Some people are unable to sleep unless it is quiet; others need background noise. Because of their nature, sleep problems almost always need relaxation techniques (discussed in Chapter 13) as well as stimulus control.

LOW-AWARENESS HABITS: A SPECIAL CASE

Low-awareness habits include chewing fingernails, lips or objects such as pencils; picking or pulling at skin or hair; slouching, fidgeting or grimacing; making noises such as grunts; and knuckle-cracking. Some of these habits have health consequences that are obvious. Nail-biting can lead to deformed nails, infections and the spread of disease. If other people in the vicinity find these habits odd, funny or unpleasant, they all can lead to lowered self-esteem and associated problems with emotions. Almost always, the trick is to make the individual aware of the habit while it is occurring. Usually, once the person becomes aware, they are motivated enough to quit. There are quite a number of ways of making people more aware of these habits. Most of you will be familiar with the idea of painting fingernails with a foul or bitter substance to keep children from biting them. This combines stimulus control (the bitter taste signals that the low-awareness habit is occurring) with reinforcement (the taste is unpleasant). This technique works quite often, but sometimes it does not, perhaps because the habit has too many positive reinforcements associated with it, because the habit is too strongly established, or because the taste is not regarded as being that unpleasant. Also, as this approach is based in part on punishment, it shares all of the problems of punishment.

Other signalling methods can be used with low-awareness habits. Tying string around a finger to remind oneself of something is a type of stimulus control, but anything that interferes with carrying out a behaviour could be used. A fingernail biter will not be able to perform their habit if each fingernail is covered with a bandage—although they may have to do a lot of explaining to others. Slouching can lead to muscular pains or aggravate stomach or bowel problems, and most people are not aware when they are slouching. Techniques that have been used to raise the awareness of slouching include wearing wide belts inside or outside of clothing that dig into the individual when they slouch, but are comfortable when they are sitting up straight. (Again, this includes punishment.) A high-tech version of this, a computerised strain gauge worn vertically around the body, has been used to prevent the worsening of, or to improve, scoliosis (curvature of the spine) in young people who are developing this disorder. This gauge uses sound or vibration signals to tell the individual when their spine is not being held straight; the signals can be graded to be more obvious if the spine is not straightened within a particular period of time.

The role of others in providing surveillance for low-awareness habits raises a number of issues. Although friends and family may be concerned about the habit and be willing to let the person know when it occurs, they may be reluctant to do so under some conditions. Suppose a person who picks at their earrings and causes irritation and infection asks friends to tell them when the behaviour occurs. If the behaviour and reminder happen in a public place, it may cause embarrassment for one or both parties. Verbal signals could not be used in public places such as classrooms without problems, but the main problem with surveillance is that the person being watched may come to resent it. Even long-time friends or married couples may find their relationship is strained by what can come to be seen as nagging. Still, surveillance can be used to good effect in many instances.

PAUSE & REFLECT

Earlier in this chapter, you were asked to think about health behaviours you would like to change. Pick one of them. Which stimulus control methods might be appropriate to changing that behaviour?

CHANGING BEHAVIOUR BY CHANGING REINFORCEMENTS

This section deals with changing motivation related to problem behaviours, and this involves changing reinforcements. Reinforcements follow a behaviour to make it more or less likely to happen again. We eat because afterwards we feel more satisfied or because the tastes during the meal are pleasurable—these are reinforcements. Another way of thinking about reinforcements is in terms of gains and costs. Talking to people about why they do not exercise as much as they should, they will often list the gains ('It makes me feel good and I sleep better') followed by the costs ('but it takes too much time, and I feel too tired afterwards'). In any attempt to change behaviour, it is useful to look at the reinforcements and whether they can be changed. Nicotine patches or chewing gum are two of several ways that the reinforcements of smoking can be changed by reducing the costs of not smoking that are related to nicotine withdrawal.

CROSS-REFERENCE
Reinforcements are discussed in detail in Chapter 6.

The longer it has been since we ate or drank, the more likely it is that we will feel hungry or thirsty. When we eat or drink, the reduction in tension is reinforcing (negative reinforcement). Whether we wish to lose weight or not, we do not want to eliminate eating entirely. Modifying eating means changing the way we eat, not the fact that we eat. The addictive nature of nicotine—as with other drugs—produces an increasing need as time passes. Satisfying this need is not essential for survival, so we can eliminate it without risk.

The general principle of reinforcement, then, is to reduce the costs and/or increase the gains of desired behaviour, which may also involve increasing the costs and/or reducing the gains of undesired behaviour. A person who wishes to include more fibre in their diet may find that the foods that they like do not contain a lot of fibre, and that the ones that do contain fibre do not appeal to them. They could increase the gains of eating fibre by finding attractive foods that are higher in fibre (increasing the gains of the desired behaviour) or in some way adding fibre to the foods they like (decreasing the costs). Alternatively, they could use punishment: not eating desirable but low-fibre foods (reducing the gains of avoidance) or putting money into a charity jar when they do not eat fibre (increasing the costs of avoidance).

POSITIVE REINFORCEMENT APPROACHES

In general, any behaviour that is followed by positive consequences will increase in frequency. Training a child to use a toilet involves making the consequences that follow positive ones. We try to make the process pleasant by having a comfortable seat for the child to sit on, and by giving praise and cuddles when the child uses the toilet. All of these are intended to—and usually do—increase the behaviour of using the toilet.

The giving of positive reinforcement is one of the essential methods of behaviour change. If a person wished to do more exercise, they could arrange for a direct payoff by having a nice meal or snack immediately afterwards, have someone praise them for exercising, or have someone give them money.

Part of the problem with exercise—and this is true of many health behaviours—is that the direct benefits are long term, while the costs are short term. Once people have exercised for a period of time, they are fitter, probably look better, almost certainly feel better and sleep better, and have better general health. For most people, these gains tend to be a bit abstract compared with the short-term costs of effort, getting sweaty, missing out on television or drinking time, and paying for equipment or facilities. This means that ways need to be found to make the rewards more immediate—or to reduce the costs.

One very useful technique involves making the payoffs part of the behaviour itself (*enjoyable* in the SAME model). Instead of sacrificing time with friends for exercise, they could exercise with their friends. Most people who do exercise regularly report that part of the reason is social. They spend time with others, make friends, gain public respect for their skills or effort, and have a network of people who share interests and values with them. Solitary exercise purely for the sake of fitness does rather poorly by comparison. The greater success of weight-loss groups over solitary weight-loss programs is primarily related to the social gains involved in having others who not only know and value what you are trying to do, but who also understand the difficulty involved in the process because they share it.

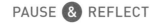

PAUSE & REFLECT

How would you go about changing the costs and gains of studying? Answering this will require that you think about exactly what motivates you to study in the first place.

The **schedule of reinforcement**—when and how you get reinforcement—is also important. When beginning to reinforce a behaviour (when the behaviour is new and relatively unlikely to occur), it is important to reinforce it frequently. If you wanted a friend to smile more, you could give him a sweet every time he smiled. Once smiling became common, the sweets might be coming so fast that they lost their appeal for your friend, or even became a punishment by making him feel sick from overeating. As time passes, the schedule of reinforcement needs to change to a less frequent one.

| **Schedule of reinforcement:** the pattern on which reinforcement is given; this may be continuous (every behaviour) or intermittent (less than every behaviour). |

Occasional reinforcement makes a behaviour harder to get rid of than does constant reinforcement, largely because the lack of reinforcement is not so obvious. Problem gamblers find this a particular difficulty. They win just often enough to keep them gambling, in spite of the fact that overall they lose a great deal more than they win. They keep thinking that the next win will eventually come along and that it could be big enough to make up for all the losses. The immediate gains of a big win is enough of a lure that they lose sight of the cost of even a large number of small losses. Dealing with this kind of problem involves making the gambler more aware of the overall costs: not just the loss of money, but also of the things that the money could have bought, as well as the loss of respect of others, family problems, and so on.

On the other hand, this knowledge about schedules of reinforcement can be used to produce positive changes by starting out with frequent rewards and gradually expecting more before a reward is given. Imagine, for example, that an individual wants to exercise three times a week and decides to use money as a reinforcement. At the beginning, they might put aside money to buy a small item of clothing each time they exercised. Once they have begun to develop the habit of exercising, they might only provide money if they have reached a particular target, such as running a certain distance within a set time. Ultimately, the goal is to have the reinforcements that arise from the behaviour itself replace outside rewards. People who continue to exercise report that the feeling of well-being that results is addictive, and that they miss that feeling badly when they do not exercise.

There are many reinforcements that can be used in behaviour change; for example, money, punishment, food, praise, time off work, fun and other people. Most of the techniques discussed below are simply well-established ways of using those common reinforcements. One of the most important is self-reinforcement.

SELF-REINFORCEMENT

Everyone wants to have a good opinion of themselves: to feel that they are good, strong, worthy, interesting and attractive. This makes self-esteem—how good a person feels about themselves—a powerful reinforcement. There is a variety of ways in which this can be used to modify health behaviours. The simplest is for the individual to praise themself when they perform the desired behaviour, which tends to happen anyway: we feel good when we have done something that we are proud of. A difficulty arises when we are doing things that are considered to be good for us. We are more likely to feel bad when we have not done them than we are to feel that we have done anything praiseworthy when we have done them. Most of us do not pat ourselves on the back when we remember to brush our teeth before going to bed—we think of it as just basic sanitation—but will feel bad if we forget. So often the trick with self-reinforcement is to recognise that a worthy behaviour deserves reinforcement.

PAUSE & REFLECT

When do you use self-reinforcement? Is it mostly when you have been successful in your work? Do you ever reinforce yourself when you have had a successful study period? When you eat food that is good for you?

Self-efficacy: the perception on the part of the individual that they can influence and control their own outcomes.

CROSS-REFERENCE
Self-efficacy is also discussed in Chapter 7.

Self-reinforcement does not simply involve feeling good about oneself. It can include reinforcement with other desirable elements such as money, time, fun and social activities. The control over these reinforcements is in the individual's own hands. They decide when and how much reinforcement, and do not rely on others. Achieving for oneself often means more than achieving for someone else, and the main area of gain is **self-efficacy**. Self-efficacy refers to the sense of being capable that a person develops: they are able to control their actions and determine their own limits. It has long been recognised as a key component of successful change (Bandura 1977a). As the person succeeds in producing a small change, they not only gain small rewards but also an increase in self-efficacy. This is a powerful reinforcement, in part because it motivates the individual to go on changing.

The gambler who has made a number of attempts to quit gambling without success will have a low sense of self-efficacy, at least in this respect. Suppose that gambler sets themself the target not of quitting and never gambling again, but of limiting the amount of money gambled on a given day. Most gamblers find a proportional change such as this fairly easy to achieve. It can be regarded as a success if the gambler chooses to praise or otherwise reward themself for it; and self-efficacy is increased for an attempt to further reduce expenditure. The setting of progressively more difficult targets is very useful, because it allows regular reinforcement and because it increases self-efficacy with regard to the target behaviour.

CASE STUDY

DANIELLE (CONT.)

The process Danielle has gone through is not unlike motivational interviewing, in that she has been trying to reduce her ambivalence about hand washing by clarifying her motivations. Next, she decides that for the change in her behaviour to succeed in the long term, she needs to look at the reinforcements of the behaviour. She concludes, after looking at the clinical setting, that placing a dispenser in a more convenient location, and using quick alcohol hand-wash techniques, could decrease the costs of hand washing. Thinking about the potential harm that could result from passing an infection to a patient, or to herself, could increase the costs of not washing. Praising herself when she remembers to wash could increase the gains of washing and increase her sense of self-efficacy (which adds esteem needs to her motivation). So could seeing others follow her lead and wash their hands at the same time. These are self-reinforcements, and policy changes at the clinical placements would probably be required for any extrinsic reinforcements of this particular health behaviour.

1   What policy changes can you think of that would be likely to improve hand hygiene in health-care settings?

2   How effective would it be to begin punishing people for not hand washing; for example, by docking their pay if they are caught not washing their hands between patients?

PUNISHMENT

It is always important to remember that punishment has drawbacks: it does not give any information about desired behaviour, it tends to produce avoidance of the whole situation and negative reactions to whoever is doing the punishing, and it can generalise to desirable behaviour that just happens to be associated with the undesired behaviour. If we want someone to eat less because they are fat, then reminding them that they are fat will simply make them feel angry towards the person doing the reminding; it will also lower their self-esteem and reduce their sense of self-efficacy. The overweight person is very likely to start avoiding that person. Whenever you use punishment in behaviour change, it should be combined with positive reinforcement.

CROSS-REFERENCE
The drawbacks of punishment are discussed in Chapter 6.

GOOD BEHAVIOUR BONDS

One technique that is often used very successfully in behaviour change is the **good behaviour bond**. Usually, this is a sum of money that is set aside and returned only if the behaviour change program is successfully completed. On the surface, this may look like punishment since failure to change results in losing money, but these bonds are very useful in motivating people to stay in programs, even if behaviour does not necessarily change very much or change at all.

Good behaviour bond:
A sum of money (or equivalent goods or services) that is set aside to be returned only if a behaviour change program is successfully completed.

A common example is provided by weight-loss programs. It is very common for psychologist-run weight-loss programs to involve each participant in paying an up-front bond equal to one week's salary. If the participant sticks with the program until its conclusion, they will get their money back. If not—and this is vitally important—the bond is forfeited, but never to the person running the program because the person running the program must not be seen to have a vested interest in failure on the part of the participants. Some programs give the money to charity, others use it to fund future programs or give it to recipients chosen by the participant. Some behaviour change experts feel that the bond is most effective if the money goes to a cause that the participant hates; that way, the participant cannot take comfort in the fact that although they have lost their bond, at least it is doing some good.

Bonds are often most effective when used to enforce participation and not achievement. If the participant attends all sessions, keeps all the appropriate records, and still does not modify their weight, they nevertheless get their money back. In this way, they at least leave the program with a knowledge of the methods and a sense of self-efficacy, both of which can be useful in future attempts to lose weight. It is probably more common to link bonds to performance goals. This can be progressive. Each time the individual loses a certain amount of weight, they recover a portion of the bond. This gives immediate reinforcement during the program and keeps the individual from feeling that it is an all-or-nothing outcome. Sometimes programs mix performance and participation rewards—so much for attending, so much for weight loss etc.

Bonds do not have to be money; they can also involve goods or services. An individual could buy themselves a desirable object, but put it in the hands of someone else to keep or give away if behaviour change goals are not reached. Where money is a problem, the bond could consist of time or work. The individual could, say, agree to provide twenty hours of unpaid work for someone and recover the hours through participation or performance. Bonds can also be used in support of a variety of other approaches.

SUMMARY OF REINFORCEMENT METHODS

- Specific and clear targets should be set that need to be reached before reinforcement occurs.
- A number of smaller targets that can be reinforced progressively is usually better than one big, far-away target.
- Reinforcement must be reliable; that is, if the individual reaches the target, reinforcement must be given.
- Success builds self-efficacy, which in turn encourages further change.
- Punishment should only be used in support of positive reinforcement.
- Reinforcement should occur frequently at first, then less frequently as behaviour changes. Intermittent reinforcement is best for maintaining behaviour.
- Reinforcements that arise directly from the behaviour change are the best kind—such as the good physical feeling that follows exercise, or social contact from programs with others or as part of a group.
- A reward that can only be used if change is successful (such as a dress that will only fit if a certain amount of weight is lost) can be useful, but can also cause problems if, for instance, the target is too hard to meet.

MANAGING LAPSES

Lapses are likely to occur with any behaviour change program, and often result in the attempt to change being abandoned (Marlatt & Gordon 1985), which means that it is always a good idea to have plans for managing lapses. The most important of these is to ensure that lapses are not seen as failure. If a person thinks smoking that first cigarette means they are a hopeless case, without willpower or permanently addicted, then it will be hard to keep up the behaviour change program. If they see it as a momentary lapse—that is, not desirable but predictable, and to that extent acceptable—they are more likely to continue to try.

A lot of specific techniques exist for dealing with lapses, including procedures for preventing them, minimising the damage they cause, or relabelling them as part of the change process (Marlatt & Gordon 1985). Weight-loss programs often use averaged changes, or trends in change, to avoid the perception of failure if there is a temporary lack of weight loss or a short-term weight gain.

In exercise programs, injury represents a cause of relapse that must be foreseen and dealt with. If the person quits exercising completely during the time of an injury, the gains that have been made in general fitness, as well as in time management and other benefits, can quickly be lost. As a result, it is a good idea to keep the individual involved in some appropriate exercise that will not aggravate the injury until they are fit enough to return to the original program. Injury is usually not seen as a failure on the part of the individual, and so the consequences for self-efficacy will be less. If they continue to participate in some kind of limited exercise program, injury may not be seen as a lapse at all.

As we age, we may have to change exercise to suit changes in the body. If these changes are accomplished gradually, they usually do not affect the individual's view of themselves as a fit person.

'SANDY' SUM AND GAMBLING MOTIVATION

CASE STUDY

'Sandy' is a 32-year-old temporary migrant. He entered Australia as a trained machinist to work in the mining industry in Western Australia. His main reason for coming was to allow him to support his extended family in Cambodia. His workmates call him Sandy because they had trouble pronouncing Sakngea, his real name. At first, he felt very isolated as the only Cambodian working on a rural mine site, but gradually became more comfortable as his English improved, and as he took a greater part in social activities—which mostly involved gambling, particularly at mealtimes. He found playing cards with his workmates exciting, and he generally didn't lose or make much money.

Problems arose, however, when the company transferred him to Perth, where he didn't know anyone, and felt very isolated again. While wandering around the city, he went to the casino and discovered that the excitement of gambling on cards made life more enjoyable, as well as filling his empty weekends. Gradually, he discovered that he was spending most of his weekends in the casino, and didn't feel nearly as isolated or bored. However, he was losing far more money than he had realised at the time. Once, when he didn't have enough left from his pay cheque to make the usual transfer to his family, he borrowed the money from a workmate. Luckily, he managed to win enough the next weekend to pay this back, but eventually fell so far behind that he took out a bank loan to cover his debts. Although his financial problems were getting out of hand, he was unable to resist the excitement of gambling, and believed that he would eventually make a big win that would pay off everything and get him back on track.

When he discovered that he couldn't afford to make the payments on his bank loan and still send money home, he applied for several credit cards, and began to gamble using credit obtained that way. All the time, he hoped to make a big win so that all of his troubles would be solved.

Finally, Sandy's financial problems became so bad that he regularly began to miss the payments to his family. He was spending so much time trying to win back what he had lost that he was going without much sleep on the weekends, and was too stressed to sleep even if he stayed away from the casino. This made him feel so bad that his work was affected, and eventually he had to tell his boss about his situation.

His boss had seen gambling become a problem for other workers in the mining industry, so he put Sandy in touch with a counsellor through Gambling Help WA. His counsellor began working with Sandy to deal with his gambling behaviour, and also provided access to financial advice to take some of the pressure off his finances. The first step was getting Sandy to recognise that his gambling had become an addiction, and that a variety of strategies would be needed to help him deal with it.

One of the first steps to help Sandy to restrict and then stop his gambling was to have a good look at the things that triggered gambling, and changing or controlling some of those triggers (stimulus control). Since Sandy did not have many other activities to fill his weekends and cope with his isolation, he was put in touch with a local Cambodian community group. This group gave him a social network, involved him in projects that would fill his time and gave him a sense of self-worth through helping others. Together with his counsellor, he also worked on developing strategies to stay away from the casino and other gambling situations. He developed a plan of easy steps to deal with the emotional loss he felt from not being able to gamble. This consisted of a series of rewards (reinforcements)—mainly self-administered—when he managed to accomplish each step. Financial planning allowed him to postpone some debts, and this allowed him to resume making his full payments to his family. This again gave Sandy the feeling that he could contribute, and his sense of self-efficacy improved.

He also decided to recruit some support from his workmates, by admitting that he had a gambling problem and asking them to help him stay away from at-work gambling situations. They decided to move their usual lunchtime card games to out-of-work hours, and to include Sandy in alternative social activities at lunchtime instead. As his boss had been trying for some time to improve the fitness of his workers, they jointly developed—with Sandy participating—a lunchtime exercise program.

Because Sandy occasionally found himself drawn back to the casino, his counsellor also helped Sandy to develop a 'relapse management' plan, so that if he did slip it was only a small one. It was also not seen as a failure of his behaviour change, but only a momentary hitch in his progress. Over time, Sandy found his involvement in the workplace social network, and in the Cambodian community, met all his social needs, and left him with little time (and no desire) to return to gambling.

1 Voluntary pre-commitment schemes—where gamblers are required to identify up front how much they are prepared to lose—are being debated in many places. How would these schemes be classified as behaviour change strategies?

2 Can opponent–process theory be used to explain Sandy's excitement and pleasure in gambling?

3 All of us know smokers who have given up many times, only to return to smoking. How would relapse management be used to help them quit?

4 How does the slogan 'Never give up giving up' fit with theories of relapse management?

Points to consider

The first step in dealing with problem gambling tends to be to get the person to recognise that their gambling has become an addiction, and that a variety of strategies are needed to help them deal with it. This involves helping the person to have a good look at the things that triggered gambling, and changing or controlling some of those triggers (stimulus control). These can include alternative activities to fill things like spare time, and to provide for social needs. Sandy was put in touch with a local Cambodian community group. This gave him a social network, and involved him in activities that would fill his time, as well as giving him a sense of self-worth through helping others. A counsellor would work on developing strategies to help the problem gambler to stay away from the casino and other gambling situations. A plan of easy steps to deal with the emotional loss would involve a series of rewards (reinforcements)—mainly self-administered. Financial planning is often needed to postpone or refinance some debts. Finding social support is also important. If the problem gambler is able to admit to having a gambling problem, social contacts can be helpful in changing conditions that involve gambling. A 'relapse management' plan is also very useful, so that if there is a slip, it is only a small one—and not seen as a failure of the behaviour change but only a momentary hitch.

CHAPTER SUMMARY

- Understanding motivation—the factors that arouse, sustain and direct behaviour—is important in changing behaviour. Motivation has genetic, biological and cognitive components, but is also strongly influenced by learning.
- Primary drives are based on the biological needs of the organism. Acquired drives arise out of experience with the environment.
- Opponent–process theory and optimal level theories suggest that the organism is motivated to maintain balance as well as to satisfy needs.
- Successful strategies for behaviour change involve picking appropriate behaviours and methods, not expecting too much, giving methods a chance to work, and recognising that methods may be failures but people are not.
- Awareness of antecedents and reinforcements of behaviour are necessary before change can occur. Stimulus control techniques involve modifying the effects of antecedents.
- Low-awareness habits require the behaviour to be made more salient before it can be changed.
- Reinforcement, particularly if it is controlled by the individual, needs to be part of behaviour change strategies. The schedule of reinforcement that will be most effective differs at different stages of the change process.
- The use of good behaviour bonds is a method for increasing the costs of not changing a behaviour and increasing the gains of changing it. Lapses are common, so planning ahead to deal with them is an important part of behaviour change.

SELF TEST

1   According to Maslow's motivation pyramid, belongingness or affiliation needs would have to be satisfied before the individual seeks to satisfy:
    a   safety needs
    b   physiological needs
    c   esteem needs
    d   basic needs.

2   Which of the following statements about motivation is false?
    a   Most of human behaviour seems to be based on instincts.
    b   The head shape and proportions of a baby may serve as a releasing stimulus.
    c   Some primary drives result from deprivation and some from stimulation.
    d   Incentives may produce motivated behaviour in the absence of a need.

3   Dr Ong believes that opponent–process theory is the best explanation for gambling addiction. She would have most confidence in a treatment for gamblers who tried to:
   a   increase the primary process in existing problem gamblers
   b   decrease the secondary process in new gamblers
   c   increase the secondary process in existing problem gamblers
   d   decrease both the primary and secondary process.

4   Dr Pollack believes that patients who successfully change a health behaviour will gain a greater sense that they control their own health outcomes. Dr Pollack is referring to a gain in:
   a   self-esteem
   b   self-efficacy
   c   lapse management
   d   actual control.

5   A good behaviour bond as part of a weight-loss program should:
   a   go to the organiser of the program
   b   not be returned to the patient unless the amount of weight agreed is lost
   c   be large enough that its loss would be significant
   d   be returned only if the individual becomes thin.

FURTHER READING

Carver, C.S. & Scheier, M.F. (1999) *On the Self-Regulation of Behavior.* Cambridge: Cambridge University Press.

Fishbein, M. (2008) A reasoned action approach to health promotion. *Medical Decision Making*, 28, 834–44.

Martin, L.R., Haskard-Zolnierek, K.B. & DiMatteo, M.R. (2010) *Health Behavior Change and Treatment Adherence: Evidence-Based Guidelines for Improving Healthcare.* New York: Oxford University Press.

Ornish, D. (2007) *The Spectrum: A scientifically proven program to feel better, live longer, lose weight, and gain health.* Ballantine: New York.

USEFUL WEBSITES

Change health behaviour with a gentle nudge (MedPageToday):
www.kevinmd.com/blog/2011/02/change-health-behavior-gentle-nudge.html

Cognitive Behavioral Therapy for insomnia, part 2: stimulus control (*Psychology Today*):
www.psychologytoday.com/blog/sleepless-in-america/200905/cognitive-behavioral-therapy-insomnia-part-2-stimulus-control

Lifescripts (Department of Health):
www.health.gov.au/lifescripts

Strategies for preventing relapse (*Drug and Alcohol Recovery Magazine*):
www.drugalcoholaddictionrecovery.com/?p=120

09 A COMPLEX EXAMPLE: ACTIVITY, EATING AND BODY

CHAPTER OBJECTIVES

By the end of your study of this chapter, you should be able to:

- see activity and eating as behaviours, and recognise the differences between these behaviours and the outcomes of the behaviours—such as weight, fitness and body image
- identify individual genetic, biological, psychological, social and cultural factors that influence energy balance
- describe an ecological perspective on overweight and obesity
- understand the role that body image plays in how individuals view themselves and their ability to control their behaviour and health
- apply general principles of health behaviour from previous chapters to development and modification of eating behaviour and activity.

KEYWORDS

acute illness
bariatric surgery
Body Mass Index (BMI)
comfort food
ecological model
fitness
food pyramid

obesity
obesogenic environment
overweight
physical activity
settling point theory
stimulus control

ACTIVITY AND EATING AS BEHAVIOURAL HEALTH ISSUES

The aim of this chapter is to try to bring together many of the ideas from the previous chapters to examine a particularly complex grouping of health behaviours. It addresses the nature of these behaviours, the motivations for them, and the risks and gains associated with them, and looks at how the general principles of behaviour change might be utilised.

Overweight: a label for a range of weight that is above that considered to be healthy.

Much of the world is experiencing what has been called an epidemic of **overweight** (Zimmet & James 2006). It has been noted that over half of adults in Australia are classified as overweight or obese (ABS 2008). While these are the most recently available data, rates are almost certainly going to be higher when the next survey results become available in 2012. The average body weight of Americans has increased by 3.5 kilograms over the past 15 years. Over the last few years, it has been estimated that overweight and **obesity** have replaced smoking as the number-one modifiable health risk in developed countries (Taylor 2006). As one author put it:

Obesity: a label for a range of weight that is significantly above that considered to be healthy, and regarded as presenting a serious risk to health.

> The table fork is by far the deadliest weapon created by humans. Each year, this humble utensil abets the deaths of millions of people by conveying into their bodies all kinds of fatty foodstuffs known to cause heart attacks, cancers, strokes, diabetes and other diseases. According to the World Health Organization, approximately 17.5 million people died of cardiovascular disease alone in 2005, making up 30 per cent of all deaths globally. (Balcombe 2010)

This extreme statement was intended to make a point, but the health risks associated with obesity are real, and significant (Haslam & James 2005).

PAUSE 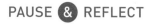 REFLECT

Think about the people around you, among your family and friends. Do they seem to you to be generally overweight? Is this a topic that you frequently discuss with other people? It has been noted that university students are generally less likely to be obese than other people of the same age. Does this seem reasonable to you? Why do you think this might be the case?

MEASUREMENT OF BODY MASS

Body mass index (BMI): an approximate measure of the amount of body fat, frequently used by health professionals because it is easy to calculate.

The most common way of estimating body fat—due mostly to its ease of calculation—is the **body mass index (BMI)**. This has been recognised for some time as a good estimator of whether someone's weight is 'healthy' for one's height (Keys et al. 1972) and is frequently used in determining the extent of overweight and obesity in an individual or group. The measure involves dividing the individual's weight (measured in kilograms) by the square of their height (measured in metres).

Common suggestions are that the healthy range of BMI for adults is 18.5–25. Both overweight and underweight have been shown to have negative health consequences. Overweight is commonly defined as being between the top of the healthy range and 30, while being over 30 is categorised as obese. Use of the BMI with children is not considered to be appropriate unless corrections for the age of the child are used (Centers for Disease Control and Prevention 2011). There are also national differences in how BMI is applied, with lower BMIs being regarded as healthy in many Asian countries, due to differences in body structure between Asians and Caucasians.

There are problems with this simple measure, however. Many elite athletes, such as football players, have BMIs well above 26—largely due to the high levels of (relatively heavy) muscle mass for their height. There is even some evidence that the mildly overweight range (26–30) may not result in higher mortality than the defined healthy range (Flegal et al. 2005). However, BMI is extremely useful in considering the general case; that is, when looking at how weight can affect the health of people within a particular group.

MELISSA HESS AND EXERCISE

CASE STUDY

The aim of this case is to look at the elements involved in changing a health-related behaviour: physical activity.

Melissa Hess is a 19-year-old university student who lives with her parents. When she was in high school, she played several sports and got plenty of other exercise by walking to and from school. She now notices that she is not exercising any more. She drives her car everywhere, even down to the shop. As a result, she is aware that she is feeling unfit and is beginning to gain weight. She also feels tired much more often than she used to, and is not sleeping as well. She does not like the changes that have happened to her appearance, particularly the 'spare tire' developing around her middle. She decides to examine the antecedents for her exercise behaviour as a first step to increasing her activity levels.

1   Why do you think Melissa got so much exercise during her school years?
2   Why do you think Melissa's exercise behaviour has changed so much in a relatively short time?

HEALTH ISSUES IN OVERWEIGHT AND OBESITY

The most obvious evidence of a concern with overweight in public media in recent years has been the frequency with which weight and weight loss are discussed. It has been estimated that there has been a 100 per cent increase reporting about obesity since the late 1990s and that it is now the number-one media topic (Thomas & McLeod 2011). This is particularly the case in media directed at women, where virtually every issue of women's magazines, every lifestyle television program and every newspaper section devoted to health tends to include discussion of weight loss and methods for achieving it. The Australian data on the proportion of each gender that is overweight, and on the health consequences of overweight, suggest that media aimed at men should be even more focused on weight loss, but this is not the case at all. The reason usually offered for such a discrepancy is that other people, such as partners and health professionals, worry about men's overweight primarily because of its impact on health, while women worry about their own, primarily because of its impact on appearance.

Recent surveys in many countries have shown a particularly troubling increase in overweight and obesity in children—even the very young. Olds et al. (2010) note that the rates of overweight and obesity in Australian children are worryingly high, although there may be some evidence that they have reached a plateau. It is possible that this is linked to media attention given to the problem. With high rates of overweight and obesity have come worrying increases in risk factors such as high blood pressure, raised blood sugar levels and type 2 diabetes among children (Daniels et al. 2005). Obesity and overweight have also recently been linked to poorer quality of life in adolescents (Keating, Moodie & Swinburn 2011).

Reductions in the rates of overweight would result in greatly increased disease-free years later in life, due to reductions in the rates of coronary heart disease, bowel cancer, diabetes, strokes and even arthritis. Changes to energy balance—that is, modification of diet and exercise patterns—in children and young adults could have an enormous impact on the costs of health care, and extend the healthy and active years of life for each person.

The issues involved in this idea of energy balance are extremely complex, however, and this complexity is often overlooked. There is a tendency to confuse behaviours (such as 'I will walk for 20 minutes' or 'I will eat smaller portions'), where intentions are reasonably good predictors, with outcomes (such as 'I will get fit' or 'I will lose weight'), where intentions are much poorer predictors (Fishbein 2008).

Most of the attention on energy balance tends to be focused on restriction of intake: limiting the amount or the kind of food that the individual eats. This is often unpleasant for the individual concerned, with social, emotional and even serious health consequences. Another consequence has been the search for a 'magic bullet': some simple, quick and painless way of restricting intake. The major result of this has been a massive increase in weight reduction products offered. Many of these are based on the idea of replacing normal meals with filling but low-kilojoule shakes, soups or bars. Although these products are being improved in terms of dietary balance, fibre, vitamins and minerals, it is likely that their main value is short-term (Egger 2006). Few of them offer anything that could not be achieved by choosing lower kilojoule foods. One of the main objections to them is that the individual does not learn a great deal about eating behaviour over the long term.

Many of the 'magic bullets' are totally fraudulent, offering no-pain weight loss through untested, unproven and even dangerous methods in exchange for large amounts of money. One of these products—SensaSlim, an oral weight-loss spray—has had its approval by the Australian Therapeutic Goods Administration withdrawn on the grounds that its claimed research support was faked (Medew 2011). The claims for this product were supposedly backed by a Geneva-based research group. Investigation showed that the pictures of the group's executives had actually been copied from the website of an American lung clinic, which had nothing to do with SensaSlim—or even with weight loss. Sadly, the product (and its supposed 'scientific' support) is still available on the internet. The US Federal Trade Commission (2004) states that ads that claim you can lose large amounts of weight quickly by taking a pill, putting on a patch or rubbing in a cream 'are almost always false'.

Bariatric surgery: surgery aimed at weight loss in the obese that works by reducing the size of the stomach, either by mechanical devices (lap bands) or removal of part of the stomach.

A different type of rapid weight loss treatment involves **bariatric surgery**, such as bypass operations or lap-band surgery (where the size of the stomach is reduced by the placing of a band around the stomach to restrict the amount of food that can be eaten). Such surgical procedures can have dramatic effects (Colquitt et al. 2009). Surgery is considered a last choice option after other approaches to weight control have failed and is used only with moderate to severe obesity. It can place the patient at serious risk of after-effects such as infections and surgical complications, and side effects such as gastric upset and ongoing heartburn. Surgery is only suitable in extreme cases of clinical obesity where the health risks of doing nothing are immediate and severe. If surgical procedures such as lap-bands need to be reversed, weight tends to be regained quickly. Even surgery needs to be combined with long-term changes in eating behaviours if long-term weight loss is to be achieved and maintained.

In reality, overweight is not just about how much food is taken in. It is also highly dependent on the kind of food—and other intakes such as alcohol—as well as the output side of the balance, such as work and exercise (Scarborough et al. 2011). Environmental and biological factors also play a role in this complex system. Figure 9.1 presents an **ecological model** for understanding obesity (Swinburn, Egger & Raza 1999).

Since part of the complexity comes from the confounding of the issues, topics are discussed separately later in this chapter. As it is in many ways the simpler side of the intake–output equation, activity will be looked at first.

Ecological model: a model proposing that overweight and obesity are based on biological, behavioural and environmental factors rather than just food intake.

Figure 9.1   An ecological model for understanding obesity

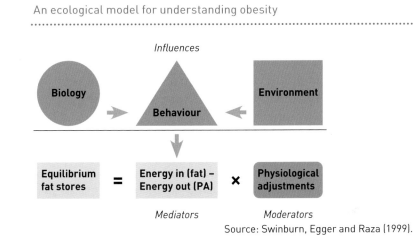

Source: Swinburn, Egger and Raza (1999).

MELISSA (CONT.)   CASE STUDY

Melissa decides that part of the difference is that several things that used to trigger exercise—a school requirement that she play sport, the fact that her friends played sport, and special times during the day set aside for exercise—no longer happen. Now she has a part-time job, and her studies take up a lot of time. When she is not studying, she likes to talk to her friends on the phone, or meet them at the pub or coffee shop to talk. She also notes that exercise makes her feel tired now, that there never seems to be enough time and that she does not particularly like to get sweaty.

Melissa realises that the antecedents for her behaviour need to be changed. Apart from triggers, there also used to be a number of stimuli that no longer occur: having someone tell her that it was time to exercise, having exercise clothes with her, having easy access to a place to exercise, and remembering to exercise. Melissa decides that she will set aside specific times for exercise each week. She will make it hard to forget these by marking them in her diary and leaving herself notes. She asks her parents to remind her to exercise, washes her exercise clothes as soon as she finishes exercising, and places the clean clothes in her sports bag ready for the next scheduled exercise. On days when exercise is scheduled, she leaves the sports bag at the front door as a reminder. These are all examples of stimulus control.

1   Can you think of any other ways Melissa might control the stimuli that trigger exercise behaviour, or that you could use to trigger your own?

2   How might Melissa use reinforcements to modify her behaviour?

PHYSICAL ACTIVITY

Messages encouraging increased physical activity are everywhere. Schools and worksites frequently run programs explaining the benefits of activity, and the risks associated with a sedentary lifestyle. One entire Australian city—Rockhampton—undertook a program to encourage everyone to take 10,000 steps each day (Brown et al. 2006). A lot of the attention being given to exercise, however, fails to explain the differences and similarities of incidental exercise (such as effortful work, and exercise involved in daily activities such as walking, stair-climbing and house or garden work) and intentional exercise (effortful activity undertaken solely for the purpose of getting fit, or fitter). Even the latter needs to be subdivided by purpose, as individuals may exercise for goals related to three Fs: fatness (or size), fitness (or function) and figure (or fashion).

SIZE (FATNESS)

There is evidence that suggests that adding exercise to diet can be faster, more effective and have greater health benefits than dieting alone (Grundy et al. 1999). The debates about the merits of eating less versus exercising more are complicated by the fact that eating less on its own only removes weight (with health benefits primarily limited to areas where risks arise from too much body fat), while exercise changes the nature of the weight (with health benefits that can arise from better cardiovascular, respiratory and musculoskeletal fitness as well). However, exercise has several drawbacks when the aim is to decrease body size, and these are increased when the individual is already obese. For the morbidly obese individual, even limited exercise may be very difficult, extremely uncomfortable and even seriously dangerous.

Media presentations focusing purely on weight lost, such as *The Biggest Loser*, may present a very biased view of how effective exercise (and dieting) can be in reducing body size. Firstly, the contestants are selected to have generally good health (other than being obese) so that risks of acute health problems occurring during the program are limited. When injuries or cardiovascular or respiratory problems do occur, they tend to be edited out of the program, or at least minimised in the presentation. Contestants are also devoting their full time to losing weight: a luxury that very few people can afford either in time or loss of earnings. The payoffs—monetary prizes, fame and publicity—are very great motivators (in the short term), and these payoffs are not available to the average obese individual. Finally, the duration of benefit is not considered. What do the biggest losers look like, and how is their health, a year after the program, or two years? Without a full consideration of all the issues that lead to their serious obesity in the first place, it is difficult to determine whether any long-term benefit—other than weight loss—has resulted from the program.

A problem that is often encountered by people who increase their exercise purely as a way of losing weight is that they may initially convert fat weight to heavier muscle weight, meaning

CROSS-REFERENCE

Motivation is discussed in Chapter 8.

that they may start by gaining rather than losing weight. This can be discouraging in the short term, and needs to be recognised as a benefit rather than a disappointment. Clearly, the best outcomes occur—as usually happens eventually—when the individual begins to enjoy the exercise for its own sake. This becomes a much more straightforward motivation than potential weight loss, and is more likely to lead to long-term sustainable exercise patterns.

PAUSE & REFLECT

Have your exercise and physical activities changed over the past few years? If so, why do you think this has happened? If not, what has maintained your behaviour?

FUNCTION (FITNESS)

The least discussed, but in health terms often the most significant, effect of **physical activity** is improved function. The term '**fitness**' is used mostly when the benefits are spread across a number of body systems. Increased activity—even at low levels—has been shown to help cardiovascular and respiratory function, to increase tolerance to effort, and to make individuals feel better (Shaw et al. 2006). However, these benefits may be seen in a number of different body systems. For example, even limited activity such as regular walking may reduce high blood pressure, reduce the occurrence of chest pain in patients with existing cardiovascular problems, and reduce the occurrence of asthmatic attacks, headaches, muscular pain, and depression and anxiety.

What is often overlooked is that activity can be specifically targeted towards the particular health outcomes that are most important to the individual. Gentle movement activities, such as stretching, ta'i chi, yoga and Pilates, may produce major benefits in flexibility, aiding problems such as muscular or joint pain, movement restriction, headache and negative emotions, but do little for cardiovascular/respiratory function or strength. Weightlifting may build muscle mass, increasing strength and flexibility, but do little for general fitness. Vigorous, high-impact exercise such as running, dance-based exercises (like Zumba), tennis, football or some martial arts may produce great benefit in terms of cardiovascular/respiratory function and the effectiveness of specific muscle groups, but can place individuals at greater risk of injury or **acute illness** events. This is particularly true of older people, or those with pre-existing health conditions. It is always wise to consult a doctor before beginning any strenuous exercise program, or significantly changing activity patterns.

FIGURE (FASHION)

It has been noted that men often exercise primarily for issues having to do with body shape; that is, to build up muscle and to reduce body fat levels so that that muscle is more evident. At the same time, the majority of men—regardless of their weight and shape—are satisfied with their appearance. This seeming contradiction underlines the significant gender issues in the energy-balance equation. The majority of women are dissatisfied with their shape, and yet are not nearly as concerned with musculature as with size. Where most men would like to convert fat to muscle, women are most concerned with simply getting rid of the fat and having a thinner shape (McDonald & Thompson 1992). Some women may even avoid strenuous exercise out of a fear of becoming too muscular rather than fashionably thin.

Physical activity: bodily movement produced by skeletal muscles that requires energy expenditure.

Fitness: a condition of health or physical soundness, which may be general or related to the ability to meet a specific demand ('fit for purpose').

Acute illness: a single episode of illness (or disease), generally severe and over a limited period of time.

CASE STUDY

MELISSA (CONT.)

Melissa decides that she can increase the gains and reduce the costs of exercise by making an effort to change the way she thinks about exercise. Although she does not like getting sweaty and tired, she recognises that these are short-term costs. So she focuses on the gains. After she has exercised, and then showered, she feels 'tingly' and relaxed. Being tired has a positive side, in that she sleeps better and feels more awake during the day. This allows her to get more done in less time, and because she is becoming fitter, she has more energy to bring to all her tasks. The increase in exercise also changes her thinking about her fitness and figure, and she finds this very rewarding. Finally, because she is enjoying the change to her activities, she persuades a friend to exercise with her, and together they join a netball team that plays once a week. Exercising with a friend makes it a social activity as well as a physical one, and replaces some of the lost social time. The amount of time that Melissa spends on study and work appears to be a big factor in the decrease in her exercise. She does note, however, that there is a lot of wasted time in her typical day, and this is where she can fit her exercise without losing out on more valuable activities.

1   The costs of exercise are often immediate, while the gains are long-term. How could this problem be overcome?

2   Can you think of some ways that Melissa could better organise her time to make room for exercise?

EATING

The determinants of what we eat, when we eat, how much we eat and why we eat are far more variable than are often recognised (Ogden 2007). They include childhood learning and developmental factors, social and cultural influences, and many psychological factors. The variety of these influences can be seen in what is sometimes called 'food porn': television, internet and printed media presentations of the most exotic, delicious and attractive foods that can be produced by expert chefs and duplicated in your own home.

The existence of the huge number of sources of information about food indicates that we clearly do not just eat to survive. Hunger is only one small part of our motivation to eat. We also eat for pleasure, for social interaction, for our own emotional reasons (comfort, relaxation and stress reduction) and even to impress others. Have you ever bragged about what, where or how much you have eaten?

One easy way to think about the complexity of the issues is to separate what we eat from how much we eat, and why we eat.

WHAT WE EAT

Food pyramid:
a triangular-shaped figure divided into segments to indicate which food groups are more or less desirable as proportions of diet.

School programs in many countries teach children about '**food pyramids**' or 'food pies'. These indicate the various food groups, and how much of each we should eat for health reasons. The smallest section of these graphic representations is always the section for fat. The diet in developed countries is characterised by including too much fat, and much of the health-related information about diet is focused on reducing the amount of fat as a proportion of food intake. This can have the unfortunate consequence of making some children fat-phobic, and extreme low-fat diets can be hazardous to the health of children because of fat's role in growth and development. The fact that many of the favoured foods of children are classed in the fat category can make other children simply tune out the balanced diet message.

The reality is that what children eat is usually not under the children's control at all (Ogden 2007). The decisions about what food to buy and prepare are commonly under the control of their parents or other carers. There is some evidence that parents—particularly mothers—may pay more attention to how healthy their personal food intake is than to how healthy their children's food intake is.

As the above discussion suggests, what we eat is under a great deal of **stimulus control**. Because of prior experience, we find certain types of food attractive and others unattractive. Salty, sweet and fatty foods unfortunately tend to be very attractive to all of us. Other stimulus characteristics of food—colour, texture, shape or thoughts about the source—can be highly important in determining attractiveness. For example, a person may have no problems with eating beef, lamb or pork because the meat comes in large, anonymous chunks, but be unable to eat chicken or fish because they are smaller and therefore look more like animals.

> **Stimulus control:** changing behaviour by changing its antecedents.

Children quite often have aversions to certain kinds of food; for example, vegetables. Research has shown that they can be brought to increase their intake of these foods simply by exposing them to other people—including peers, role models or even strange adults—eating those vegetables (Ogden 2007). Food that is strange in colour, texture or flavour may be less desirable than familiar foods. So-called 'picky eaters' are common among children, but this restriction in willingness to eat novel foods often is found among adults as well.

PAUSE 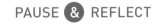 REFLECT

Have you, or someone in your family, ever had a food aversion? Or a fad for eating a particular kind of food very frequently? Did your family have an explanation for this that you shared with one another? Did this aversion or fad have an effect on what the other members of the family ate?

Culture and media are very important in educating people about what is desirable and undesirable food. Many novel ingredients—including Asian staple foods such as lemongrass, bok choy and varieties of chillies—are now easily available in supermarkets in Western countries. Australasian customers have a very diverse range of foods available because of the multicultural nature of their populations, and dramatic changes in the sources of immigrants and refugees over the past few decades. Cookery shows also introduce viewers to a new range of ingredients and preparation methods. However, some foods that are regularly eaten in some places may even be illegal foodstuffs in others—such as dogs and cats in most Western countries.

HOW MUCH WE EAT

Another learned component of the food intake equation is how much food is appropriate. Most people in the older generations were raised on the principle that we 'should' eat everything on our plate. This ethical dimension of 'not wasting good food' made good sense during a depression or war when the amount or kind of food available was limited. However, in most of the developed world, food is now easily available, and quantities are seldom limited by any factor other than affordability. For the majority of the population in Western countries, affordability is also not a problem.

Learning to identify appropriate portion and meal sizes follows very similar patterns as learning what to eat. During childhood, parents make available what they believe are appropriately sized meals, and children are still expected to eat those meals. If the child asks for more food, or a particular kind of food, it is seen as appropriate to provide it. There is again an ethical dimension, in that depriving a growing child of 'enough' to grow on is frowned upon. It is quite common for a family, or restaurant goers, to keep eating until all the food is gone, even if this leads to a feeling of being overfull, or bloated. Hunger is clearly not motivating this eating. If this is a regular experience, learning that the appropriate portion size is very large can result. An experience often noted by travellers to the US is that the meal sizes in restaurants seem to be aimed at the largest eaters, not the average, and that often significant portions of the meal have to be left behind.

This means that an important part of helping both children and adults to maintain a healthy weight or body shape is stimulus control; in this case, portion control (Clark et al. 2010). Instructions that an appropriate size for a meat portion is 'the size of a deck of cards' gives the individual more immediately accessible information than saying 'about 200 grams'. Reducing portion sizes—even without changing any other aspect of a meal—can be a very effective strategy for helping maintain a healthy weight, or lose unwanted weight.

WHY WE EAT

CROSS-REFERENCE

Motivation is discussed in Chapter 8.

The most important, and complex, issue with regard to eating is motivation. The easiest assumption to make about eating is that people eat when they are hungry and stop when they are not. This is not a very accurate description of the eating patterns of most people. Eating tends to take place at mealtimes, in places where food is available even when it is not mealtime, and in the presence of attractive food in the environment. Stimulus control may be as important, or more important, than needs and drives where eating behaviour is concerned.

An interesting—and perhaps counterintuitive—finding regarding stimulus control of eating is that overweight people are less likely than underweight or normal weight people to eat because they are hungry. The overweight person may be, in fact, more likely to be triggered to eat by the presence of food, by the approach of a mealtime or by an emotional state than are others (Schachter 1971). It has been suggested that this happens because of early experience with food, which becomes associated with certain times, with social interaction or with comfort. As a result, some people may fail to regulate their eating by sensations of hunger, and eat when they are lonely, when they are stressed or simply when they are in the presence of food.

Food restriction diets simply fail to take these factors into account, leading dieters to feel unsatisfied—not because they are still hungry but because they have not had their usual diet. They may also feel isolated because they cannot eat as others are eating, or stressed because they have not eaten things that have been associated with pleasant tastes or emotional comfort.

Comfort food: food eaten primarily for positive emotional reasons rather than hunger—often with traditional or nostalgic connections.

Such **comfort food** is typically high in sugar and/or fat, and it has been noted that while it can relieve some stress, it also tends to add to abdominal fat stores (Dallman, Pecorato & la Fleur 2005). Overeating among dieters is quite common, and has been connected with theories of disinhibition (or the 'what the hell' effect) in the presence of food cues, along with regulation of mood by eating, escape from stress or the relapse violation effect (Ogden 2007).

Ogden (2007) also discusses how control influences eating or overeating. An individual may believe that they cannot control their eating for a wide variety of reasons. They may, for example, believe that their weight is genetically determined, so efforts to change eating will not work. On the other hand, if they feel that many elements of their life—for example, stress, other people's behaviour or work—are out of their control, they may believe that eating is one thing that they do have direct control over. Our beliefs about where control of our eating lies may have a quite significant effect on how we go about trying to change, or whether we make the effort to change at all.

Focusing simply on the individual and his/her motivation also ignores a range of other very important factors. Swinburn, Egger and Raza (1999) have referred to modern conditions of living in developed countries as '**obesogenic environments**', with many elements of the environment tending to encourage behaviours that lead to excess intake and inadequate outputs, and far fewer elements that encourage healthier behaviours. Dealing with these elements requires making changes to the environment, perhaps through education, restrictions on advertising, better labelling of food or regulations about availability. One example of the latter is limiting unhealthy choices in school 'tuck shops' and workplace cafeterias.

This does not mean that there may not also be biological or genetic influences that exert some control over eating. Set point theory suggests that there may be brain mechanisms that 'defend' our current body fat content, so that if we eat too little—as in a restriction diet—our body tries to defend our current fat levels by making us hungrier. It also suggests that if we eat too much, our body will make us less hungry (Kennedy 1953). In a major review, Speakman et al. (2011) identify some basic problems with this theory. It does not really account for the environmental controls on eating discussed above, or explain why there should be an 'obesity epidemic' occurring. They discuss some alternative balance models. **Settling point theory** suggests that when either inputs (eating) or outputs (activity) change, the balance may settle at a new equilibrium point, and then remain relatively stable at that point until either the inputs or the outputs change again. This agrees nicely with the idea of the 'obesogenic environment': any obesity epidemic could result from either increased accessibility to food or a decrease in the need for physical activity, as a result of societal change. There are some problems with this model as well, however. Probably the biggest one is simply the question, 'Why don't we all get fat?'

In Chapter 6, we talk about person–environment interactions as basic to understanding human behaviour, and what is needed here is a theory that takes account of both environmental influences and individual predispositions or vulnerabilities. Such models exist (Speakman et al. 2011), but are beyond the scope of the current discussion. Regulation of eating and activity behaviours are quite complex—relying on a variety of systems at a variety of levels—but what is clear is that any approach needs to involve both psychological and biological aspects.

BODY IMAGE AS A HEALTH ISSUE

Given that overweight and obesity have become such a health pandemic (ABS 2008), it is informative to look at what people think about their bodies. Sadly, there are extremely high levels of body dissatisfaction, and substantial evidence that this dissatisfaction is causally linked to a wide range of psychological and physical health problems. In one particularly disturbing report, Nichter and Nichter (1991) surveyed teenage girls about what the 'ideal' body for a teenage girl should be. The result was that the ideal girl was seen to be 1.7 metres in height, but weighing only a little over 45 kilograms. Such a body would not only be nearly impossible to achieve for most girls, but with a Body Mass Index of under 16, it would also be extremely unhealthy if not actively dangerous—in the anorexic range.

The strongest evidence is that there is a definite link between dissatisfaction with one's body and disordered eating. Disordered eating includes, but is not restricted to, clinical eating disorders such as anorexia and bulimia nervosa. It also includes crash dieting, so-called 'yoyo'

CROSS-REFERENCE
Locus of control is discussed in more detail in Chapter 13.

Obesogenic environment: an environment (including culture, physical structures and other elements) that encourages overeating and/or inadequate physical activity.

Settling point theory: a theory that suggests that changes in energy balance become habitual, and remain at the new level.

CROSS-REFERENCE
Learning is discussed in Chapter 6.

dieting—where weight gain and loss alternate—and eating a severely unbalanced diet resulting in dietary deficiencies.

PAUSE 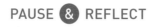 REFLECT

Are you dissatisfied with your body? Given the discussion in this chapter, it would be quite likely that you are—particularly if you are female. What factors do you think contribute to you being satisfied or dissatisfied with your body?

Research has linked numerous influences to the development and maintenance of weight-related problems. These include teasing (by peers, parents or others), early physical maturation, negative emotions, stress, developmental challenges, academic pressures and social comparison, and particularly images presented in the media (Thompson & Heinberg 1999). This includes not only the presentation of fashion models and media stars who are uniformly thin, but also a relative scarcity of not only obese but also normal, healthy-weight characters in the media. For girls, the correlation tends to be between attractiveness and thinness, while for boys it tends to be with strength and low body fat levels as well.

Periodically, media will attempt to defend themselves from criticism that they are contributing to a society-wide body image problem by running special features on 'normal' size models, or restricting their use of very thin, or very young, models. These defensive activities are often short-lived, or undermined by other media who continue to use unhealthy models or the retouching of pictures to increase their market share at the expense of the more responsible media. However, the use of those same media to change perceptions about what is healthy weight, and desirable shape, should not be overlooked (Thompson & Heinberg 1999).

INTERVENTION

CROSS-REFERENCE
Behavioural change is discussed in Chapter 8.

With the issues being as complex as they are, it would be unreasonable to expect simple solutions. Clearly, behavioural interventions at the individual level have an important part to play. These interventions—either on their own or together with pharmacological treatments, dietary substitutes and even surgery—can be effective in many cases. Other approaches being tried include meal replacement programs, internet- and telephone-based interventions, and a more active role for health professionals in supporting the individual in their pursuit of a healthy weight (Berkel et al. 2005). However, as overweight and obesity are issues for society as well as for the individual, it is important not to neglect intervention at the level of the family, the community and even globally (Swinburn, Egger & Raza 1999).

CASE STUDY

DONALD JOHNSON AND OBESITY

The aim of this case is to look at factors that may be involved in encouraging and maintaining obesity in an individual.

Donald Johnson is a 43-year-old security guard at a suburban shopping centre in Adelaide. He was born in a 'town camp' outside of Alice Springs to a young Indigenous woman who herself was clinically obese. When Donald was 18 months old, his mother was hospitalised with complications of respiratory disease, and Donald was fostered to a white family in Adelaide. This family discouraged members of his mother's family from having any contact with Donald, and when his mother died in hospital, they ceased all communication. These foster parents were themselves overweight, and Donald was raised on a diet that was heavy on potatoes, bread and other starches, and large portions of fried food. He received little attention from his foster parents, as he was one of four children they were caring for, and most of the attention was at mealtimes.

When he was aged 6, these foster parents decided that they could no longer care for so many children, and for the next four years Donald was shuttled from institution to foster home to institution. Food was always plentiful, and sweets and fatty foods were often given as treats, because Donald 'always seemed to be hungry'. At age 10, he was placed with an aunty living in a small Indigenous community in western Queensland. She made an effort to see that Donald was never hungry, but fresh food was hard to get and very expensive, so his diet was high in starch and processed food. Other children at school made fun of him for being so fat, and he gradually found that his only friends were other overweight children.

When he reached high school age, Donald started associating with other 'unpopular' kids, and was introduced to beer. Eating and drinking beer gradually became his primary source of comfort against the teasing that he received, and the pressure from teachers and some other adults that he should lose some weight for his own health. Donald left school before finishing high school. Because he was big and strong, he was able to get labouring jobs. However, labouring—particularly in hot weather—was very stressful for him, and he got out of breath easily. It was common for him to join other labourers on building sites for large fatty lunches accompanied by several beers, and to wind down at the end of the day at the pub for more fatty food and beer. As his weight continued to increase, he had to leave several labouring jobs, and began to drift from place to place.

Eventually, Donald returned to Adelaide, and obtained his job as a security guard at a shopping centre. He lives alone in a rented room, so he eats at the shopping centre or in the pub on the way home. His job involves little physical activity other than walking, and considerable time sitting. Because he was always thirsty, and had to take more and more frequent breaks to urinate, his boss sent him for a medical evaluation and he was discovered to be suffering from type 2 diabetes. The doctor gave him a printed diet to control his symptoms, but Donald could not find the time or energy to follow the diet very often, and he found it hard not to just eat whatever looked good at the shopping centre's food court. He did manage to cut out drinking, however, but seemed to be hungrier after giving up alcohol. In the last month, Donald has begun to have increasingly severe chest pain when he climbs stairs at work, and has started to use escalators and lifts instead.

1   What are some possible biological and social elements contributing to Donald's obesity?

2   Why do you think Donald's weight received so little attention as a behavioural problem during his childhood?

3   What are some of the reasons why giving up alcohol has had so little effect on Donald's obesity?

4   What factors make a typical suburban shopping centre an obesogenic environment? What might be done to make it less so?

Points to consider

Many components are involved when an individual has developed a pattern of excess eating behaviour. In this case, there were cultural and social class factors, ranging from being removed from his mother, family and culture at an early age, through the instability of early life, lack of educational opportunities and a variety of other issues linked to deprivation. More about how social factors impact on health is discussed elsewhere in this book. There are also several individual behavioural issues in this case, such as a lack of self-efficacy, and the fact that established health problems have already appeared that might have been avoided with early interventions. Behaviour change can be vital at any stage, but community development, education, governmental programs and basic help for the disadvantaged are also needed.

CHAPTER SUMMARY

- The relationship between weight and health has become a major focus of attention in the area of health behaviour. High rates of overweight and obesity, and low levels of physical activity, have been identified as significant public health issues—particularly in developed countries.
- Although the health problems associated with overweight and lack of activity are greater for men, concern with body weight and shape are greater for women.
- The issues are complicated, and a focus on just one aspect of the activity–eating interaction can produce an unbalanced picture of possible solutions.
- The reduction in physical activity has been related to an increase in the number of sedentary jobs and sedentary leisure pursuits, such as television and computers.
- The behavioural issues in eating are more complex, as consideration needs to be given to what we eat, how much we eat and why we eat. A variety of theories has been advanced regarding how individual eating is regulated, and why overeating occurs—even when the individual is consciously attempting to eat less.
- There are also elements of the environment and society that contribute independently to the problem of overweight in society, and a broader ecological model helps with understanding this issue.
- Body image is an important part of the equation, with high levels of body dissatisfaction raises issues making the activity–eating interaction even more difficult to understand, and creating a need for more comprehensive solutions to the public health problem.

SELF TEST

1 Which of the following statements about the Body Mass Index (BMI) is false?
   a It is the most commonly used measure of weight in public health.
   b There are slight differences is what is considered the healthy range for men and women.

    c   Anyone with a BMI over 25 or 26 is unhealthy.

    d   BMI is more useful in considering the health of a group than of an individual.

2 Overweight and obesity have not been linked to:

    a   risk of heart disease

    b   lung cancer

    c   quality of life in adolescents

    d   type 2 diabetes.

3 According to the ecological model of obesity, the major influences do not include:

    a   biology

    b   behaviour

    c   finances

    d   environment.

4 Portion control intervention is most likely to affect:

    a   what we eat

    b   why we eat

    c   when we eat

    d   how much we eat.

5 Interventions to deal with obesity over the long term:

    a   always need to include behavioural aspects

    b   should be directed at outcomes such as becoming thin

    c   work best if they include crash diets

    d   always need to include bariatric surgery.

FURTHER READING

Clark, A., Franklin, J., Pratt, I. & McGrice, M. (2010) Overweight and obesity: Use of portion control in management. *Australian Family Physician*, 39(6), 407–11.

Hardman, A.E. & Stensel, D.J. (2009) *Physical Activity and Health: The Evidence Explained* (2nd edn). Routledge: London.

Ogden, J. (2007) Eating Behaviour (chap. 6). *Health Psychology: A Textbook* (4th edn). Open University Press: New York.

Pool, R. (2001) *Fat: Fighting the Obesity Epidemic.* Oxford University Press: New York.

USEFUL WEBSITES

Bathroom scales don't tell the whole story (MedicineNet):
www.medicinenet.com/script/main/art.asp?articlekey=56830

Going for the gaunt: How low can an athlete's body fat go? (Scientific American; read the Editor's note at the bottom):
www.scientificamerican.com/article.cfm?id=athlete-body-fat

Is your brain making you fat? (ABC Science):
www.abc.net.au/science/articles/2010/01/21/2798024.htm

Stress feeds the need for comfort food (WebMD):
www.webmd.com/balance/news/20030909/stress-comfort-food

PART 3

PSYCHOPHYSIOLOGICAL ASPECTS OF HEALTH

IS IT ALL IN YOUR MIND?

So far, the focus of this book has largely been on behavioural and cognitive factors as they impact on health, while the issue of emotion has hovered somewhere in the background. Emotion has been mentioned frequently, but up to now has not been dealt with directly or in depth. Yet anyone who thinks about what health means will be aware that emotions make up a critical component. To take one example, the media are full of stories about stress: the effects of stress on how people feel and behave, and the effects of stress on their health. Invariably, stress is thought of as existing within the emotional domain or the individual. This part of the book begins the examination of this domain and how it is linked to the concepts that have been discussed up to this point.

So, why is it titled 'psychophysiological aspects'? This is intended to get you to think of the psychological (mental) and the physiological (bodily) elements of the person as inseparably connected with one another. Western patterns of thinking have often tried to separate the mind from the body, as if the two could operate in isolation from one another. One of the main aims of this part of the book is to challenge those patterns of thinking. What needs to be considered, particularly when we think about health and illness, is the whole person. In Chapters 4 and 5, we discussed in some detail how illness affects the whole person, not just limited elements of them. In the next few chapters, we focus on how the whole person, with a mind and a body, experiences their emotional world.

The first place to start is with an understanding of what emotion is and how it works. Chapter 10 examines the interactions between the elements of the whole person that give rise to the experiences we call emotion. It looks at the importance of the brain and nervous system, along with other systems of the body, as well as at the importance of thought processes on the operations of these systems. The role of faulty regulation of emotions in mental illnesses such as anxiety disorders and depression is considered. An integrated perspective is vital to the understanding of how emotional states can produce health effects in key systems of the body, such as the cardiovascular and immune systems; these are also considered.

Pain is often thought to be a condition of the body. Chapter 11 examines how this most common of all symptoms is also an emotional and cognitive condition of the individual. The diagnosis and management of pain constitutes a large part of the work of health professionals, but is often based on incomplete understandings of where pain comes from, why it persists as it does, and what can be done about it.

Chapter 12 shifts the focus to stress. Again, this is a very common concept in discussions of health, but frequently is poorly understood. The total process that we refer to as stress involves elements of stimulus and response. Whether we experience our situation as stressful is dependent on judgments that we make about the significance of several aspects of that situation, such as our appraisal of how much the situation demands of us and whether we have capabilities or the resources to meet those demands. The effects of the most extreme level of demand—traumatic events—are also considered.

Fortunately, stress is neither inevitable nor irresistible. Chapter 13 looks at coping strategies that are adopted to deal with the experience of stress, including naturally occurring ways that we cope with stress; it also introduces some strategies that can be adopted to help with stress management.

In this part of the book, the idea of the individual as a whole person is more of a focus than it has been up to this point. We encourage you to think back to earlier parts of the book from this holistic viewpoint, as this will make it easier for you to understand all of the links between health and human behaviour.

10 UNDERSTANDING MIND AND BODY INTERACTIONS

CHAPTER OBJECTIVES

By the end of your study of this chapter, you should be able to:

- understand interactions between psychological and physical states
- understand the functions of different areas of the brain and the role the autonomic nervous system plays in emotion
- apply the principles of emotion to explain interactions between mind and body, and how these impact on health
- apply an integrated understanding of health to issues such as cardiovascular disease, cancer, mental illness and functioning of the immune system.

KEYWORDS

attribution theory of emotion
cytokines
dysregulation of emotions
emotions
holism
psychoneuroimmunology
psychophysiology
psychosomatic illness
type A (coronary prone) behaviour pattern
type C (or cancer prone) behaviour pattern
type D (distressed) personality

INTRODUCTION

Even though the link between feeling bad in a psychological sense and feeling bad in a physical sense is well recognised, Western philosophy has traditionally regarded the mind (psyche) and body (soma) as separate domains (known as mind–body dualism). Traditionally, the mind and body were viewed as parallel and independent; only some disease states were thought to involve both. The discipline of psychology challenged mind–body dualism. Sigmund Freud (1856–1939) suggested that individuals could convert unconscious psychological conflicts into physical symptoms, and in so doing reduce the anxiety associated with the conflict. Indeed, in response to highly stressful events, there are reported cases of individuals suddenly losing their ability to speak or hear, or developing some form of paralysis. In the late nineteenth and early twentieth centuries, such cases were labelled 'conversion hysteria'.

Subsequently, personality rather than a single specific unconscious conflict was proposed as a contributing factor to the development of ill health. Researchers such as Flanders Dunbar (1947) and Alexander (1943) argued that psychological conflicts produce anxiety and, over time, prompt associated physiological changes to take place via the autonomic nervous system. It was proposed, for example, that repressed anger associated with a frustrated need for love and attention increased secretion of digestive acids that eroded the stomach lining and produced an ulcer.

Psychosomatic illness: an outdated term reserved for a few specific conditions—such as bronchial asthma, neurodermatitis and gastric ulcers—that were regarded as being caused by worry.

The term '**psychosomatic illness**' was reserved for a few specific conditions—such as bronchial asthma, neurodermatitis and gastric ulcers—that were regarded as being caused by worry. Over time, other diseases were added to the list, including hypertension (high blood pressure) and arthritis. Still, there was no genuine consensus about what constituted a psychosomatic illness.

Ideas proposed during the early psychosomatic movement are still popular today, despite widespread criticism (associated with the poor methodological rigour of earlier experiments and its applicability to a very restricted range of conditions). Moreover, medical advances have proven some of these earlier notions to be incorrect and further shaped our thinking. In contrast to psychosomatic models of the role of worry as the single cause in the development of gastric ulcers, for example, two Australians, Barry Marshall and Robin Warren, received the Nobel Prize in 2005 for their discovery of the *Helicobacter pylori* bacterium as the cause of most stomach ulcers and gastritis. This does not mean, however, that emotions such as worry play no part in the development or aggravation of ulcers. We now know that the onset of disease is associated with a variety of factors, including genetic predisposition, environmental factors, early learning experiences, current stressors, cognitions and coping strategies (Consedine & Moskowitz 2007).

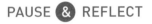

PAUSE & REFLECT

Some people are reluctant to accept that both mind and body interact in health and illness. Why do you think this might be the case and what arguments could you make for a more integrated approach?

Holism: from the Greek, meaning entire or total.

Holism, or holistic health care, is a broad, integrating concept that takes into account cognitions, emotions, and social and spiritual awareness, in addition to traditional physical or biomedical knowledge. Holism attempts to bridge the gap between the physical and mental aspects of patients' suffering. In a health sense it means that all the properties of health or illness cannot be explained by adding up each element. Complementary and alternative health practitioners have subscribed to this idea for hundreds of years and have sought to understand health and illness in the wider context of an individual's life (Bell 2006; Chummun 2006; Julliard, Klimenko & Jacob 2006).

This chapter explores interactions between the mind and body, with particular emphasis on the role of emotion and physiological functioning on health. We investigate the interplay between emotion and different areas of the brain, arousal states and cognitions, as well as factors influencing the expression of emotion. The chapter also discusses how poor regulation of emotion is linked to adverse mental and social consequences for individuals. We also apply our understanding of psychology and physiology (psychophysiology) to cardiovascular conditions, cancer, mental illness and immune responses.

EMOTION

Emotions are such a common component of our experience that it is difficult to imagine life without them. Because an understanding of emotion is critical to an understanding of so many aspects of health and illness, the following section examines emotion in detail.

Emotion is an adaptive, goal-defining aspect of experience, associated with changes across multiple response systems (Mennin et al. 2007). An emotion may, for example, influence decision making, produce behaviour such as crying or smiling, and generate automatic bodily changes such as sweating or a pounding heart. Emotions can be natural, or unlearnt, responses to stimuli that have affective (feeling-producing) properties, such as when an individual accidentally burns their hand on the stove and screams out in response to the pain. Emotions can also be learnt responses to stimuli that have personal value, such as feeling a surge of happiness when you see a loved one after time apart. As such, emotions involve multiple appraisal processes that judge or assess the significance of stimuli in terms of what it means to the individual, with responses modified accordingly.

Emotions: positive or negative responses to external stimuli (situations, events, things and people) and/or internal mental representations (thoughts, dreams and ideas).

MARTIN O'CONNOR AND IRRITABLE BOWEL SYNDROME

CASE STUDY

The aim of this case is to examine the experience of an individual with a physical problem that is closely linked with psychological experience.

Martin is a 17-year-old completing Year 12. As the year has gone on, he has coped well with schoolwork by studying harder than ever, but has begun to experience a range of uncomfortable abdominal symptoms. Some days he will be constipated, but feel his bowels are full and bloated. He has sensations of nausea at times, while at others he just has rumblings in his stomach, accompanied by feelings of bloating and pressure. The following day, he is frequently awakened early in the morning by an urgent need to have a bowel movement, and when he does, he is likely to experience strong pain followed by a rush of diarrhoea. On these days, he tends to have additional attacks of diarrhoea all day—often having to leave class to rush to the toilet. He also has a lot of wind on these days, which he finds very embarrassing.

1 What emotional experiences are likely to be linked to Martin's condition?
2 How do physical and mental factors interact in these emotions?

PHYSIOLOGY OF EMOTION

The physical side of our experience of emotion is basically under the control of the autonomic nervous system (ANS), which regulates the body's internal environment. The ANS has two divisions: sympathetic and parasympathetic. The sympathetic division operates to promote energy expenditure when the body is under demand. This happens when, for example, we are startled or find ourselves in a dangerous situation. Sympathetic nervous system activation produces the 'fight or flight' response. Activation of the sympathetic division is associated with the experience of strong emotion. Characteristics of sympathetic nervous system activation are:

- increased heart rate, speeding delivery of oxygen and nutrients to skeletal muscle
- deeper and more rapid breathing to increase available oxygen, with the pancreas secreting glucagons to increase sugar release into the bloodstream and to muscles
- constriction of blood vessels leading to the gastrointestinal tract so as to shut down digestion; dilation of those vessels leading to muscles
- secretion by adrenal glands of the hormone epinephrine to sustain a number of reactions, resulting in tremor (butterflies in stomach), dilation of pupils (increasing visual acuity), shutdown of salivary glands (causing dry mouth), increased sweating (better heat dissipation) and contraction of surface muscles (goosebumps).

In contrast, the parasympathetic division of the ANS operates during relaxation to promote energy conservation. Once the emergency situation is over, the parasympathetic nervous system takes over to reduce energy loss and provide appropriate conditions for acquisition of energy (such as digestion).

The physiological responses described above are fairly easy to measure using a variety of electronic or chemical sensors, and many efforts have been made to try to understand emotion by studying physiology. Our understanding of emotional control entered a new phase with the advent of functional magnetic resonance imaging (fMRI) studies, which enabled higher mental processes in humans to be detected. Cognitive neuroscientists continue to investigate the 'hot' control of emotions as well as the 'cold' control of attention and memory (Ochsner & Gross 2005). However, fMRI studies can only tell us part of the story. For example, we know that some individuals can manipulate the results of lie detector tests. The polygraph measures small changes in a number of physiological variables, such as heart rate and sweating; but people can change their test results by changing their thought patterns.

The influence of the brain and cognition on emotions is discussed in the next section.

EMOTION AND THE BRAIN

CROSS-REFERENCE
Vulnerability and capability are discussed in Chapter 4.

Emotional reactions may be most easily observed in the body's responses to sympathetic activation, but overall coordination of emotion is conducted by the brain, in particular the cortex, hypothalamus and limbic system, including the amygdala. Electrical stimulation of parts of the hypothalamus, for example, can lead to sympathetic activation and emotional behaviour (such as rage or terror) in laboratory animals.

The role of the limbic system in emotions, particularly violence, has raised the possibility that psychosurgery can alter behaviour, though the ethics of such operations are highly questionable. In laboratory studies with animals, destruction of tissue in a part of the limbic system called the amygdala produced docile behaviour. Any alterations to the brain tend to result in widespread behaviour effects and the use of psychosurgery in humans remains highly controversial.

Emotions are regulated by a range of cognitive processes that vary from attentional mechanisms (such as ignoring emotional stimuli and choosing to focus on something else) to cognitive change (such as reinterpreting the meaning of stimuli). When this happens, the behavioural and neural processes that normally accompany an emotion are also inhibited. It seems that paying less attention to emotional stimuli affects emotional appraisal systems in the amygdala, although research evidence on this is mixed. In terms of cognitive change strategies to control emotions, studies have shown that emotional appraisal is related to neural control systems in the cortex, and to cingulate control systems (Ochsner & Gross 2005). The amygdala is associated with generating emotion and the prefrontal cortical regions with regulating emotion (Burroughs & French 2007).

The dominant hemisphere of the brain is associated with positive emotions, while the non-dominant hemisphere involves negative ones. Recently, research identified different types of emotion in specific areas: the left forebrain with positive feelings, approach behaviour and affiliative (group interest) emotions; and the right forebrain with negative affect, avoidance and survival (or self-interest) emotions (Craig 2005). Clearly, the cortex plays a significant role in emotion.

AROUSAL AND EMOTION

Links between arousal and emotion are well recognised. James (1890) proposed that an exciting event leads to physical arousal, and our perception of this arousal is emotion. It was assumed that different emotions resulted from the perception of different patterns of arousal. This theory, elaborated by Lange, and called the James–Lange theory, placed emphasis on arousal, which preceded the experience of emotion, determined the nature of the emotion experienced and, when it faded, led to the disappearance of the emotional experience.

Cannon (1932), in his critique of the James–Lange theory, proposed several limitations. He suggested the following:

1   Separation of the brain from sensations in the body (in the case of spinal lesions) did not eliminate emotional behaviour.
2   The same bodily changes appear to occur in response to a range of emotions, making it difficult to see how we could perceive one emotion over another.
3   There is a poor correlation between bodily changes and changes in emotional experience.
4   Bodily changes are fairly slow compared with the speed of emotional experience.
5   Artificial induction of bodily changes (by an injection of epinephrine, for example) does not produce emotion.

Although some of these criticisms, such as points two and four, have not been completely supported by subsequent research, the other points reveal crucial flaws in the James–Lange theory.

Cannon (1932) offered an alternative view of emotion, called activation theory (now known as the Cannon–Bard theory). This theory proposed that the perception of an exciting stimulus leads to disinhibition of the midbrain, and results in a general sympathetic nervous system discharge, which produces the physiological arousal and experience of emotion. Unfortunately for Cannon, this theory did not actually meet all of his own criticisms of the James–Lange theory. First, measures of physiological arousal do not compare well with one another. The presentation of a stimulus, for example, may produce an increase in heart rate and a particular emotion, but a repeat presentation of the same stimulus may produce the same emotion but with a decrease in heart rate. Activation theory still does not explain why artificial induction of physiological arousal does not produce emotion. It also fails to explain the richness or variety of emotions we experience. It took another thirty years for the next step to be taken in unravelling the puzzle of emotion.

COGNITION AND EMOTION

Schachter (1964) proposed a two-factor theory of emotion. Although he agreed that arousal was basic to emotion, he proposed that cognitions about arousal is the other element on which emotions are based. For individuals to really experience emotion, they must have both a state of arousal and an appropriate set of cognitions that label the experience as emotional. This was demonstrated in a classic experiment by Schachter and Singer (1962), which is worth describing in detail here. (It should be noted that this study involved deception of participants, and would almost certainly be regarded as unethical within current understanding of the ethics of psychological research.)

Participants were male university students recruited to a study of 'the effects of vitamins on vision', which enabled the experimenter to give participants an injection without telling them either that the experiment concerned emotion, or that they might be receiving an injection of epinephrine. When participants arrived for the experiment, they were given a description of a fictitious vitamin compound called Suproxin, with which they were to be injected. They then were given an injection of epinephrine and one of three sets of instructions. The 'Informed' participants were told, correctly, that the Suproxin might produce shaking of the hands, pounding of the heart, and a warm and flushed feeling. The 'Ignorant' participants were told nothing about side effects. To determine whether mentioning side effects alone might alter response, 'Misinformed' participants were told, incorrectly, that the Suproxin might produce numbness of the feet, itching and slight headache. As a control condition, a group of different participants were given a placebo (a saline injection) and either Informed or left Ignorant. It was expected that Informed participants would have a good explanation (the injection) for their experienced state and would not report emotion. The Ignorant and Misinformed participants would not have a good explanation for their experienced internal state, and so would begin looking for one. The researchers arranged to give them an emotional explanation.

Participants were placed in a waiting room with someone they were told was another participant in the vision experiment, but who was actually a stooge: a paid confederate of the researcher. This stooge then proceeded to act either euphorically or angrily. The results showed that physiological arousal was not sufficient to produce emotional experience:

1   The Informed group did not indicate feeling euphoric or angry, nor did they act as if they were. They showed that cognitions were not sufficient on their own to produce emotion.
2   The Placebo group reported little emotion in the presence of the stooge (although enough to suggest that the experience of receiving an injection is in itself arousing).
3   Both the Ignorant and, to an even greater extent, the Misinformed participants reported feeling either euphoric in the presence of a euphoric stooge or angry in the presence of an angry stooge, and proceeded to act emotionally as well.

Schachter (1964) proposed that participants attributed their arousal to emotion in the presence of appropriate cognitions, which he called the **attribution theory of emotion**. Attribution theory suggests some interesting possibilities. It should be possible, for example, to begin an emotional experience with either physiological arousal and have emotional cognitions follow, or with appropriate cognitions and have arousal follow. The theory underlying this research was that arousal (excitation) from one source ought to be transferable to another emotion if appropriate cognitions were present. One study looked at athletes who had just finished exercising and had some residual physical arousal remaining. If they were angered, they became angrier than when they did not have that residual arousal, which would suggest that arousal produced by another emotion, such as fear, might also transfer to anger. In line with this, studies of police officers found they were more likely to use weapons against either offenders or innocent bystanders when their arousal levels were high.

> **Attribution theory of emotion:** the idea that emotion results when physiological arousal and emotion-related cognitions about that arousal exist at the same time.

Another influential two-factor (physiological arousal plus cognitions) theory of emotion is Arnold's appraisal theory (1960). She proposed that it is not the events (situational or physical) that produce emotional responses, but the individual's appraisal of those events. Consider the effect of walking round a corner and coming face to face with a lion. An initial reaction to this might be a startled response, but before you experience a true emotional response you would be influenced by whether the lion was in a cage or out, whether it was alive or stuffed, and whether it was a picture or genuine. Genuine experience of emotion, therefore, depends on our appraisal of events: their meaning, their relationship to us as individuals, and our needs and wants.

PAUSE & REFLECT

What is the role of appraisal in the experience of emotion? How could this explain why we like to watch things in movies that we would hate to watch in real life, such as a kind person dying slowly from disease?

Consider what your reaction would be to a film that showed a boy undergoing a tribal initiation rite that involved having the underside of his penis slit open. Lazarus and Alfert (1964) found that people who saw this film as a silent film appraised it as real and reacted with high levels of arousal and expressed emotion. Others, who heard a soundtrack that told them that the film was staged using special effects and that the boy was not really being operated on or hurt, experienced much less physiological arousal in the face of the same scenes. Individuals who heard the soundtrack before they saw the film were even less aroused. Apparently, their appraisal had been completed before the events started, and could exert greater control over their responses. Thus, appraisal about what we might encounter in the future allows us to predict, and even exert control over, what we will experience when we encounter the expected events.

> **CROSS-REFERENCE**
> The importance of appraisal regarding stress is considered again in Chapter 12.

MARTIN (CONT.)

CASE STUDY

Emotions are likely to be both a cause and an outcome in Martin's condition. While it is not clear what might have caused Martin to develop this particular condition at this particular time, there are nervous system connections between the brain and the bowel. During times of strong emotion, sensory signals from the bowel may be interpreted differently by the brain, and signals from the brain may cause the bowel to squeeze more, leading to both pain and changes to bowel habits. Martin's symptoms are not constant—sometimes he will go for a week without a bad episode—but as the year progresses, the constipation and diarrhoea become more frequent, so Martin makes an appointment to see his doctor. His doctor suspects from the description of the symptoms that Martin has Irritable Bowel Syndrome (IBS). However, there is really no test that can diagnose IBS. The tests the doctor is running are to eliminate the possibility of conditions with similar symptoms, such as coeliac disease, Crohn's disease or intolerance of dairy products. In this case, all of the tests indicate no other condition. When he learns about IBS from his doctor, Martin is not at all happy to hear that the cause of his problems is not clear, but much happier to learn that there are things that can be done to help him.

1   Is there any illness or disease that is not affected by emotional issues?
2   How does understanding and managing emotions affect the kind of illness that an individual may experience?

EXPRESSION OF EMOTION

The most widely studied medium of emotional communication is facial expression. Charles Darwin proposed that much of our facial communication is innate: that the communication of emotions by facial expression has evolutionary value. By warning others of our intention to act in a particular way, we enable them to respond to an intention without the need for the act itself. A fearful expression may signal to friends that they should prepare for flight. An expression of sadness signals the need for support.

Similar expressions are universal; that is, found across all cultures. A study of New Guinea highlanders, who had experienced little contact with Westerners, showed that they were easily able to recognise and label emotional expressions on the faces of Westerners they encountered (Ekman 1980). When asked to express the same emotions themselves, they were able to display them in a way that was understood by Westerners. Other evidence for the generality of expression has come from studies of emotional expressions of infants.

In general, facial expressions play an important role in emotions. One small body of research suggests that socially anxious individuals show negative biases in interpreting the facial expressions of others. Anxious patients may interpret a facial expression as angry when in fact it is neutral. This finding suggests that helping patients to develop a more accurate interpretation of facial expressions could be a useful intervention in dealing with excess anxiety (Mohlman, Carmin & Price 2007).

EMOTION AND HEALTH

Emotion is a complex phenomenon. It involves internal state, mental activity, survival value and other physical and psychological elements, all of which can affect our health or our appraisal of our health, or be affected by our health.

Being ill may arouse our emotional experience by creating internal biochemical conditions characteristic of emotion (increasing circulating adrenaline, for example, or endorphins), by mimicking arousal (increasing heart rate, or sweating) or simply by producing negative cognitions. Such experiences are commonly recognised. Someone who is, say, overactive or irrational may be described as 'feverish'. This is not surprising, since very high temperatures can cause delirium. Diseases that depress the body's processes, such as the common cold or glandular fever, may make people feel emotionally flat or depressed. A number of physical illnesses are known to cause mood change, with AIDS (Clucas et al. 2011) and cancer (Banks et al. 2010) being just two examples. Similarly, drugs taken for physical conditions can produce or modify some of the physiological or mental characteristics of emotional states. It is known, for example, that treatment for hepatitis B can lead to depression, or that a class of drugs prescribed for hypertension (beta-blockers) are sometimes taken by musicians to reduce symptoms of stage fright without interfering with dexterity. The use of drug side effects to modify emotion or its consequences can, however, be quite dangerous.

In contrast, emotions may create sensations we interpret as illness. Consider the example of emergency workers at a major disaster. They may experience long periods of physiological arousal during the rescue. After the rescue, the threat is removed and they may expect to feel relieved, but because they have depleted bodily resources from the constant state of high alertness they feel emotionally flat and physically unwell. Any prolonged stressful experience can produce similar effects. Conversely, happy experiences or the experience of support from those around us can lead to positive health outcomes. This might operate through facial feedback, biochemical means or many other pathways. There is clear and substantial evidence that links optimism, social support and even an aggressive fighting attitude with improved outcomes for various health situations, such as recovery from surgery, response to infection and cancer. One study of over 1000 patients showed that hope (positive emotion) was associated with lower chances of developing disease (such as hypertension, diabetes mellitus or respiratory tract infection) and curiosity with lower likelihood of hypertension and diabetes (Smart Richman et al. 2005). Improvements of physical and mental health have also resulted from treatment aimed at increasing self-confidence, assertiveness and optimism.

REGULATION OF EMOTION AND MENTAL ILLNESS

Various aspects of emotion play a role in different mental disorders. Individuals suffering from a major depressive or anxiety disorder demonstrate difficulty managing their emotions. One variable of interest is overall emotionality, which involves feeling intense positive or negative emotions. In anxiety and depressive disorders, there may be low levels of positive emotion such as happiness, and/or high levels of negative emotion such as fear and sadness. Intense emotions are not dysfunctional in themselves, but it is the overall greater occurrence and strength that can render them pathological.

Another variable of interest is the **dysregulation of emotions** (or poor management of emotions). Dysregulation involves three elements:

1 poor understanding or insight
2 negative reactivity
3 ineffective or maladaptive coping intelligence (Mennin et al. 2007).

It is more difficult for individuals to regulate their emotions if they do not recognise or understand what they are feeling, or if they have negative reactions to what they are feeling. Such

Dysregulation of emotions: poor understanding or insight, negative reactivity, and ineffective or maladaptive coping intelligence.

CROSS-REFERENCE
Emotional
intelligence is
discussed in
Chapter 2.

individuals may fear their emotions, or believe they are powerless to control their emotions. Poor coping or maladaptive management means not being able to take action to soothe anxiety, calm down anger or use other regulation strategies to control impulses. To a certain extent, emotional dysregulation is the opposite of emotional intelligence. It appears that emotional dysregulation is directly connected to mental health symptoms independent of our negative emotions; that is, symptoms are not just being reported because people feel bad (Bradley et al. 2011).

Emotions can also have an indirect influence on our mental well-being and daily functioning. Possessing an optimistic or pessimistic outlook on life, for example, affects our perception of the likelihood of a good outcome, and therefore alters the way we make decisions, the kind of risks we feel are worth taking, and the amount of effort we will expend to achieve a certain goal. Emotion can also affect health-related behaviours such as drinking alcohol, smoking cigarettes, exercise, diet and even the way we drive our car.

CASE STUDY

MARTIN (CONT.)

The recommendations that Martin receives from his doctor are about treating his symptoms. For example, he is advised that he can add fibre to his diet if constipation is the main problem, and that there are over-the-counter medications to relieve constipation and reduce attacks of diarrhoea. To help him deal with the causes, he is also given lifestyle advice, such as avoiding caffeine (limiting coffee, tea and cola drinks), not eating large meals, and noting if there are any specific foods that trigger his attacks and then limiting these. However, as IBS tends to differ between individuals, the doctor tells Martin that the best general advice tends to revolve around psychophysiological triggers such as stress. Martin is advised that regular exercise and sleeping patterns—both the timing of sleep and the amount of sleep (at least eight hours per night)—are really important. Martin has been neglecting both exercise and sleep during the year because he felt it was more important to spend his time studying. Importantly for Martin, he was also told that while IBS can be upsetting, it does not cause permanent damage to the intestines or lead to more serious disease.

1 How could the principles of behaviour change (see Chapter 8) benefit Martin?
2 How important is good time management to maintaining health during stressful times of life?

PSYCHOPHYSIOLOGY

Psychophysiology:
the study of the
interactions between
the physiological
and psychological
aspects of a situation
as experienced by an
individual.

Psychophysiology enables us to better to understand individual experiences at both physiological and psychological levels. Often, both arise from the same underlying causes and occur together in response to the same stimuli. The combined response is important.

There are specific areas in which knowledge gained from psychophysiology has made an enormous difference to the way health and illnesses are considered, and, subsequently, the way in which health professionals assess and care for patients (Andreassi 2006). These differences are primarily, but not exclusively, related to emotion. The following sections examine psychophysiology in regards to cardiovascular function, cancer and immune function.

CARDIOVASCULAR PSYCHOPHYSIOLOGY

Heart disease and stroke–diseases of the cardiovascular system–are two major causes of death. Though there is a traditional belief in the link between the heart and emotions, it appears that the heart is more a victim of emotions than the seat of emotions.

There are many studies of short-term physiological responses to behavioural demands that include physiological responses. These include changes in adrenaline and noradrenaline levels that affect cardiovascular function and alter heart rate, rhythm and electrical activity, blood pressure and cardiac output (how much blood is being pumped). People who, for example, are involved in a problem-solving task show faster heart rates and higher blood pressure when working under time pressure than when working at their preferred pace. Similarly, students display striking elevations of cortisol (a physiological measure of stress) when sitting a major exam (Jones, Copolov & Outch 1986).

Long-term responses—including changes in blood pressure, heart rate and rhythm; cholesterol levels in the blood, blood coagulation and platelet aggregation; and adaptation patterns such as hyper-reactivity—have been noted in response to either severe or prolonged stress. High stress periods at work are accompanied by increases in serum cholesterol, a risk factor for heart disease due to an increased likelihood of blocked arteries. Even minor stresses (hassles) that continue over a long time span have been shown to result in relatively enduring changes in cardiovascular functioning. Other research has linked characteristics of the individual to heart disease. Bunker et al. (2003) reviewed this literature and found strong and consistent evidence for links with depression, isolation and a lack of quality social support. There are established relationships with social factors such as education, social class and job type, but there is some debate about whether these differences might be related to lack of control or other psychosocial factors (Skodova et al. 2008).

Research has attempted to link personality and heart disease, including seemingly stable personality characteristics such as anger or hostility, competitiveness, stoicism or optimism. **Type A (coronary prone) behaviour patterns** have been shown to double the risk of having a heart attack in some individuals. There has been much criticism of the type A concept, and more recent evidence shows little support for the concept (Bunker et al. 2003). However, a tendency to become angry often, particularly if that anger is directed at the self, has been predictive of clinical events such as a heart attack (Spindler et al. 2007). It is likely, though, that these relationships are mediated by arousal changes over a long period of time and the associated physiological effects of arousal damage to the body.

The **type D (distressed) personality** is an emerging construct to help explain links between behaviour and disease. Individuals with type D personality have a tendency to feel negative emotions (such as depression and anxiety) combined with a reluctance to discuss these feelings with others (negative affectivity combined with social inhibition) to avoid social disapproval (Pedersen et al. 2007; Spindler et al. 2007). A man may, for example, feel anxious or depressed about a lack of meaningful satisfaction in his highly paid position, but deliberately choose not to tell his wife or work colleagues about it. Mols and Denollet (2010) have reported that type D represents a general vulnerability for both mental and physical health.

A ten-year study of over 5000 people showed that happy people tended to stay happy over a long period of time and miserable people tended to stay miserable. Individuals who tend to have a more negative emotional style (that is, persistently miserable) were at greater risk for illness than those with a positive style (Rosenkranz et al. 2003).

Type A (coronary prone) behaviour pattern: the idea that individuals who show a pattern of competitive achievement striving, an exaggerated sense of time urgency, and aggressiveness and hostility are at greatly increased risk of heart attack.

CROSS-REFERENCE
The type A behaviour pattern is also discussed in Chapter 4.

Type D (distressed) personality: a tendency to feel negative emotions combined with a reluctance to discuss these feelings with others that increases the probability of disease.

Some studies have examined life events as causes of acute cardiovascular events. There is an apparent link between bereavement and death from pre-existing heart problems. For many people the most likely time for death from heart attack is Monday morning: the beginning of the work week. One interesting line of research has shown that deaths from all causes are lower than expected in the month before important events such as birthdays and anniversaries, and higher than expected in the month following them. Again, such results could possibly be explained by short-term physiological responses.

Depression and anxiety may worsen the outlook for a positive outcome for stroke and can influence the course of diabetes in complex and reciprocal ways. People with depression and diabetes are more likely to report poor control of their blood glucose levels and suffer a range of physical complications (Raphael, Schmolke & Wooding 2005). Among patients with coronary artery disease, around sixteen to twenty-three in one hundred will have depression (Raphael, Schmolke & Wooding 2005). Depression is linked to nearly double the risk of death in such patients. Myocardial infarction (heart attack) is preceded by depression in around one-third to one-half of patients. The Australian National Heart Foundation recently concluded that depression is a serious independent risk factor for heart disease. Patients who are hospitalised for severe depression have a higher risk of clinical events than their level of risk (indicated by, for example, blood pressure and cholesterol) would predict. Anxiety also increases risk of repeat heart attack and death in cardiac patients, and possibly should be considered a risk factor in its own right (Spindler et al. 2007).

Linking disease-specific physical symptoms with a patient's underlying depression and anxiety may avoid unnecessary treatment. A patient with a cardiovascular condition, say, may have continuing chest pain due to anxiety rather than the physical symptoms caused by the condition. In response to the reported symptoms, health care providers may escalate the cardiovascular disease medication regime and order more invasive tests, without realising that anxiety may be a contributing cause (Katon, Lin & Kroenke 2007).

PAUSE 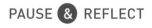 REFLECT

As a future health professional, how might you distinguish between disease-specific physical symptoms and those engendered by emotion?

CANCER PSYCHOPHYSIOLOGY

Type C (cancer prone) behaviour pattern: the idea that a passive and emotionally repressed personality style is associated with higher rates of cancer occurrence and death from cancer.

As was the case for heart disease and type A personality, some researchers proposed a **type C (cancer prone) behaviour pattern** linked to cancer (Eskelinen & Ollonen 2011). Although several studies have shown that a passive and emotionally repressed personality style is associated with higher rates of occurrence and death from cancer, serious questions exist about type C research. It is likely that passivity and emotional repression come with, or after, a diagnosis of cancer. These traits are just as likely to be the result of the diagnosis as to be present before diagnosis. Other studies have shown that a passive coping style can lead to shorter survival times for cancer patients, while an aggressive coping style is associated with longer survival. How much this has to do with behavioural differences—such as aggressive patients getting more or better care as a result of demanding it, while passive patients ignoring symptoms until it is too late—is not clear. The idea that psychological factors can cause cancer is not well supported by the research, but in some cases such factors can be related to differences in cancer survival rates, or how distressing the experience is for individuals (Raphael, Schmolke & Wooding 2005). In one quality-of-life study, women with cancer believed their spirituality had a positive impact on their illness and that being sick had meaning, and saw it as a challenge for personal development and as a sign to change their lives (Bussing, Ostermann & Matthiessen 2005).

PSYCHONEUROIMMUNOLOGY

Psychoneuroimmunology (PNI) is concerned with communication between the brain and immune system. At first, the idea that there was crosstalk between the brain and the immune system was rejected by many immunologists, who regarded the immune system as autonomous. It is now known not only that people are more susceptible to infections and other illness at times of stress, but also that stress measurably alters immune functioning.

Mechanisms by which stress alters immune function have only recently been understood, and this has emphasised the importance of knowledge about PNI for understanding the biopsychosocial aspects of health (Lutgendorf & Costanzo 2003).

Molecular and cellular systems in the brain are geared to represent dangers occurring in various parts of the body monitored by the immune system. The immune system provides immediate and short-term defence against infectious agents in the blood and body tissues. When pathogens trigger the immune system, **cytokines** are produced.

Pro-inflammatory cytokines fight disease by producing fever, inflammation and tissue destruction, and eliciting behaviours such as nausea and tiredness, as well as symptoms of depression, requiring the person to rest. Anti-inflammatory cytokines have healing effects. These cytokines work through several phases to a point where B-cells manufacture antibodies to fight foreign invaders (Graham et al. 2005).

The immune system may also be sensitised by other stressors, such as repeated activation (that is, recurring stressors) or prolonged activation. Once the brain is sensitised in this way, it is less likely to turn off when the threat has passed and is more likely to be activated by non-immune stimuli (Anisman & Merali 2003; Dantzer 2005). A study of family members providing care to a relative with dementia found some had still not recovered normal levels of immune function two years after ceasing that role (Christian et al. 2006). Stress in patients predicts a range of adverse clinical outcomes, such as slower wound healing, lower production of antibodies to flu vaccine, and more rapid progression of immune disorders (Kiecolt-Glaser et al. 1991).

On the other hand, positive emotions have also been shown to have a variety of health benefits (Richman et al. 2005). Positive emotions may improve immune function, and psychological interventions of various sorts have been shown to lessen the risk of infection, reduce the need for antibiotic treatment, and even double survival times in individuals with cancer. Interestingly, laughter is linked to immune function, with a number of reports showing reduction in clinical symptoms and improvement in immune markers in a variety of conditions. These health consequences of prolonged stress and ways of coping with the consequences are discussed in more detail in following chapters.

Psychoneuro-immunology: the study of the communications between the brain and the immune system.

Cytokines: a group of proteins and peptides that work as signalling compounds, enabling cells to communicate with each other; they regulate the body's response to infection, inflammation and trauma.

PAUSE 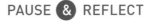 REFLECT

Think about how the mind communicates with the immune system. What are the implications of this in terms of strong or prolonged emotion and the risk of disease?

CASE STUDY

ANNA LEE AND ANXIETY

Anna Lee is a 37-year-old mother of three children. As long as she can remember, she has had problems with anxiety. At school, she used to feel sick to the stomach, sweaty and trembling any time that she had to speak in class. During recess periods, she tended to stay on the edge of play—sitting with one or two friends and talking rather than actively being involved in games. She came to feel that she was awkward and unskilled, and finally asked her parents to have her excused from physical education on medical grounds: that she was prone to palpitations, shortness of breath and headaches if required to exercise. Outside of school, however, she was quite active. Since she lived on the edge of a small rural town, she could easily ride her bicycle into the countryside, and enjoyed the experience of hard physical exercise. Although she was very shy in class, she worked hard at her schoolwork and did very well. It was only speaking in class that caused her problems. She knew she was smart and hardworking, but also thought that there was something wrong with her body or her mind because she always felt so frightened in social situations.

She found puberty very difficult because she developed later than most of the girls in her class. She felt like a child around the more physically developed girls, and this contributed to her being embarrassed in classroom situations. Even though there were less developed girls, and she caught up with most of the others a year later, she continued to feel immature and out of things. Her anxiety became worse in social situations outside of school, and she became more of a loner.

During high school, she became interested in how the brain and body worked, and did extremely well in her science subjects. She could begin to see that there were some patterns to her own anxiety. First of all, a lot of her relatives—including her parents—had problems with anxiety or depression. One of her uncles drank heavily, and was unable to keep a job. Anna realised that he was not bad, but that he drank to deal with his anxiety. Although nobody in the family talked about anxiety, there were a number of other signs that it was a problem for many of her family members. Her younger sister—two years her junior—became depressed during high school. She was placed on antidepressant medication and started to see a counsellor. Anna considered seeing someone about her own anxiety, but always avoided it because she thought she should be able to handle things by herself. She thought that being smart and physically fit should give her enough resources to handle things.

Because her high school required her to do some kind of sports, she took up tennis, worked hard at it and became quite skilled. However, she became very anxious before any kind of competition, so she never did well in those. It became common for her to be physically sick before any competition, and while playing she would feel dizzy and uncoordinated. However, she did meet a boy who, like her, enjoyed playing tennis but not competing. After more than a year of being friends, they started dating—not so much because they were strongly attracted to one another, but just to have someone to be with in social situations.

During university, her anxiety problems became somewhat worse, and she missed a lot of lectures because of anxiety attacks. Her boyfriend had chosen the same university, and they both were doing the same science subjects, so he helped her with notes, and they worked together at studying and assignments. Even though she had a lot of trouble at exam time—she always seemed to catch cold or injure herself, and would be sick before and sometimes during tests—she completed her degree.

She felt very relieved when her boyfriend asked her to marry him, as that took the pressure off her to work full-time. They decided to postpone having children until they could set themselves up, and she took a job working in a laboratory for a pharmaceutical company. It was very routine work and didn't pay much, but it allowed her to work on her own, and the company was understanding about her frequent sick days.

As soon as she fell pregnant, she stopped work and began to spend almost all of her time at home. She took a lot of pride in her house, and in the meals she prepared for her husband, but hated entertaining because it made her feel shaky and unwell. Gradually, they stopped socialising with other people.

After the birth of her third child, her paediatrician suggested that she might be suffering from an anxiety disorder, and her GP referred her to a psychiatrist. Anna has now begun taking medication to limit the physiological symptoms, and is seeing a psychologist to help her with the psychological and social impacts.

1   What genetic, biological and social factors might have contributed to Anna's family being subject to anxiety problems?

2   How did Anna's cognitions about her physiological states during her school years contribute to her emotional difficulties in young adulthood?

3   What where some of the interactions between her emotions and her choices about her lifestyle?

Points to consider

Social phobias are the most common type of phobia, and most of us know someone who suffers to a greater or lesser degree from anxiety related to social situations. This can range from mild nervousness in stressful interactions—something we all experience—to inability to leave home under any conditions. People with extreme social phobias are often undiagnosed partly because they don't leave home, and so are not observed by other people. This can make the whole process of treatment difficult, as patients often miss appointments or find excuses to avoid seeking treatment at all.

CHAPTER SUMMARY

- The separation of mind and body as part of Western philosophy has affected our thinking about health, how illness arises and approaches to treatment.
- A more integrated view has highlighted the importance of emotion to health and well-being. Emotion results from the combination of physiological arousal and emotion-relevant cognition.
- The appraisal that the individual makes of their situation determines what, and how much, emotion they will experience. The close integration of physiological and psychological factors in health has led to the development of a large body of research linking the two.
- Cardiovascular psychophysiology looks at interactions between psychological events and the workings of the heart and circulation. The psychophysiology of cancer is less

well researched, but significant links have been found with occurrence and progression of cancer.

- Psychoneuroimmunology examines the connections between psychological experience, the operations of the nervous system and immune functioning. The integration of physiological and psychological factors provides a background for the understanding of stress and coping.

- It is now recognised that emotional health is relevant to maintaining good physical health and aids in recovery from physical illness. Emotional health also enhances an individual's capacity to lead a fulfilling life, study, work, pursue leisure interests and optimise day-to-day functioning.

- Disturbances to emotional well-being, such as anxiety and depression, compromise these capacities, often in debilitating and ongoing ways.

- Conceptualising health and illness in a holistic way has produced different approaches to understanding, assessing and treating illness.

SELF TEST

1   Which of the following is not a common criticism of the concept of psychosomatic illness?
    a   There is no consensus as to what a psychosomatic illness is.
    b   This concept has no clear theoretical basis for causation of illness.
    c   The number of illnesses identified as psychosomatic is limited.
    d   The concept suggests that all illnesses could be affected by psychological factors.

2   Sympathetic nervous system activation involves:
    a   decreased heart rate
    b   decreased release of sugar into the bloodstream
    c   dilation of pupils
    d   dilation of blood vessels in the gastrointestinal tract.

3   The part(s) of the brain believed to be most associated with cognitive control of emotion is the:
    a   prefrontal cortex
    b   orbitofrontal cortex
    c   cingulate control system
    d   all of the above.

4   Which of the following statements about cardiovascular psychophysiology is false?
    a   Stress may have both short-term and long-term effects on cardiovascular responding.
    b   Patients with depression show more clinical events than their level of risk would predict.
    c   There are no demonstrated relationships between positive emotions and cardiovascular health, although negative emotions are related.
    d   Stressful periods at work are associated with increased levels of cholesterol in the blood.

5   Which of these statements about the brain, immunology and depression is true?
    a   There is no association between immune function and depression.
    b   Depressed patients have too much serotonin.

   c Depressed patients are capable of preventing emotions from interfering with goal-directed behaviour.

   d There is a pathway from the immune system to depression.

FURTHER READING

Andreassi, J.L. (2006) *Psychophysiology: Human Behaviour and Physiological Response* (5th edn). Mahwah, NJ: Lawrence Erlbaum.

Hassed, C. (2000) *New Frontiers in Medicine: The Body as the Shadow of the Soul.* Melbourne: Hill of Content.

Lutgendorf, S.K. & Costanzo, E.S. (2003) Psychoneuroimmunology and health psychology: An integrative model. An Invited Review. *Brain, Behavior and Immunity*, 17, 225–32.

Schachter, S. (1964) The Interaction of Cognitive and Physiological Determinants of Emotional State (pp. 49–80). In L. Berkowitz (ed.) *Advances in Experimental Social Psychology* (vol. 1). New York: Academic Press.

USEFUL WEBSITES

Emotion rules the brain's decisions (USA Today):
www.usatoday.com/tech/science/discoveries/2006-08-06-brain-study_x.htm

How the brain controls emotions (Medical News Today):
www.medicalnewstoday.com/releases/52415.php

Mind/body connection: how your emotions affect your health (Family Doctor):
http://familydoctor.org/familydoctor/en/prevention-wellness/emotional-wellbeing/mental-health/mind-body-connection-how-your-emotions-affect-your-health.html

Psychoneuroimmunology (PNI): understanding how the mind and body work together (*In Touch*: The official magazine of the MS Society of NSW/Vic):
www.mssociety.org.au/documents/intouch/intouch-autumn08.pdf

The biology of emotion—and what it may teach us about helping people to live longer (Harvard School of Public Health):
www.hsph.harvard.edu/news/hphr/chronic-disease-prevention/happiness-stress-heart-disease

A COMPLEX EXAMPLE:
UNDERSTANDING PAIN

11

CHAPTER OBJECTIVES

By the end of your study of this chapter, you should be able to:

- understand the nature of pain
- understand the physiology of pain and how it is measured
- appreciate the clinical implications of acute pain and chronic pain
- understand the use of various pain control techniques in clinical practice
- understand factors related to the management of chronic pain.

KEYWORDS

acute pain

biofeedback

cognitive techniques

culture

endogenous opioid peptides

gate-control theory

hypnosis

nociceptors

pain control

pain management programs

persistent (chronic) pain syndrome

relaxation

reporting pain

stigma

A BROADER UNDERSTANDING OF PAIN

We live with minor pain all of the time; indeed, low-level pain is critical to our survival. Low-level pain provides feedback about the functioning of our bodily systems and informs the unconscious adjustments we make to our posture and body position. An extremely small number of individuals are born with insensitivity to pain, which is known as congenital analgesia (Borigini 2012). Not only are they at risk from accidents, but may also unknowingly damage themselves through an inability to recognise when they are hurt. Pain that is more intense gains our attention, but is usually acute and the experience disappears in hours or weeks. Other forms of pain may persist for several months, worsen over time and become chronic. Pain is the most common reason why people seek medical care. The Cochrane Pain, Palliative and Supportive Care Group (2012), for example, lists 266 topics on pain prevention and management on its website.

Interestingly, the prospect of uncontrolled pain is the most feared aspect of illness by individuals (Taylor 2006). It is usually assumed that pain arises in predictable and measurable ways from tissue damage, but attempts to determine a precise relationship between the extent of tissue damage and pain have been only partly successful. Further, many people experience pain in the absence of any observable physical damage. There is no evidence that pain without physical damage (psychogenic) or unclear origin (idiopathic) is any less real to the sufferer than pain with associated tissue damage (organic) (Wicksell, Melin & Olsson 2007).

Unfortunately, there is a tendency for health professionals to make judgments about the person with pain symptoms. If a physical cause (for example, a bulging disc, arthritic condition of the spine or neuropathy) cannot be found for the pain, then there is an overwhelming tendency to assign psychological causes (Gustafson 2000). This judgment leads to treating people with psychogenic pain differently from those with organic pain, particularly when the pain is reported to persist over a long period of time. Judgments by health professionals may result in not providing narcotic medication for someone complaining of migraine pain, for example—a decision that could be medically and ethically unsafe.

Given the propensity of health professionals to misjudge the pain experience, it is essential for you to develop a good understanding of this issue. This chapter explores how pain is reported or expressed, the physiology and neurochemical basis of pain, and how the body works to inhibit perceptions of pain. Psychological factors that increase pain sensations—such as anxiety, stress, depression and focusing attention on the pain—are discussed, along with recent developments in pain control and management of chronic pain.

CROSS-REFERENCE

The interplay of physical symptoms and emotion is discussed in Chapter 10.

ANDREW SERJKIN AND AMPUTATION

CASE STUDY

Andrew Serjkin is a 44-year-old motor mechanic who loves riding his motorcycle. He belongs to a recreational motorcycle club, where he enjoys the social side of the club as well as hands-on maintenance and design of motorcycles. He recently built his own model of motorcycle, specifically designed to be comfortable for him personally on long rides. Sadly, as a result of a serious accident in which he was speeding and lost control on a slippery road surface and slid underneath a car, he had his right leg amputated just above the knee. All of his other injuries were minor, and after being fitted with an artificial limb, he was able to return to his normal work and family commitments. However, the loss of his leg meant that he could no longer safely ride a motorcycle.

Andrew's reactions are on several levels: physical (immediate severe pain), behavioural (changes to his lifestyle), cognitive and emotional. He experiences many and varied emotions, which are to some extent dependent on his cognitions about his loss. As he realises that his careless riding was responsible for the loss of his leg, he directs his anger inwardly. Frequently, he feels churned up inside about the unfairness of his situation, but also guilty and stupid. He can't blame the driver of the car, and wishes he could, because this would give him a direct target for his anger.

1   What factors would determine the severity and nature of Andrew's pain?
2   How would being able to blame someone else make Andrew feel differently about his pain?

REPORTING PAIN

Pain is fundamentally a psychophysiological experience. The International Association for the Study of Pain (IASP; 2011) defines it as 'an unpleasant sensory and emotional experience associated with actual or potential tissue damage, or described in terms of such damage'. The IASP emphasises that 'pain is always subjective'. This means that it is internal to the specific individual, and cannot be linked to external judgements about what is causing it, how bad it is or what it feels like. The extent of pain and the level of incapacity caused by pain in daily life depend in large part on how it is interpreted and the context in which in occurs. Natural labour and childbirth, for example, are associated with a great deal of physical pain and yet women are often able to cope without any analgesia because of the release of natural endorphins, the joy attached to the experience, the knowledge that it is acute and will be of (relatively) short duration, and the support offered by others. Similarly, some players in contact sports such as various codes of football have diminished pain sensitivity and continue playing a game despite grievous injuries. These joyful or challenging contexts differ from an office worker who is under stress to meet a deadline and suffering lower back pain. In this situation, stress aggravates the experience of pain, narrows the individual's focus and intensifies the pain experience.

Pain is an imprecise science (Daniel & Williams 2010), which means there are a number of challenges associated with providing an accurate description of it. There are many common words used to describe pain—words and terms that can be a useful source of information for health professionals attempting to understand the complaint. The nature of pain may be described as throbbing, shooting or a constant dull ache. It is important, too, to determine the intensity of pain. This is often achieved by asking the person to describe their pain on a scale of 0 (no pain) to 10 (worst pain imaginable). When assessing pain in young children, simple diagrams of the body can be used to locate the pain and line drawings of faces showing different expressions can be used to rate pain intensity. There are also verbal scales for assessing pain, the emotions produced by pain, and a number of other pain-associated dimensions (Daniel & Williams 2010).

Pain can also be conveyed by observing behaviour. People demonstrate pain through facial expressions or groans, by protecting the tender area, or by limiting movement that may provoke pain. When pain has persisted for some time (say, in the case of lower back pain), people change the way they stand or walk. Observation and analysis of physiological, psychological and behavioural elements of pain behaviour is important to define characteristics of different kinds of pain.

Part of the complexity of measuring pain is simply due to differences in what the individual perceives as being the most important *to them*. Often this importance is tied to the impact on their own life: the losses they experience as a result of their pain. These usually include thoughts about what their pain prevents them from doing. This could include social activities, sports and leisure, work and employment, self-care and day-to-day living; but also the meaning of these activities to the individual. Chronic pain might mean loss of enjoyment, social networks or a sense of self-worth. It may also mean the occurrence of emotional distress such as depression, frustration, anger, anxiety or fear. If the individual's pain requires them to use visible supports (such as canes or frames) or noticeable supports (such as pain-relieving medications that may cause sleepiness, inability to operate machinery or unusual amounts of resting), the individual may experience **stigma** from their disability. In many senses, chronic pain shares these characteristics with other chronic illness (see Chapter 5).

Stigma: a mark of disapproval that may be attached to an individual who differs from social or cultural norms.

PAUSE & REFLECT

Think about the worst pain you have experienced. What words would you use to describe that pain? Think about the cause of that pain. How did the experience differ from pain generated by other causes?

FACTORS AFFECTING THE EXPERIENCE AND REPORTING OF PAIN

However it is measured, the reporting of pain is influenced by many factors, such as age, gender, context, attention, fatigue, previous experience of pain, and coping style. Of particular importance to the delivery of effective health care to our diverse communities is an understanding of how culture can influence differences in the meaning attached to pain and how it is experienced and expressed. Although there are no racial differences in the ability to discriminate painful stimuli, **culture** may influence pain tolerance and how intensely pain is reported. Culture also influences the extent to which it is appropriate (or inappropriate) to express pain. Failure to groan, cry out, grimace or thrash does not mean that the person is pain free; it may be a reflection of cultural values. People from different cultures who have difficulty communicating in English report miscommunication and a lack of information sharing by health professionals. A recent study (Kalauokalani et al. 2007) with cancer sufferers from fifteen different ethnic minority groups tested the effectiveness of a twenty-minute individualised education and coaching session compared with standard information on controlling pain. Patient coaching was found to increase knowledge of pain self-management, redress personal misconceptions about pain treatment, and reduce racial or ethnic disparities in pain control.

Culture: the total way of life shared by members of a group.

Individuals may be reluctant to ask for pain relief for different reasons. As identified by Kalauokalani et al. (2007), individuals from culturally and linguistically diverse backgrounds may have difficulty communicating their needs. Some may not know the options available to them for pain relief and so attempt to tolerate the pain or suffer in silence. People from some Asian cultures may place the needs of others before their own, believe that the needs of others are more important, or may not wish to disturb the person in authority (that is, the doctor or nurse). Some people may hold strong views about their innate ability to cope without pain-relieving drugs. Others may be afraid of taking drugs because of adverse side effects or a fear of becoming dependent on medication.

PHYSIOLOGY OF ACUTE PAIN

Nociceptors: nerve endings in the peripheral nerves that identify injury and release chemical messengers that pass to the spinal cord and into the cerebral cortex.

Acute pain sensations generally arise when injured tissues release chemicals that activate nerve endings called **nociceptors** to send pain signals through the spinal cord to the brain. The cerebral cortex identifies the site of injury and acts to block the pain (muscle contractions) or change bodily functions (such as blood flow or breathing).

There are three kinds of pain perception: mechanical (tissue damage), thermal (exposure to temperature) and polymodal (which triggers chemical reactions from tissue damage) (Taylor 2006). Two major types of peripheral nerve fibres are involved in nociception. A-delta fibres are small, myelinated fibres that transmit sharp pain in response to mechanical or thermal pain. C-fibres are unmyelinated nerve fibres involved in multimodal pain that transmits dull or aching pain. Myelination increases the speed of transmission, so sudden and intense pain is rapidly conducted to the cerebral cortex. The difference in conduction speed explains why pain seems to occur in two distinct waves. A painful stimulus first causes a sharp localised pain, followed by a dull diffuse pain.

Sensory aspects of pain are determined by A-delta fibre activity in the thalamus and sensory areas of the cerebral cortex. The motivational and affective elements of pain are influenced more strongly by C-fibres. Processes in the cerebral cortex are involved in cognitive judgments about pain such as the evaluation of its meaning. Pain sensation, intensity and duration interact to influence pain perception, its negative consequences and related emotions through a central network of pathways in the limbic structures and thalamus to the cortex. The affective dimension of pain (or secondary affect) relates to feelings of unpleasantness, negative emotions and concern for the future (Taylor 2006).

Gate-control theory: the idea that that the brain controls the experience of pain by influencing the amount of pain stimulation that is allowed to pass a sensory gate at the level of the spinal cord.

An important advance in our understanding of pain resulted from the **gate-control theory** of Melzack and Wall (1982). This theory proposed that the brain exerts 'downward' control over the experience of pain by influencing the amount of pain stimulation that is allowed to pass a sensory 'gate' at the level of the spinal cord. The amount of pain experienced by the individual is related to the amount of information that gets through the gate to the brain. This, in turn, depends on:

1   the amount of activity in the peripheral pain fibres; that is, where the pain starts
2   the amount of activity in other peripheral fibres (that carry non-pain information and may compete with pain information to get through the gate)
3   messages coming from the brain.

This theory helps to explain why pain experiences can vary according to the physical, emotional or mental conditions at a given time. Inappropriate physical activity, anxiety or boredom could open the gate, while medication, relaxation and interesting life events could close it. This theory is supported by evidence that the brain exerts downward control over other sensory information as well. Paying close attention to only one kind of input inhibits the reception of other kinds of input.

CASE STUDY

ANDREW (CONT.)

As well as the immediate damage to tissue and nerves, Andrew has experienced a sense of loss after his accident. He was initially very depressed by his amputation, and retreated into social isolation. Since he lives alone, he felt less embarrassed and different if he stayed on his own. To make matters worse, Andrew feels pain and itching in the missing foot. He finds this very distressing, especially as it is genuinely an itch he can't scratch. His doctor explains the experience to him. Some of the long nerve cells in Andrew's leg were damaged, but not destroyed, by the amputation. These nerves formerly carried information from the foot and lower leg to the brain via the spinal cord, and input from these cells are still being interpreted by Andrew's brain as coming from the foot. Some of these signals are pain signals, so, as far as Andrew's brain is concerned, that pain is in the foot. This phenomenon is known as phantom pain.

Much depends on how Andrew experiences pain in the short and long term. Loss of activities, and negative emotions associated with loss, may lead Andrew to focus attention on his bodily sensations. Even boredom is associated with increased awareness of, and sensitivity to, pain.

1 What kinds of experiences might change Andrew's pain experience, including his phantom pain?

2 How could the concept of self-efficacy help in understanding how Andrew feels about the loss of his leg and his pain?

NEUROCHEMICAL BASIS OF ACUTE PAIN

Pain motivates us to take quick action to relieve an injury. As discussed, the brain can control the amount of pain experienced by blocking transmission of pain signals. A landmark study by Reynolds (1969) pursued a different line of thinking and demonstrated that electrical stimulation in a rat brain produced such a high level of analgesia that abdominal surgery could be performed without anaesthetic on the animal. Subsequently, Akil et al. (1984) discovered that the neurochemical basis for this effect was related to **endogenous opioid peptides**. These peptides, known as endorphins, are a group of amino acids that function as neurotransmitters that, when released, suppress pain.

Endogenous opioid peptides: opiate-like neurochemical substances, produced in the body, that act as an internal pain regulation system.

Opiates, such as morphine and heroin, are plant-based drugs that help control pain. Endogenous opioid peptides are opiate-like substances produced by the body as part of its internal pain regulation system. There are several forms of opioid peptides, such as beta-endorphins, which vary in potency, receptive action and other characteristics. Endogenous opioid peptides are found in the adrenal glands, pituitary gland and hypothalamus, and are released in response to stress. Opioids, which have a powerful analgesic effect, are used to treat chronic pain.

Unfortunately, opioids have a number of serious drawbacks. In the short term, they cause drowsiness and interfere with mental function, and cause changes to other bodily processes (for example, constipation). If used for any length of time, they are physically addictive and produce psychological dependence. Their use needs to be carefully considered, and detailed guidelines have been issued by a panel of pain experts (Chou et al. 2009).

A recent review of addiction to opioids in chronic pain sufferers found that prevalence varied from zero to 50 per cent in studies with chronic non-malignant pain patients, but only ranged up to 8 per cent in studies with cancer patients (Hojsted & Sjogren 2007). Opioids also produce an increased sensitivity to pain, so that greater amounts are needed (see Chapter 8 for discussion of opponent–process theory). They also play a role in depressing immune functioning and cardiovascular control, but we are yet to understand their full function (Taylor 2006).

PSYCHOLOGICAL RESPONSES

Acute pain: pain that is more intense and gains our immediate attention, but usually disappears within hours, days or weeks.

Chronic pain, in comparison to **acute pain**, involves complex interactions between physiological, psychological, social and behavioural components (Fordyce 1984). Chronic pain interferes with activities of daily living and persists despite the best efforts of the individual to control it. Depression, anxiety and frustration (or anger) are common among chronic pain sufferers (Pincus, Santos & Morley 2007).

Depression reflects the feelings of despair that can often accompany chronic pain. When pain persists for a long time, depressed pain patients are more likely to be preoccupied with the pain, believe that the pain will never stop and, indeed, get worse (Pincus, Santos & Morley 2007). Maladaptive coping strategies such as catastrophising or wishful thinking about the condition can magnify the distress, complicate treatment and contribute to illness behaviour. Chronic pain requires individualised, multiple techniques for its management.

CROSS-REFERENCE
Illness behaviour is discussed in Chapter 4.

Persistent (chronic) pain syndrome: a subtype of abnormal illness behaviour that can occur if an individual experiences pain over a lengthy period of time.

When an individual experiences pain over a lengthy period of time, it is not uncommon for some fairly dramatic behavioural changes to occur (see Chapter 4). These include favouring the site of the injury out of fear of aggravating the pain, using medication (pain killers), feeling unhappy and helpless, and complaining about the pain. All of these behaviours are predictable in the short term, but may become habitual, leading to a subtype of abnormal illness behaviour called **persistent (chronic) pain syndrome** (Addison 1984). Peck (1982) refers to four traps in this syndrome: 'Take it Easy Trap', 'Medication Trap', 'Depression Trap' and 'Complaint–Resentment–Guilt Trap'. Recent media campaigns in Australia have urged back pain sufferers to avoid the first of these by increasing their levels of activity. Medication can be a serious problem for sufferers of long-term pain because the drugs used are either addictive (such as opioids) or have other serious side effects. Depression needs to be managed as a psychological illness, whether it occurs in reaction to an obvious loss or without such a visible cause. Complaining is a natural behaviour when one is in pain, but can develop into a habit, which causes resentment in others if it goes on too long. This, in turn, can lead those others to feel guilty. It can also lead the complaining individual to feel guilty about the burden they place on those around them. These characteristic traps of persistent pain syndrome may produce secondary gains and so exacerbate the behaviour. The individual may be excused from normal duties and responsibilities, receive drugs and be served by family and/or professionals.

The process of learning to cope with persistent pain involves a wide range of behavioural techniques (Peck 1982), not just medication. Perhaps the most basic of these (Daniel & Williams 2010) is simply the provision of information about pain. If the pain is understood only in terms of tissue damage, then logic suggests rest, avoidance of activity and pursuit of healing as the only appropriate responses. Over an extended time, the similarity of this list to the persistent pain syndrome should be obvious. Alternative ways of thinking about pain are required. These are frequently based on the idea of acceptance of chronic pain, and responding to it as a changed (but not sinister or dangerous) condition of the individual. Control of the pain—that is, learning ways to live with it instead of chasing ways to get rid of it—then becomes possible.

CASE STUDY

ANDREW (CONT.)

Andrew has experienced an initial period of time when he feels overwhelmed by his pain and loss. His doctor is concerned that he may be developing persistent pain syndrome. However, Andrew finds that the pain in his right foot is less severe after he is fitted with a prosthesis (artificial leg). About the same time, some of the members of his motorcycle club decide to seek him out, and begin to drop by his house to talk, and specifically to ask for his advice about design issues. Andrew gradually becomes interested in design enough that he returns to the club for meetings. He still remains very unhappy about his inability to ride. One of his friends offers to take him for a ride on his bike, and as soon as Andrew returns from this ride, he reports to the doctor that his pain is gone. He proceeds to build a specially designed motorcycle, which he has modified so that he doesn't have to use his right foot, and rides it everywhere.

The provision of a prosthesis for his leg and a new motorcycle have enabled Andrew to regain something approaching his former image of himself, as well as recover favoured activities and regain friends who may have drifted away while he was not able to walk or ride. These changes have enabled him to experience more positive emotion and less negative emotion. The result is an improvement not only in his mental health but also in his acceptance of and adaptation any residual pain.

1   What is the difference between tolerating pain and accepting pain?

2   How do theories of grieving (see Chapter 3) help in the understanding of a loss of function such as Andrew's loss of his leg?

PAIN CONTROL TECHNIQUES

This section briefly introduces several different **pain control** techniques. Controlling pain can mean different things. Treatment could result in the person no longer feeling anything in the injured area (for example, by inserting drugs into the spinal cord to block sensation), feeling sensation but not pain (for example, through sensory control techniques), feeling pain but not being concerned by it, or still feeling pain but be able to cope with it (Taylor 2006).

The most common form of pain control is through drugs that affect neural transmissions locally, to the spinal cord or to higher brain regions. Antidepressants, for example, aim to improve mood and reduce anxiety, but also affect the downward pathways from the brain that modulate pain. Medication is usually sufficient and successful in managing acute pain, but may not be effective in the longer term.

Pain control: the ability to reduce the experience of pain, report of pain, emotional concern about pain, inability to tolerate pain or presence of pain-related behaviours.

PAUSE 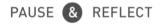 REFLECT

Cancer pain management guidelines are concerned with the fact that pain may be undertreated by health professionals because of fear of addiction. If fears of addiction are emerging, how can health professionals monitor a patient's response to pain and intervene?

Biofeedback training provides biophysiological information to a person about a bodily process such as heart rate or blood pressure. The bodily function is tracked by a machine and converted to a tone. While listening to the tone, individuals are taught how to modify the function through techniques such as concentration, relaxation and slow breathing. Eventually, some individuals can become proficient at slowing their heart rate or increasing circulation in an area without

Biofeedback: the control of internal processes through conditioning, using mechanical devices to make those internal processes perceptible.

feedback from the machine (Taylor 2006). There is growing evidence on the effectiveness of biofeedback techniques (Nestoriuc & Martin 2007), even though the specific method of action is unclear. It could be, for example, that effects are largely a result of relaxation, enhanced self-control or a placebo effect rather than the biofeedback technique per se.

Relaxation training is widely used and enables individuals to put their body into a low state of arousal by progressively relaxing sections of the body and taking deeper and longer breaths. Such techniques are very useful during labour and childbirth. Similarly, meditation can be used to achieve relaxation by focusing attention on a simple and unchanging stimulus. Relaxation is relatively successful in cases of acute pain and can be useful in managing chronic pain in conjunction with other treatment.

Hypnosis requires the person to enter a deep state of relaxation. Once in a trance-like state, individuals are told that their pain will reduce, and are instructed to think differently about the pain (altering the meaning attached to the pain). The exact mechanism by which hypnosis works is unclear, but several studies have used it successfully for pain associated with different injuries, illnesses and conditions.

Relaxation: the placing of one's body into a low state of arousal by progressively relaxing sections of the body and taking deeper and longer breaths.

Hypnosis: a deep, trance-like state of relaxation.

PAUSE & REFLECT

Many case studies and several controlled clinical trials have indicated the effectiveness of hypnotherapy for some medical conditions; however, because of the inadequacy of some research designs, hypnotherapy, like many complementary therapies, is still criticised for not having strong scientific evidence to support its claims. Would you recommend this approach to pain sufferers? Why?

BEHAVIOURAL REACTIVATION

An increasingly common approach focuses on behavioural reactivation; that is, getting the individual to return to 'lost' activities by gradually increasing those that produce enjoyment. As the enjoyable activities are regained, the individual often discovers that pain doesn't increase, and the gains in enjoyment and function are worth the costs of pain.

Pacing is an approach that aims at achieving specific staged goals of behavioural reactivation (Birkholtz, Aylwin & Harman 2004). This approach has a considerable amount of appeal to individuals with chronic pain—that is, it seems sensible and achievable—but it is really more of a cognitive perspective than a single method, and the evidence for it is spotty as a result (Gill & Brown 2009).

Pain management programs: programs that address concerns associated with chronic pain, with strong emphasis on patient education.

Pain management programs have been developed to primarily address concerns associated with chronic pain. These programs include many of the techniques outlined previously, with a heavy emphasis on patient education and closer attention being paid to all aspects of living, such as sleep, diet, exercise, and social and family engagement, as well as specific goal setting (Filoramo 2007).

Cognitive techniques assist people to control pain by thinking positively about their experience and ability to manage. With the use of coaching strategies, individuals develop an expectation of success and reconceptualise their role as competent and resourceful, which promotes feelings of self-efficacy. Individuals also learn to monitor negative, maladaptive thoughts, feelings and behaviours. Through positive self-talk and skills training (such as relaxation), people begin to attribute their success to their own efforts and minimise the likelihood of relapse into maladaptive patterns of behaviour. It is increasingly being recognised that an important component of cognitive approaches is acceptance that pain is not a danger signal, but a part of a person's normal life experience.

JUNE CHAN AND LUNG CANCER PAIN

CASE STUDY

June Chan is a 59-year-old Chinese woman born in Hong Kong. When she completed her commerce degree, June was employed by an Australian import/export company and eventually became regional manager for their Asian division. June's position was demanding: she often worked under a tight schedule, travelled a great deal and regularly entertained potential clients for business development. She found cigarette smoking relaxing. Her father and older brother had smoked when she was growing up, and many of her Asian clients also smoked.

June is at high risk for lung cancer because of her gender, her history of smoking and (more currently) her exposure to secondary smoke from being around people who smoke (both in her family of origin and in her business life). Furthermore, her lifestyle is stressful and sedentary.

When she was in her mid-forties, June was feeling the consequences of smoking (such as breathlessness when walking quickly) and decided to quit. Life continued to go well for her, but six months ago June contracted the flu and had respiratory distress. She was in bed for three days, and found it difficult to fully recover. After two months, she was still experiencing fatigue, had a dry persistent cough and one night started to cough up blood. She spoke to her doctor who ordered a chest CT scan, which revealed moderate emphysema and dark spots on her left lung. A biopsy determined lung cancer. June was referred to an oncologist and commenced chemotherapy. Over time June experienced considerable neuropathic pain, which is a common consequence of chemotherapy. She took extended sick leave from work.

A year later, June was diagnosed with secondary cancer (metastasises) in her spine. She continues to experience neuropathic pain. Neuropathic pain as a result of nerve damage from a tumour is usually less responsive to opioids (such as morphine) or requires higher doses. June suffered many side effects from taking the medication over a long period of time. She went online and found some useful information about coping with pain. She read that people have certain coping predispositions that they use when faced with a stressor such as pain. An individual's coping style not only influenced the specific coping strategies they might use to deal with stress but also their responses to that stress (for example, increased pain or depression). Information on the website prompted June to reflect on how she tends to cope with stress.

June believed that she could tolerate the cancer pain. She realised that she also had a tendency to be in command of her feelings and rarely expressed negative feelings. This belief in being stoic and coping silently was taught to her from a very young age by her Chinese father and grandmother. For interest, June decided to complete an online questionnaire on coping styles (see below).

1   What factors placed June at risk of developing lung cancer?
2   How might have June reacted to her experience of persistent pain and its impact on her work and lifestyle?
3   What might be the benefits of a repressive coping style for June in coping with cancer pain?

Points to consider

When faced with persistent cancer pain, individuals show varied responses. Some people seem to cope well, report low to moderate pain, and appear to show little psychological distress. In contrast, others cope poorly, report high levels of pain and feel depressed. Given June's international lifestyle and work demands, she is likely to grieve the loss of these activities, and negative emotions associated with loss may lead her to focus attention on her pain. As noted previously, even boredom is associated with increased awareness of, and sensitivity to, pain.

The Coping Strategies Questionnaire has 50 items and responses are made on a seven-point Likert scale (0 = never to 6 = always). The items assess five cognitive and two behavioural strategies for coping with pain (Wilkie & Keefe 1991). The cognitive strategies include coping self-statements, catastrophising, diverting attention, reinterpreting pain sensation and ignoring pain sensations. The behavioural strategies include praying/hoping and increasing behavioural activities. June's score indicated that she had a 'repressive coping style'. People with this coping style are particularly prone to rely on two specific strategies: intentionally not paying attention to their pain; and engaging in active behaviours or thoughts to maintain a positive mood or to distract themselves from a negative mood.

A repressive coping style is potentially adaptive. It may allow June to develop a high pain tolerance through her belief that she can cope and minimising sensitivity to her pain by diverting her attention to other things. She is likely to reinterpret her pain sensations to be positive messages from her body to take care, and ignore pain sensations. Consequently, she is less likely to experience anxiety and depression as a result of the pain. She is also less likely to perceive the pain as a catastrophe than someone who is highly anxious. Catastrophising generally is a maladaptive cognitive coping strategy as the person tends to think the worse about their condition and their ability to cope.

CHAPTER SUMMARY

- Pain is a significant and complex aspect of illness that involves an interplay of physiological, psychological, social and behavioural factors.
- There is greater understanding about the transmission of pain and the role of neurochemicals such as endogenous opioid peptides in regulating pain.
- In contrast to acute pain, chronic pain is long term and not necessarily related to a specific disease or injury.

- Chronic pain is difficult to treat because of adverse and pervasive effects on daily activities and development of maladaptive coping strategies. Treatments can involve pharmaceutical drugs (such as morphine) and alterations to the sensory pathways involved in pain transmission.
- Increasingly, psychological interventions such as biofeedback, relaxation, hypnosis and cognitive–behavioural strategies are having some success. Nevertheless, chronic pain requires a comprehensive program to minimise pain and enhance the likelihood of adaptive coping strategies.

SELF TEST

1 The most essential step in providing pain management for an individual is a:
   a comprehensive pain assessment
   b comprehensive health history
   c written plan of care
   d familiarity with prescription medications often used for pain control.

2 A comprehensive pain assessment includes:
   a type of pain
   b duration of pain
   c medication
   d all of the above.

3 Which of the following are potential barriers to pain assessment?
   a language and culture
   b diet and exercise
   c site and duration of pain
   d client education.

4 Which of the following scales is appropriate to measure pain in a 3-year-old child?
   a linear scale marked 1 through 10
   b a faces-of-pain scale illustrating happy through crying
   c a linear scale with printed words describing pain
   d a verbal scale with words describing pain.

5 Andrew's management of pain from his amputation is likely to have involved:
   a being less aware of his pain
   b new information from the stump closing the gate on the pain
   c his brain has learnt what the signals from the nerve cells in his leg mean
   d all of the above.

FURTHER READING

Daniel, H.C. & Williams, A.C.D. (2010) Pain (chap. 24). In D. French, K. Vedhara, A.A. Kaptein & J. Weinman (eds). *Health Psychology* (2nd edn). Chichester, UK: BPS Blackwell.

Scholz, J. & Woolf, C.J. (2002) Can we conquer pain? *Nature Neuroscience*, 5(Suppl.), 1062–7.

Thernstrom, M. (2010) *The pain chronicles: cures, myths, mysteries, prayers, diaries, brain scans, healing, and the science of suffering.* New York: Farrar, Straus and Giroux.

Wall, P.D. & Melzack, R. (1996) *The challenge of pain.* New York: Penguin Books.

USEFUL WEBSITES

Acute Pain Managment: Scientific Evidence (ANZCA):
www.anzca.edu.au/resources/college-publications/Acute%20Pain%20Management/books-and-publications/acutepain.pdf.

Anatomy and physiology of pain (Nursing Times):
www.nursingtimes.net/nursing-practice/1860931.article

Pacing: what's the evidence for it? (Health Skills):
http://healthskills.wordpress.com/2008/11/24/pacing-whats-the-evidence-for-it

The girl who can't feel pain [congenital analgesia] (ABC USA):
http://abcnews.go.com/GMA/OnCall/story?id=1386322

The management of persistent pain (Medical Journal of Australia):
www.mja.com.au/public/issues/178_09_050503/gou10286_fm.html

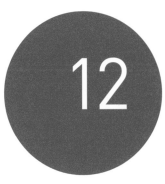

12 STRESS AND TRAUMA

CHAPTER OBJECTIVES

By the end of your study of this chapter, you should be able to:

- understand the differences between viewing stress as a stimulus and as a response, and as a process that links the two
- know how concepts of stress, appraisal and coping are linked
- describe and compare demands and resources, and describe how these affect the experience of stress
- use a goodness of fit model to explain differences in individual responses to stress and coping
- understand the effects of traumatic events as an extreme form of the stress process.

KEYWORDS

allostasis
allostatic load
catastrophising
chronic strain
fight or flight response
goodness of fit
hassles

post traumatic stress disorder (PTSD)
primary appraisal
secondary appraisal
stress
stress response
stressor
tend and befriend

WHAT IS STRESS?

Stress has been a popular topic in the media over the past two decades. Much has been made of whether the stresses of everyday life are greater now than in the past, and whether stress is the disease of the twenty-first century. It is widely accepted that stress has a significant negative impact on health and that the successful management of stress will prevent that negative impact. One major German insurance company offers lower rates for people who regularly practise meditation on the grounds that these people will make fewer claims based on stress. To evaluate whether stress affects health and, if so, how much, it is necessary to clarify what stress is. Such clarification is complicated by the fact that stress is often thought of as an event, and often as a response of an individual to events (Fisher 1986).

STRESS AS A STIMULUS

When describing stress, many people tend to think of specific events (stimuli) that have produced the experience for them or for others. Examples include examinations, bereavements, natural disasters, illness, relationship breakdown, accidents and so forth. Holmes and Rahe (1967) developed a life events scale that attempted to classify how stressful certain events were for people by assigning the events a weighting based on a survey of a large sample of people. Not surprisingly, the events rated as most stressful were major personal losses such as the death of a child or long-time spouse or partner. More surprisingly, positive events—such as being promoted, getting married or buying a new car—were also weighted as producing stress.

PAUSE 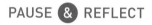 REFLECT

Can you recall a positive event in your own life that was stressful for you? What were the characteristics of that event that made it stressful? Would everyone else in that situation have felt the same amount of stress that you did?

CASE STUDY

EDUARDO MOIO AND HARD WORK

The aim of this case is to examine an individual's experience of stress and some of the consequences that may arise from it.

Eduardo Moio is a 28-year-old male working as the manager of a paper products company. Eduardo enjoys his work and would very much like to continue to move upward in his career. Due to difficulties in the industry, he has been working up to 18 hours a day during the week and additional hours on weekends. He has been eating irregular meals, often does not see his wife for more than a few hours each day, and sometimes does not see his two children at all, except for short times on the weekends. Although she understands why Eduardo works as hard as he does, she still complains from time to time about his absence from home.

In recent years, Eduardo has found it necessary to make some significant changes to his life. He does very little exercise, partly due to a lack of time, and partly because he and his wife gave up their memberships in a gym to save money. After the birth of their second child, they moved to a larger house, which meant taking on a substantially larger mortgage. It also meant moving further from the city where Eduardo works, which means that he has to spend more time commuting. He drives to and from work, and often spends considerable amounts of time stuck in traffic.

1   Is Eduardo experiencing stress?

2   What things in your life produce stress for you?

There are major problems with the view that some stimuli are inherently stressful. Events that are stressful for some—such as jumping out of a plane—can be recreation for others. It is hard to see a woman who has been brutalised by an abusive husband having the same level of reaction to the death of her spouse as a woman who loved her husband. Another problem arises from the observation that some people may not perceive major life events as being relevant to stress at all—or only at some times. This suggests that there is a threshold for stress, and that a particular stimulus must register above that threshold before it is perceived as standing out from the background of stimuli. Consider the individual who makes a career out of performing in public. If there is a lot at stake in a particular performance, that person may experience stress, but if the performance is simple and routine, they may not.

Just looking at the events themselves does not make it possible to understand the difference between a stress and a challenge. We often seek out activities that produce excitement, or that make us feel elation when we have successfully completed them, and this is very difficult to explain using a stimulus definition of stress. The stimulus should always be stressful or not stressful. The impact of any given stimulus is based on the fact that it requires adaptation on the part of the individual. Stress is, then, being thought of as 'an extreme level of everyday life' (Fisher 1986: 7). Adaptation to any extreme requires mobilisation of resources on the part of the individual, and this changes the individual's internal physiological state.

It is generally more productive to refer to events as **stressors**, which may vary in terms of their likelihood of producing a response within the individual.

Stressor: an event that appears likely to an observer to produce stress.

STRESS AS A RESPONSE

When stress is conceptualised as a response of the individual, the focus is placed on the physical and mental reactions that result. The mental component includes thoughts, ideas and beliefs. Most of the research in this area has focused on physical arousal and how it relates to outcomes such as performance, coping and health, rather than on the mental component.

A well-known principle in psychology is the curvilinear or inverted-U relationship between arousal and performance (see Figure 12.1). This Yerkes–Dodson Law (based on Yerkes & Dodson 1908) indicates that there will be some optimal level of arousal for performance of any task. If arousal is too low, the organism will be unmotivated to perform. As arousal increases, motivation will increase to a point where the individual is focused and energised. As arousal increases past that point, errors will increase until ultimately the organism's behaviour becomes panicky and disorganised. The arousal–performance curve will be different for each task and each organism. It has been established that well-known tasks are much less prone to breakdown than novel ones. This is basically why we practise skills. The presence of arousal increases the

CROSS-REFERENCE
Optimal level theories
of motivation are also
discussed in Chapter 6.

occurrence of dominant—that is, more probable—responses. For a new task, these will be errors; for a well-known one, these responses will be correct.

Figure 12.1   The arousal–performance curve

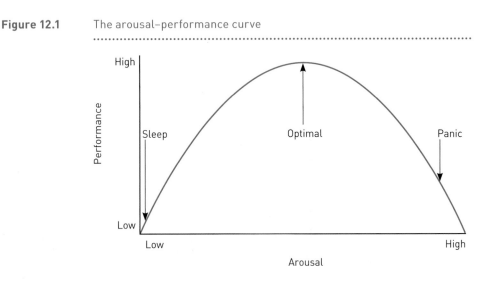

Sometimes, the term 'eustress' (Selye 1978) is used to describe arousal that is at the optimal level for performance, and that provides motivation and direction for the individual's behaviour. The word 'eustress' means good stress, and can be distinguished from distress—bad stress—by its effects on how the individual acts and feels. It is likely, however, that an individual will not really think of an optimal level of arousal in terms of stress at all. For most people, the concept of stress implies 'bad', so the idea that it can be good is confusing.

Stress response: a
pattern of physiological
and cognitive reactions
that an individual
experiences to a
situation.

The nature of the **stress response**, a pattern of physiological and/or cognitive reactions to a situation that are experienced by an individual, is obviously going to be quite variable. Cannon (1932) described the **fight or flight response** eighty years ago, based on the release of catecholamines, which prepare the organism for action. But whether the organism will fight or turn and run cannot be explained by what is going on in the body. Although the release of catecholamines may be similar, if not exactly the same, the cognitions that go with running and those that go with standing to fight are very different. It is now generally recognised that there is not a single generalised response to environmental demand. Not only do individuals differ in the likelihood that they will be flooded with catecholamines, but also in the effects that those hormones will have on their behavioural and physical responses.

**Fight or flight
response:** the release
of catecholamines,
which prepare the
organism for action.

PAUSE **&** REFLECT

How do you know when you are under stress? Do you respond to stressors in your life in a typical way? Is your response primarily physical or mental?

STRESS AS A PROCESS

Stress: a perceived
imbalance between
demands and
resources.

It is much more useful to conceptualise stress as a process involving a complex interaction between the individual and the situation. Figure 12.2 shows a biopsychosocial model of **stress** (Frankenhaeuser 1991). Because the process takes place within the individual, stress is a subjective experience, and it is impossible for an outside observer to look at the situation and the person, and determine exactly what is going to happen.

Figure 12.2   A biopsychosocial model of stress

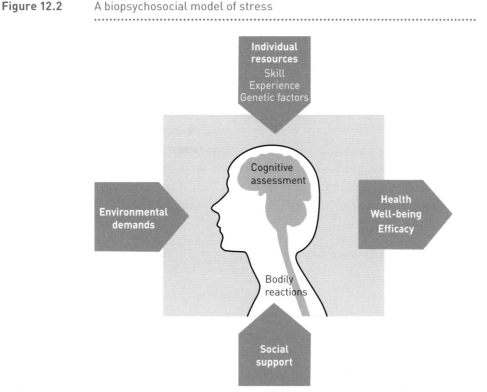

Source: Frankenhaeuser (1991).

The key element of interactive stress models is the balance between the individual's appraisals of the environmental demand and individual resources for dealing with the demand. Lazarus and Folkman (1984) presented a detailed model of how these appraisals take place, and what their impact is on the experience of stress.

Typically, in the presence of an environmental demand, people first assess or appraise the severity of the demand. This is referred to as **primary appraisal**. With everyday demands, where the resources of individuals are more than adequate to cope, the demand is appraised as being not a significant threat to well-being; that is, as something that can be dealt with routinely. In the case of severe demand, where either the harm or loss already experienced or the threat of future loss is great, individuals may need to make additional, non-routine resources available to deal with it. Then the primary appraisal will be that the situation is stressful. The primary appraisal could even be that the demand is irrelevant and can safely be ignored. This might be the case if, for instance, we heard a dog barking viciously but could see that the dog was locked up.

The next appraisal that individuals make is about their own resources; this is called **secondary appraisal**. This appraisal can range from no resources (time to panic) to plenty of resources (no sweat). It could even be that no resources are needed; that it is safe to ignore the demand completely. Primary and secondary appraisals don't necessarily occur at the same time, and each of them can change over time. Even so, they are usually very closely linked. In an emergency, we may make an instantaneous appraisal of demand and react. Later, when we have

Primary appraisal: the idea that in the presence of an environmental demand, individuals first assess or appraise the severity of the demand.

Secondary appraisal: the appraisal that individuals make about their own resources.

time to do the secondary appraisal, we might be surprised at the outcome. For example, a person who has reacted quickly and managed to avoid an accident may think, 'How did I get out of that?'

The process of appraisal is highly individual. Not only do the resources of individuals differ, but so do the appraisals they make of them. We are often surprised by which individuals cope with a severe stress and which do not. A physically strong person may be less able to deal with a prolonged physical demand than a weak person, not because their resources are depleted more rapidly but because they appraise them as being inadequate and give up sooner. The individual may **catastrophise**, telling themselves that the situation is impossible for them to cope with when in fact it is not. People also differ in their ability to adopt new roles in the face of demands. Many victims of Nazi concentration camps during World War II died during the first days in the camp because their resources were not adaptable to such extreme demands. Those who survived—often for amazingly long periods of time—were able to divert resources towards survival by redefining themselves, or living for each day, or living for the single goal of being a witness to the atrocities at the end of the war. So, there is another way of defining stress: the appraisals by the individual that the resources they can call on are not sufficient to deal with the demands placed on them.

Catastrophising: the appraisal by an individual that a situation is impossible for them to cope with when in fact it is not.

PAUSE 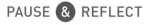 REFLECT

What are some of the advantages of thinking about stress as a process rather than a series of events or responses to events? How would this be helpful in thinking about why a school teacher might experience burnout from their workload?

When stressors are being appraised by individuals, there are several important characteristics that affect their impact.

1   *Clear versus ambiguous*—If we know exactly what the demand is and how to deal with it, it will have a different effect than if it is ambiguous. Research by one of the authors (Jones 1970) with industrial foremen showed that major conflicts with superiors were not as stressful when there were clear conflict resolution procedures as were minor conflicts in the absence of those procedures.

2   *Acute versus chronic*—Time-limited events, such as a physical assault, will have different effects from ongoing chronic stressors, such as disability or unemployment.

3   *Intermittent versus continuous*—Examinations, which occur in regular, predictable cycles, will have different effects from a continuously occurring stress, such as pain following an injury or surgery; this is independent of whether the stressor occurs over a long period of time or a short one.

4   *Random versus personally relevant*—Being the victim of a natural disaster, such as a bridge collapse, would have quite a different impact from an event that we felt had relevance to our self-image or esteem, such as being fired from a job for incompetence.

5   *Limited versus pervasive*—Some events affect quite limited areas of life (for example, breaking your non-dominant arm), while others affect every aspect. Becoming a quadriplegic means the loss of far more than mobility: it may also mean the loss of sexuality and employment, and a complete change of life.

6   *Controllable versus uncontrollable*—Many theorists, such as Fisher (1986), believe that this is the most important appraisal of all. The more controllable a stressor is, the less likely it is to produce stress (see Figure 12.3).

Figure 12.3   Demands and resources

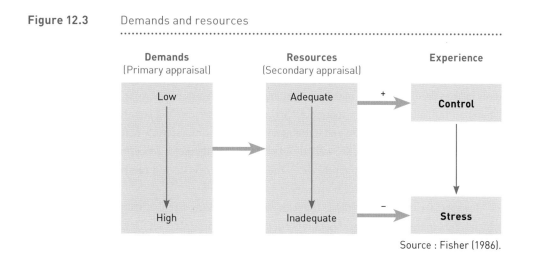

Source : Fisher (1986).

EDUARDO (CONT.)   CASE STUDY

Eduardo is exposed to a number of stressors, including working long hours, not being able to see his family and not eating regular meals. Whether this means that he is experiencing stress is not clear, however, because we don't know how his situation looks to him. Whether another person would also experience those same responses in the face of the same stressors would depend on a number of variables; a single man, for example, might find the lack of contact with family less of a problem. Someone who was less attached to their career might find the events less challenging. Whether Eduardo is stressed would depend on his appraisal of his situation.

However, he suffers from indigestion and has trouble both getting to sleep and staying asleep. This means that he is showing stress responses. They may be related to his experience of stress, but they might also be due to purely physical causes. Eduardo complains to his wife that he feels pressured at work, and that one of his superiors has been making negative comments about the quality of his work. He can't understand why he is being singled out by this person, but finds it uncomfortable to sit in meetings when that person is present. These meetings always make his indigestion worse, and he can't sleep the night before a meeting.

1   How can you use a biopsychosocial model to understand what Eduardo is experiencing?

2   What factors would be relevant to Eduardo's appraisal of his situation?

3   Would his appraisal be the same if Eduardo were Chief Executive Officer of his firm with salary and bonuses of several million dollars a year?

DAILY HASSLES

Not all of the stresses that face individuals are major. Researchers have also looked at the effects of minor stressful events on health (Kanner et al. 1981). Such events, or **hassles**, can include being put on hold during a phone call, finding that you have run out of toilet paper or having

Hassles: apparently minor events that can cause irritation, aggravate existing health problems or (in large numbers or over a prolonged period of time) affect an individual's health.

to make a small decision. Not only can these small hassles produce irritation, but they can also aggravate physical and mental health in several ways. The cumulative impact of small hassles can wear the individual down. They can also exaggerate the effects of a concurrent major life event, sometimes by being the last straw that breaks the individual's back. Research has shown that daily hassles predict to health outcomes (DeLongis et al. 1982) even where (or, possibly, *especially* where) an individual has not experienced any major life events. In a survey of undergraduate university students, Caltabiano and Caltabiano (1992) found that family matters were the most common sources of daily hassles, well ahead of time management, concerns about the future, personal failings, health and appearance, and other sources. As you can imagine, the list of things that are seen as significant stresses is quite different.

Chronic strain: the repeated or constant occurrence of a minor stressor.

One special case of minor hassle that can have particularly strong effects is **chronic strain**, which refers to the repeated or constant occurrence of a minor stressor. Usually, people become habituated to a minor stressor and so it fades as a source of stress. However, if prolonged, exposure may have the same effect as many daily stressors. Examples could include background noise at work, a personality conflict with someone who you constantly come into contact with and cannot avoid, financial problems, a poor living environment and family problems. One kind of chronic strain that has been shown to have health consequences is having a job that is high in demands but low in control. Such job situations have been demonstrated to predict psychological and cardiovascular problems (Karasek et al. 1981).

PAUSE & REFLECT

What daily hassles bother you the most? Do any of them produce chronic strain for you? If so, why do you think this happens? If not, why not?

It is a good idea to keep in mind that daily life also provides uplifts as well as hassles. Uplifts are small victories or pleasing moments that indicate that things are going well. They might include a successful interaction with someone, a job completed or finding a way to solve a problem. Uplifts have not always shown as large a relationship to health as hassles (DeLongis et al. 1982).

ANXIETY

It is not uncommon for people to confuse the concepts of stress and anxiety. Clearly, there is a high degree of relationship between these concepts, and they often occur together, but it is important to distinguish some of the differences between them. Anxiety is an emotional state and, like other emotions, consists of somatic (or physiological), cognitive and behavioural components. The somatic effects often include an accelerated heartbeat, stomach symptoms (like nausea or pain), sweating and trembling. Cognitive components can include feelings of dread, trouble concentrating or having your mind go blank, feeling irritable or jumpy, or thinking about things that might go wrong. Behavioural components can include withdrawal from the situation, seeking out comfort or doing things to damp down the feelings—such as drinking or drug use.

Unlike fear—which is usually attached to a particular object—anxiety may occur with or without a specific focus. Students frequently experience examination anxiety, for example, not because they are unprepared, or because they have appraised the demands as being greater than their resources, but because of the importance of the examinations for their future progress. It might also occur because everyone else is (or appears to be) anxious, or simply from past learning. Spielberger (1975) differentiated between state anxiety (a temporary condition) and trait anxiety (a more generalised and long-term condition of the individual). Anxiety may result from stress appraisals, and may serve to focus and activate the individual to cope. However, too much anxiety (see discussion of the Yerkes–Dodson Law above) can be disruptive, and lead to avoidance or disorganised behaviour. The occurrence of anxiety is a highly individual thing, and may be the result of a generalised biological (and possibly inherited) vulnerability, a generalised psychological vulnerability (based on early experiences of control) or a specific psychological vulnerability (where the individual learns to focus anxiety on certain events) (Barlow 2000). Where anxiety becomes a common experience, the individual may have an anxiety disorder and need to seek professional help.

There are a number of different kinds of anxiety disorders distinguished by mental health professionals. The usual categorisation includes: generalised anxiety disorder (GAD), panic disorder (PD), phobias, obsessive compulsive disorder (OCD) and post traumatic stress disorder (PTSD).

GAD is a long-lasting state of anxiety not related to a particular object or event. It typically involves continual worry about everyday matters, with ongoing symptoms of anxiety. PD, on the other hand, is diagnosed when the individual has sudden intense attacks of apprehension— often marked by considerable somatic components such as rapid heartbeat, nausea, trembling or breathlessness—accompanied by cognitions; these somatic symptoms have long-term and serious meaning for the individual's health. Phobias refer to anxiety that is aroused by specific objects or events, such as public speaking or spiders.

> **CROSS-REFERENCE**
> Phobias are discussed in Chapter 6.

In OCD, the anxiety involves ongoing and intrusive thoughts (obsessions) that can only be relieved by the carrying out of specific acts or rituals (compulsions). The relationship between the obsessions and the compulsions is not necessarily a rational one, and in severe cases the carrying out of the compulsions can interfere with normal activities of living, or affect the health of the individual. PTSD is discussed in more detail in the trauma section later in this chapter.

THE INDIVIDUAL'S RESPONSE TO STRESS

The way in which the individual reacts to a demand will depend on a number of factors, but one useful way to think about this is **goodness of fit** between the individual and the demand (Jones 2001). We have already talked about individual vulnerability and capability in an earlier chapter, and this represents one of the aspects of goodness of fit. Individuals differ in their physical strength, their immune competence, their genetic predispositions, their mental resilience, their networks of social supports, their financial resources, and so on. When a demand occurs, the individual may have the right resources—or they may not. If they have a good fit, they will cope even if the demand is severe. In the absence of a good fit, even a minor demand can be catastrophic.

> **Goodness of fit:** the appropriateness of the specific resources of the individual to the specific demands that they face.

In some cases, the individual may be able to substitute one resource for another. An individual may, for example, want to have a nice garden but not have the time or interest to work on it. If they have enough money, they can hire someone else to do the work. To take another example, if we do not know how to make two parts fit together easily, we may be inclined to try to use brute strength to force them together.

> **CROSS-REFERENCE**
> Vulnerability and capability are discussed in Chapter 4.

It has recently been suggested that there are gender differences in response to stress: that women use different resources from men. Although it has been traditional to talk about the fight or flight response as a general one (as we have done earlier in this chapter), Taylor et al. (2000) suggest that this is primarily a male response. They suggest that women are more likely to **tend and befriend** when stressed, by looking after their children or seeking social support. This theory is still controversial, but offers interesting directions for future research.

Tend and befriend: a suggestion that women, when stressed, look after their children or seek out social support in order to deal with their stress.

HEALTH EFFECTS OF STRESS

Much has been written about the health effects of stress (Jones & Bright 2001), including increased susceptibility to infections, an increased likelihood of clinical events at the same level of risk, and a decreased rate of healing. It has even been shown that stress in pregnant women affects the health outcomes of the children in later life. It is not intended to include a survey of the literature about the negative effects of stress at this point. What is more useful is a model for how the health effects may come about. Figure 12.4, taken from Taylor (2006), which can be seen as an elaboration of Figure 12.3, shows pathways to the development of physical and psychiatric illness. The fact that physiological responses to stress lead to both seems logical enough, but many authors have overlooked the behavioural consequences almost entirely. People use a variety of behavioural coping strategies that negatively affect health outcomes. These include substance abuse—smoking, drinking and drug use—which results in increased exposures to toxins. They also divert time away from healthy activities such as exercise and relaxation to task-focused activities, and divert attention from symptoms and self-care activities. The all too common strategy of substituting increased effort for increased skill leads to higher risks of accident and injury.

Figure 12.4   Effects of stress on health

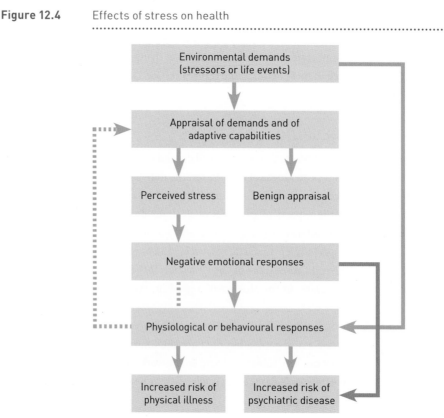

Source: Taylor (2006).

ALLOSTASIS

One theoretical approach that aims to explain individual differences in responses to stress and how they interact with health involves the concept of allostasis (McEwen 2000). When faced with a situation that is interpreted by the individual as a stress or challenge, various systems of the body are activated to protect functioning and enable the organism to operate with greatest effect and least damage. This is called **allostasis**. It can be seen that this concept relates to homeostasis: when the organism attempts to keep physiological states such as body temperature at an optimal level. Allostasis differs, however, in that is seen as a specific type of homeostasis, with the aim not of maintaining one level but finding the best level to cope with the perceived demands of a situation. There are several systems that are identified as being part of the allostatic processes, including hormonal, cardiovascular, neural and immune systems. When the process of allostasis works, then adaptation to the stressors or challenges is effective.

In some circumstances, allostatic systems can be overused, not perform normally, or fail to switch off once the demands have been dealt with. This has been called **allostatic load**. McEwen (1998) describes three types of allostatic load: frequent activation of the allostatic systems; failure to shut off allostatic activity after stress; and inadequate response of allostatic systems, which can throw excess demand on other systems that may lead to negative effects rather than adaptation. Any of these types of allostatic load can lead to problems with health. This may occur by aggravating wear and tear, by misdirecting bodily resources in such a way that the overall effect is negative for health, or by interfering with normal operations of bodily systems.

The concept of allostasis is proving useful in generating research ideas, but the similarity between the proposed mechanisms and other stress theories (see, for example, chronic strain discussed above) makes it difficult to determine the independent contribution of these concepts.

Allostasis: the process of maintaining balance in bodily systems, through physiological or behavioural means, in the face of a demand.

CROSS-REFERENCE
Homeostasis is discussed in Chapter 8.

Allostatic load: the cumulative cost to the body of allostasis.

PAUSE & REFLECT

A friend tells you that too much stress can give you cancer. What kinds of issues would you need to think about before you decided whether this could be true? How would stress produce an effect on the structure of cells so that they become cancerous?

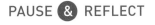

EDUARDO (CONT.)

CASE STUDY

Eduardo wants to succeed in his career and believes that he can do so. As a result, he is motivated to continue putting in long hours and to expend extra effort. Although he feels that he has the support of his wife and family, the fact that he is not home as much as they would like bothers him. Eduardo keeps reminding himself that it will all be worth it when he has a secure career. He has apparently appraised the demands as being within his resources to manage. Those resources include some that are within himself (the ability to work hard and cope with long hours) and some that are outside (support from his wife and family). His motivation to do well encourages him to continue to try to meet the demands of his situation.

However, he and his wife decide that some additional resources would help him. They decide that more exercise would help him to be more resilient, and also that he needs to eat better. He goes to see his doctor to find out if the indigestion is an indication of some kind of disease, or a response to his situation. He looks for more information about the effects of stress, and ways in which he might be better able to cope. Not much of this seems to be directly useful to him, and worrying about it actually makes him feel worse about his situation.

1   How have Eduardo's appraisals changed?
2   How would his experience of stress be different in the face of a single traumatic experience?

TRAUMA

Sometimes individuals face events that unexpectedly intrude on their lives and threaten their physical or psychological safety or integrity. The term 'trauma' is used to describe such events. These may include a natural disaster or an event such as war, violent personal assault such as rape or robbery, being taken captive or imprisoned, or being involved in an accident—and each of these places enormous demands on resources. This can be true even when individuals are not personally involved but witness such an occurrence, or hear about it happening to someone close to them.

Events of these produce very strong responses in the individual. As with illness, reactions may include physical, emotional, cognitive and behavioural aspects. Common physical reactions include nausea, shaking and sweating, which are all typical of extremely high levels of sympathetic nervous system arousal.

Common emotional reactions include fear and anxiety on the one hand, or numbness and detachment on the other. Cognitive reactions often include confusion and disorientation, poor attention or concentration, and thoughts or images of the traumatic event. Behavioural reactions can include avoidance or escape behaviours, and restlessness and searching for information. These are all normal, and usually occur most strongly during or immediately after the event.

The primary appraisals will vary quite a lot from one event to another. If a child of rich parents is kidnapped for ransom, for example, it may be a continuous and personally relevant trauma, while Alizia Selzic's appraisal of an earthquake (see the case study below) is likely to be that it is acute and random. The appraisal that most traumatic events have in common, however, is that they are uncontrollable. When events are appraised as uncontrollable, secondary appraisals are usually that resources are going to be insufficient. In both of the cases above, there will be little that the individual can do to gain control over the initial event.

As with reactions to illness, individuals may have abnormal reactions to trauma as well as normal ones, and again it is the persistence of maladaptive symptoms and responses that identifies abnormal reactions. Norris (2001) looked at studies involving 50,000 people who had been involved in disasters (most of them natural disasters) and found that the impact was greatest in the first 12 months. Only a minority of individuals remained significantly impaired after a year.

The nature of the trauma and the events that follow it have a great effect on what proportion of people show abnormal reactions. Studies have reported that the prevalence of post traumatic stress disorder (see the next section) following a traumatic event is highly variable, but the overall prevalence in the Australian population is significant (Creamer, Burgess & McFarlane 2001). If, however, there is a significant aftermath to a traumatic event (such as the continuing radiation risk in the Ukraine many years after the Chernobyl nuclear reactor meltdown), the

CROSS-REFERENCE
Sympathetic arousal is discussed in Chapter 10.

CROSS-REFERENCE
Normal reactions to illness are discussed in Chapter 4.

proportion of individuals affected will be higher than if there is little aftermath (such as being a witness to a fatal automobile accident).

POST TRAUMATIC STRESS DISORDER

When individuals have been exposed to a traumatic event and had an intense response to it, this can occasionally lead to later psychological problems. **Post traumatic stress disorder (PTSD)** is a condition that has received a fair amount of attention in the media. The important thing to remember about PTSD is that it is a response that persists, or reappears, long after the event. PTSD is considered to involve re-experiencing the traumatic event, continuing avoidance of stimuli that remind the individual of the event, and/or numbing of general responsiveness to everyday life, resulting in significant distress or impairment of functioning. Often, sufferers experience nightmares or intrusive thoughts about the event (cognitive), relive the fear and anxiety of the event (emotional), have sudden flashes of physical arousal (physical) and experience interference with work and social life (behavioural). Some of the characteristics of events that make PTSD more likely to occur are experiences that are clearly life-threatening (particularly horrific) and that result in injury and death to family and close friends, separation from family, and loss of property or dislocation. The 2004 Asian tsunami, and the 2010 Japanese tsunami and subsequent nuclear accident, for instance, have had—and will continue to have for some time—all of these effects for many of the people involved.

Post traumatic stress disorder (PTSD): a persistent pattern of symptoms, including preoccupation, nightmares and flashbacks, that some individuals experience subsequent to a major stressful event.

There is some doubt, however, as to how clear-cut a diagnosis PTSD really is (Bodkin et al. 2007; Wilson & Barglow 2009). Hundreds of studies have been carried out to determine how common it is, but given the difficulties of defining what a trauma is, and what a normal or abnormal reaction to that trauma is, it is not surprising that PTSD is controversial. Rates have been shown to be as low as 1 per cent, or as high as 100 per cent, but comparing the conditions under which these rates have been obtained is impossible.

Factors about the individual that also have an influence on long-term adjustment can include cultural differences, psychological preparedness and coping styles. While there is little that can be done to change the first, disaster managers are learning new ways to influence the others. Strategies can include having good warning systems and an understanding on the part of the population of the possibility of an event, good immediate and long-term support programs after an event, and helping people with coping. The availability of coping strategies with beneficial health outcomes is commonly overlooked. The next chapter focuses on stress management and coping behaviours.

ALIZIA SELZIC AND AN EARTHQUAKE

CASE STUDY

Alizia Selzic is a 53-year-old academic who is attending a conference on an island in Indonesia. She has been enjoying the conference discussions, lying on the beach at the end of the day, and dining with her colleagues in the evening. One evening at dinner, the ground begins to shake, the ceiling in her hotel begins to crack and fall in, and the people around her begin to scream and run. When a piece of concrete lands on the chair next to her, shattering it to pieces, she jumps out of a broken window into the street. The air is filled with a sound like thunder, there is dust everywhere and the ground is still shaking. She is thrown to the ground, and grabs hold of a lamp post with one arm and covers her head with the other.

All around her, people are running and shouting or screaming. Her own heart has begun to race, she feels sick to her stomach and suddenly realises that she is screaming too. She begins to think about the possibility that the wall of the hotel is going to fall on her and kill her, but she is too terrified to move to get out of the way. She finds that it is difficult to breathe because of all the dust that is in the air, and that she has begun to shake all over. She closes her eyes—more so that she can't see what is going on around her than to avoid the dust—and desperately wishes to be somewhere, anywhere else.

Gradually, after what seems to her to be hours, things begin to quieten down, and the ground stops shaking. She can smell burning as well as dust, but can't bring herself to open her eyes or let go of the lamp post. She pulls herself closer to the post, curling herself into a ball, but still can't get rid of the thought that the hotel is going to fall on her. She hears the sound of sirens, people screaming and crying. Although she stops screaming, she can't stop crying. She begins to think about moving to a safer place where the hotel can't fall on her, but just then there is another tremor—although it is only a small one. Still, this makes her freeze, and she continues crying.

After several minutes, she realises that one of the voices she hears is crying for help. This makes her open her eyes, and look around. It is hard to see for all the dust, which she is terrified to realise is now mixed with smoke. However, she can see that the woman calling for help is sitting in the road, and has blood streaming down her face. Alizia begins to crawl toward the woman, but then thinks to herself that this is stupid as it will take ages to reach the injured woman to help her. Standing up, she crosses to the injured woman and uses the tail of her shirt to wipe away some of the blood. She knows from experience that scalp wounds tend to bleed profusely, and this one doesn't seem too serious, so she concentrates on compressing the wound to reduce the bleeding. Because she can still smell smoke, she looks around to see if she can find the source. It seems to be limited to a small area at the back of the hotel, and she can also see that several people are working to put it out, so she turns her attention back to the injured woman. Remembering some basic first aid, she helps the woman to lie down, and checks her for other injuries, which seem to be limited to small cuts, scrapes and bruises. It is only then that she realises that she is also badly scratched, and has a few bits of broken glass embedded in her leg from a broken window. However, none of her injuries are serious, and the other woman's head wound is. She keeps the compression on the head wound, as this seems to be helping, and starts to look around for possible sources of help.

Every few minutes, there are additional small aftershocks, and each time Alizia feels her heart leap in terror, and feels like grabbing hold of the ground. Eventually, emergency services arrive and take over tending the injured woman. Alizia is too frightened to go back into the hotel, but luckily brought her handbag—containing her passport and identity papers—when she jumped out or the window. She seeks out services for herself, getting her wounds cleaned, getting some bottled water to drink and getting a sheltered place to lie down. The next morning, she is evacuated to a safe area, and is able to contact the consulate and arrange for transport to the airport and a flight home.

For the next two years, Alizia seems to experience no impact from the earthquake. However, over time, she begins to have flashbacks to the experience, with vivid images of blood and a re-experience of her initial feelings of panic. Alizia is now undergoing treatment for PTSD.

1   What are the somatic, cognitive and behavioural reactions that Alizia has experienced
     during the earthquake?
2   How would her reactions to this situation differ from her usual stress responses?
3   Once Alizia has begun to help someone else, her reactions appear to have changed
     dramatically. Why might this be the case?

Points to consider

Whether or not a given person will experience PTSD is virtually impossible to predict.
Factors that are important can include age, gender, nationality, social supports, acceptance
of the reality of the symptoms by other people and prior life experiences, as well as all of
the variables discussed above. Hundreds of studies have been carried out, but given the
difficulties of defining what a trauma is, and what a normal or abnormal reaction to that
trauma is, it is not surprising that PTSD is quite controversial. These studies may show
rates as low as 1 per cent, or as high as 100 per cent, but comparing the conditions under
which these rates have been obtained is impossible. The most important factor must be the
well-being of the person involved.

CHAPTER SUMMARY

- The topic of stress has received a great deal of attention in recent years.
- Stressors are events that have the potential to produce stress. Stress responses describe
  the ways that individuals experience stress. The term 'stress' should be reserved for the
  process by which the individual and the situation interact to produce a response that is
  experienced as stressful.
- A critical part of this process is the individual's appraisal that the demands of the
  situation exceed their resources for dealing with the demand.
- Daily hassles, as well as major life events, can produce stress for an individual. The
  goodness of fit between the individual's resources and the demands they face influences
  their appraisal. Stress leads to health effects through negative emotional states and/or
  physiological or behavioural responses. Trauma—extreme events that threaten physical
  or psychological safety—may produce particularly strong stress responses.

SELF TEST

1   Stress as a stimulus is defined as:
     a   the demands placed on people by stressors demanding adjustment
     b   an exhausting effort to process frightening experiences
     c   interactions between the person and the environment
     d   the impact of the stimulus on the individual's health.

2 Which of the following situations fits the definition of a hassle?

   a winning the lottery

   b the death of a loved one

   c getting married

   d going to work in the morning.

3 One kind of minor hassle that can have particular strong effects is:

   a post traumatic stress disorder

   b grieving

   c chronic strain

   d none of the above—minor hassles have little effect.

4 Goodness of fit refers to the relationship between:

   a stimuli and responses

   b demands and resources

   c hassles and uplifts

   d major life events and illness.

5 According to Taylor's model of stress, the critical step between environmental demands and negative emotional responses involves:

   a appraisal of the nature of the demand

   b physiological responses to the demand

   c increased risk of psychiatric disease

   d abnormal illness behaviour.

FURTHER READING

Bodkin, J.A., Pope, H.G., Detke, M.J. & Hudson, J.I. (2007) Is PTSD caused by traumatic stress? *Journal of Anxiety Disorders*, 21, 176–82.

Folkman, S. (ed.) (2010) *The Oxford handbook of stress, health, and coping*. New York: OUP.

Schulkin, J. (2007) *Rethinking homeostasis: allostatic regulation in physiology and pathophysiology*. MITPress: Boston.

Taylor, S.E. (2012) *Health Psychology* (8th edn) *Stress and Coping* (part 3). New York: McGraw-Hill.

USEFUL WEBSITES

Anxiety Disorders (ABC):
www.abc.net.au/health/library/stories/2005/06/07/1828950.htm

Types of stress (eustress vs distress) (MentalHelp.net):
www.mentalhelp.net/poc/view_doc.php?type=doc&id=15644

Veterans Voices on PTSD (Make the Connection):
http://maketheconnection.net/conditions/ptsd?utm_source=adcenter&utm_medium=cpc&utm_term=ptsd&utm_campaign=KeywordSearch

What is catastrophizing? (PsychCentral):
http://psychcentral.com/lib/2007/what-is-catastrophizing

COPING: HOW TO DEAL WITH STRESS

CHAPTER OBJECTIVES

By the end of your study of this chapter, you should be able to:

- understand the range of interventions that can reduce the effects of stress
- describe the concept of relaxation and how it relates to stress
- know how to carry out a progressive relaxation technique
- understand key elements of some of the behavioural and cognitive approaches to stress management.

KEYWORDS

arousal
biofeedback
cognitive behavioural therapy (CBT)
cognitive restructuring
coping
emotion-focused coping
FITT principle
locus of control
problem-focused coping
progressive relaxation
systematic desensitisation

INTRODUCTION

Because stress is such a common experience, it is not surprising that a lot of attention has been given to managing it. The evidence is good (Hassed 2000) that a number of skills and behaviours are helpful in dealing with stress. Most people who experience stress in the short term can find something among this range of techniques that suits them and that produces improved well-being. There is also considerable evidence that doing so produces overall health benefits as well. Attempting to manage the stress is called coping. Management does not necessarily guarantee complete—or any—success in controlling stress, and a variety of strategies can be used. These strategies can be different for different individuals and a given individual will use different strategies at different times. Sometimes we are not even aware that we are behaving strategically; we just react to circumstances we find ourselves in, but an outside observer can see the strategy if they are looking for it.

TYPES OF COPING

Coping strategies can be classified into two groups—problem-focused (or task-focused) and emotion focused (Lazarus & Folkman 1984)—and which type of strategy will be used depends on the desired outcome.

Coping: any strategy by which an individual attempts to manage the perceived discrepancy between demands and resources.

PROBLEM-FOCUSED COPING

The aim here is to modify the balance between demands and resources in a particular situation, which will clearly be more useful the more control the individual has over the situation. **Problem-focused coping** can involve decreasing or eliminating the demand or increasing the resources available to meet that demand (Lazarus & Folkman 1984).

Problem-focused coping: behaviour, such as problem solving or increased effort, aimed at modifying the balance between demands and resources in a particular situation by reducing the demand or increasing resources.

If the individual is hungry, they can reduce the demand of the situation by eating. If they have a large amount of work to do, they can complete it. If they are attacked, they can run away or fight. All of these are attempts to modify the demand. Problem-focused coping aimed at the demand commonly involves increased effort, fuelled by increased **arousal**. It can also involve problem solving that leads to meeting tasks more efficiently. It can also involve a variety of other strategies, such as modifying the task, learning new skills, deflecting the responsibility for the task onto someone else, or leaving the situation so that the demand is avoided.

Resources can also be addressed. When we know a task is coming, we prepare for it. The athlete builds up strength prior to a game. Patients are often encouraged to build up their strength and mentally prepare for surgery. Getting help from others is a very common and useful way of increasing our resources.

Arousal: the activation of the sympathetic nervous system, which produces visceral changes and provides energy for behaviour.

EMOTION-FOCUSED COPING

Coping is sometimes aimed not at dealing with the demand so much as dealing with the way that the demand makes us feel. If we are hungry, we will feel bad, but even if we have no access to food, we can attempt to do something about how we feel. Many people voluntarily go hungry to benefit others. The parent who gives their share of food to their child remains hungry, but may feel good that they are doing a worthwhile thing. If we have too much work and cannot possibly do it all, we may acknowledge that fact, but still deal with the emotion that the situation causes. We can accept that the demands are impossible to meet and stop worrying about our inability to do it. If we are attacked, and can neither run nor fight, we can still cope with the emotion of fear. These approaches are referred to as **emotion-focused coping**.

Emotion-focused coping: behaviour, such as relaxation, distraction or prayer, aimed not at dealing with situational demands but with the way that the demands make an individual feel.

Emotion-focused coping approaches to stress management can be put into three groups. The first of these includes approaches that aim to tap into existing positive emotional experiences of the individual. Because individuals vary a great deal in where they have found their positive emotional experiences in the past, these experiences can also vary considerably. Things such as humour and laughter, music and hobbies can be tools for some people. Humour can work by distracting the person from the situations that are producing stress, but also produce more direct effects on physiological and cognitive processes (Abel 1998). The same holds true for music, art and dance. Spirituality is attracting more attention as a moderator of stress, with some evidence that religious commitment is protective of physical and mental health (Matthews et al. 1998). Many people report using prayer as a stress management technique. The good feelings associated with these pleasurable experiences become a buffer against stress and reduce the effects of it on health.

The second group contains techniques aimed principally at modifying physiological arousal. These include deep breathing, muscle relaxation and exercise. These are becoming a major tool for health professionals in helping patients deal with both stress that arises from illness and stress that makes illness worse. (Several of these are discussed in more detail below.) The literature on the effectiveness of such techniques is growing rapidly, and includes post-heart-attack exercise programs that reduce risks of a further episode (Kugler, Seelbach & Krüskemper 1994) and relaxation techniques that improve immune function (Kiecolt-Glaser et al. 1985), among many others.

The third group includes techniques that are aimed at modifying the cognitions associated with the experience of stress. This can include various kinds of psychotherapy, including psychoanalysis, and a variety of cognitive behavioural approaches. The latter are often combined with relaxation and/or exercise programs to deal with both the physiological and the cognitive aspects of the negative emotions that are characteristic of stress responses. (Several techniques are discussed later in this chapter.) Much attention is being paid to the role of positive cognitions in general, and optimism has been found to predict positive health outcomes (Scheier & Carver 1985). Techniques to replace cognitive distortions with optimistic cognitions make up a significant part of such approaches to stress management.

WHICH IS BETTER?

Much debate (and, more recently, research) has been devoted to trying to determine which is more effective: problem- or emotion-focused coping. Although some of this research has indicated that problem-focused is better, the most important factor is control. The more control the individual has in a situation, the more likely it will be that problem-focused coping will be effective. Imagine that you are presented with a small ball and asked to place it in a hole that is several times its diameter. This should be an easy task—hold the ball in your hand and place it in the hole. Now, imagine that you are playing golf and the rules take some of your control away. Now you must not pick up—or even touch—the ball with your hand. You must leave it on the ground and try to roll it into the hole with a club. The rules have taken away control, so the task may become (as anyone who has played golf will testify) much more difficult and frustrating.

The concept of goodness of fit between demands and resources was introduced in the discussion of stress appraisals. Another goodness of fit hypothesis (Vitaliano et al. 1990) suggests that if there is a good match between the nature of the demand and the selected coping strategy, coping will be more effective; further, goodness of fit is more important than which coping strategy has been selected. It has been suggested that components of personality are related to what kind of coping works (Carver & Connor-Smith 2010). In reality, we usually use both kinds of coping in any given situation. If there is an examination coming up, you will almost certainly use problem-focused strategies (such as studying) as well as emotion-focused strategies (such as getting enough sleep and talking to your friends).

Individuals differ in their beliefs about where control is located. **Locus of control** theory (Rotter 1966) suggests that these broad beliefs about the main causes of events are important in the choices people make about how to behave and how they feel. People who tend to believe that they can direct their own outcomes by the choices they make and their own actions are described as having an internal locus of control. People who feel that their outcomes are not under their own control are described as having an external locus of control. They are sometimes further divided into those who believe that their life outcomes are the result of the actions of powerful other people, or the result of fate, luck or chance. Locus of control can be useful in thinking about how individuals deal with their health. Those who have an internal locus of control regarding health have been shown to be more likely to adopt positive health behaviours than those with an external locus (Steptoe & Wardle 2001).

> **Locus of control:**
> the degree to which an individual attributes the cause of events to either internal factors or external forces.

STRESS MANAGEMENT TECHNIQUES

The experience of being stressed is an emotional one. This means that the stress response is composed of physiological arousal and cognitions that are stress relevant (two-factor theory of emotion). Approaches to dealing with stress may begin with either of these components, but often involve both. Taylor's model (Figure 12.4) indicated that the critical link between stress and risks to health is physiological or behavioural responses (Taylor 2006), and this is the step for which coping may be of most use.

> **CROSS-REFERENCE**
> The two-factor theory of emotion is discussed in Chapter 10.

It is often very helpful to get professional help when learning how to deal with stress. Such help can be obtained through books, classes, video or audiotapes, or individual consultation with a trained counsellor, psychologist, or medical or other health practitioner. However, many people are able to pick up stress management techniques quickly from a brief description, or can make up their own. There is no magic involved in any one technique, and it is a good idea to look at all promises of miracle cures for stress with a critical eye. This chapter briefly talks about physical relaxation, meditation and some cognitive behavioural approaches.

The same basic principles that applied to behaviour change need to be kept in mind before an individual attempts to deal with stress using such psychological techniques. For major problems, professional help should always be sought. An appropriate aim and method need to be selected, a realistic target set, and the method must be given a fair chance to work. Again, it is important to remember that a method that does not work does not mean that the individual is a failure. A different approach may be quite successful.

STRESS MANAGEMENT BASED ON RELAXATION

Almost all behavioural approaches to the management of stress revolve around the very simple fact that most of us are not very good at relaxing our bodies or our minds. Therefore, the first step in dealing with stress involves learning and practising relaxation. A number of techniques are available that have been demonstrated to work and to produce a range of positive benefits (Benson 1989). Not all of them will work for any given person, and an individual may need to look at a variety of approaches before finding one that suits them.

The word 'relaxation' is sometimes used to describe anything we do that is not work. It can include exercise, watching sports, hobbies, being with friends or even using or abusing so-called recreational drugs. Although all of these may lead to the individual feeling more relaxed, there is no necessary connection between them and lowering stress. In fact, these recreational activities can be sources of stress in themselves, in that they burn up resources that are needed elsewhere.

PAUSE & REFLECT

What does relaxation mean to you? When do you feel most relaxed? Clench your fist as tightly as you can for about ten seconds and then relax it completely. How does the feeling in your hand compare to your previous thoughts about relaxation?

While almost everyone can remember having had a wonderful feeling of complete relaxation at some time, the trick is to develop the skill to create that feeling at will—not simply wait for it to occur. Many psychologists and psychiatrists view relaxation as so central to recovery that they encourage many (or all) of their patients to learn and use relaxation as an adjunct to medication or psychotherapy.

There are a number of conceptualisations of what relaxation is. What all tend to agree on is that relaxation is a pleasurable state; one that includes physical and mental components. At the physical level, the pleasure is primarily related to the activation of the parasympathetic nervous system, aimed at restoring resources that have been used up by activation of the sympathetic system, and there is a fair degree of commonality in individuals' descriptions of it. At the cognitive level, there is more variability. Some people talk about relaxation as the *absence* of events, using terms such as 'peaceful', 'quiet', 'at rest' or 'unworried'. Others focus on the *presence* of signs, using terms such as 'focus', 'well-being' or 'happiness'.

For many people, learning how to relax is the end in itself. With regular use, relaxation can cause improvement in a number of physical and mental areas (Hassed 2000). Almost everyone who learns how to relax finds that relaxation spreads from one area of their life to others. It is often reported, for example, that relaxation helps people to concentrate, to communicate with others, or to deal with difficult situations. Certainly, mental relaxation feeds into physical and vice versa. As with anything else in life, if an individual wants to be good at relaxation, they need to practise.

CASE STUDY

EDUARDO MOIO AND HARD WORK

Eduardo, who we first discussed in Chapter 11, finds that he is experiencing physical and mental signs of stress. He has butterflies in his stomach, and headaches and lower back pains. He is so preoccupied in thinking about the job that he finds concentrating difficult, and cannot seem to turn off his mind, which keeps him awake at night. The strategies that he adopted (mentioned in Chapter 11) can't seem to be maintained. He is too tired and sore for regular exercise, his wife doesn't seem to be as supportive as she used to be, and eating a balanced diet seems to be just too hard. As his physical symptoms get worse, Eduardo begins to get irritable, sometimes yelling at his children for being noisy when he is trying to work. Although he has never been a big drinker, he starts having half a dozen glasses of wine each night to help him relax and get to sleep.

His constant physical arousal and mental preoccupation, and his anger and drinking, are actually coping strategies that may well be effective during a momentary difficult situation, but they clearly are now being overused. The thing he needs most for dealing with his symptoms is the ability to turn these coping strategies off until they are actually needed. Remember that, in the physical world, threats tend to arise unexpectedly. In Eduardo's case, he cannot stop himself from wasting resources by responding to threats that haven't actually occurred.

1 What skills would enable Eduardo to conserve his resources until they are needed?
2 What are some other stress management approaches that he might find easier to use on a regular basis without adding to his sense of being stressed?

Relaxation is intimately related to the management of conditions associated with excess physiological arousal. Insomnia often comes from lying in bed worrying about not sleeping, and erectile impotence from worrying about ability to maintain an erection. In such conditions, stimulus control methods can do a lot for an individual on their own, but they usually work better when combined with relaxation. The latter serves to help the individual to deal with the excess physiological arousal. A relaxation skill learnt for one purpose can later be used for others as well. A variety of cognitive therapeutic techniques combine relaxation with other activities. One such technique, called systematic desensitisation, is discussed later in this chapter.

BREATHING

A very simple and effective relaxation technique involves slow and regular breathing. People who are anxious or panicky frequently breathe rapidly, contributing to the experience of anxiety. Breathing exercises interrupt this process, are easy to explain and do, and can be an effective intervention when used by individuals with little or no training. Practise taking deeper than usual breaths, breathing in for a slow count of five and out for the same. Most people find this breathing pattern is calming and incompatible with feeling anxious.

EXERCISE

Exercise is a wonderful technique for many people. It builds physical resources such as strength and agility, lowers blood pressure, and often produces physical relaxation afterwards. Everyone can gain from exercise. It is a good idea for each individual to find an appropriate exercise program appropriate for their needs. Age, gender, body type, existing levels of fitness and a whole list of physical characteristics can affect what is appropriate for the individual. An individual's goal could be cardiovascular fitness, body shaping, flexibility, comfort or achievement of a performance target.

The **FITT principle** (American College of Sports Medicine 2010) looks at four conditions that determine the appropriateness of an exercise program for an individual at a specific time. These are *frequency* (how often to exercise), *intensity* (how hard to exercise), *time* (how long to exercise) and *type* (what kind of exercise to adopt). There are many sets of recommendations available for these conditions. Injury can result in almost any exercise program and some types of exercise can result in damage to tissues over time.

FITT principle: the idea that four conditions determine the appropriateness of an exercise program for an individual at a specific time: **f**requency, **i**ntensity, **t**ime and **t**ype.

As with any other technique, what makes exercise effective is practice and participation. Many experts believe that maximum benefit from any kind of exercise requires participation for at least half an hour at least three times a week. This holds for gentle walking as much as it does for vigorous activity, such as playing tennis. While playing squash or running marathons can be good exercise for very fit people, it is not a good idea to do this kind of extreme exercise without preparing a basis of fitness and continuing to do the exercise regularly so that a high level of fitness is maintained. Too many unfit people have suffered injuries, heart attacks or strokes during unaccustomed strenuous activity for the risks to be ignored.

It is somewhat difficult to decide if yoga is a meditation, an exercise or a physical relaxation technique, and it probably fits under all of these headings. What has been established is that it can be an effective technique for managing stress (Smith et al. 2007).

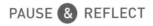

PAUSE & REFLECT

How does exercise make you feel? What are the good effects of it in the short term and in the long term? If you don't exercise enough, try to determine why not.

PROGRESSIVE RELAXATION

Progressive relaxation: a stress management strategy that involves relaxation of muscle groups one at a time so that the individual learns and remembers what relaxation feels like.

One of the simplest techniques aimed at achieving physical relaxation involves **progressive relaxation**, often combined with a program of thoughts or actions. The idea is simply to relax muscle groups one at a time so that the individual learns and remembers what relaxation feels like. As with all relaxation techniques, the key to progressive relaxation is practice and repetition. As it does for exercise, regular practice of muscle relaxation creates and maintains the skills and techniques involved.

The Jacobson Method (Jacobson 1938) uses tension and relaxation of muscles as the basis for progressive relaxation. Each group of muscles is tensed while the individual studies the sensation of tension, and then relaxed while the sensation of relaxation is studied. The comparison of the sensations increases the individual's understanding of what they are trying to avoid and what they are trying to achieve. As this kind of relaxation method is easy to describe and highly effective for many people, it will be used as an example. To practise progressive relaxation:

1 Find a private, quiet place to practise. Some of the exercises will look a bit odd to others. Intrusions will not help you to relax. Wear comfortable clothing and loosen any constricting items, such as ties or tight belts.
2 Sit upright in a comfortable straight chair or lie on a firm flat surface, such as carpet, recliner chair or an exercise mat. (As the idea is to learn relaxation, not to go to sleep, it is best to start off learning out of bed. Later, relaxation can be used to help with sleep.) It is not a good idea to practise relaxation if you are sunk too deeply into a padded chair. Close your eyes to make focusing on bodily sensations easier. Begin by breathing deeply and slowly.
3 Begin with the extremities of the body and work towards the top. Start with the toes and feet, move to the legs, then the arms, then the trunk, and finish with the neck and head.
4 Tense each group of muscles for a slow count of five and study the sensations of tension. The tighter you tense the muscles, the easier it will be to see what tension feels like (but if serious pain occurs—stop!). Then relax the muscles for a slow count of five and study the sensation of relaxation. Note that this may include feelings of heat, coolness or heaviness, depending on the muscle group and the individual. It doesn't matter what you feel, only that you learn

what relaxation of that muscle group feels like for you. When relaxing muscles that you usually keep tensed, you may even experience aches or twitches. For people who have a lot of headaches, this can occur with neck muscles; for people who have chronic back pain, with back muscles. Again, if these sensations are severe or if tension sets off a migraine or muscle spasm—stop! You may need to consult an expert.

5 Repeat that muscle group, tensing for a slow count of five and relaxing for a slow count of five, all the time studying the sensations.

6 Move on to another group. Groups may be further divided, such as working first on your lower back and then on the abdominal muscles. Face and head usually involve more than one exercise, such as forehead and scalp lifting, grimacing or scowling.

7 Some people find it useful to use images to help with the tension of muscle groups, while others do not. For the toes and feet, for example, you could imagine curling your toes down as if you were trying to touch your heels with them. For the back, press your spine into the floor as if you were trying to lift your legs, but don't actually lift them; and for the face, try to move your eyebrows to the back of your head, followed by trying to move them down to your chin.

8 It should take you at least 20 minutes to go through the whole procedure, but may take longer. Try to end each repetition with all muscle groups relaxed for a few minutes. Repeat as often as is useful. Many people do the exercises several times a day, every day; others only as needed when they feel physically tense or note a symptom coming on. To keep in practice, three times a week is probably the minimum.

Progressive relaxation techniques are often practised to the accompaniment of audiotapes, DVDs or other recordings that describe each step, and also provide a good guide to the timing of each step. The recordings may contain just spoken instructions, but they may also include soothing music or images. Once an individual has learnt and practised the method, they can choose to dispense with the recording or use it only occasionally. Recordings are cheap and widely available—many are available free from internet sites and can be useful by practically everyone who wants to become better at physical relaxation.

BIOFEEDBACK

Biofeedback, logically enough, involves feeding back information to the individual about biological processes of which they are normally not aware. This requires the use of measuring devices that might measure muscle tension, skin temperature, heart rate and blood pressure, or a number of other biological variables that are related to tension and anxiety. The aim of feeding back the biological signals using these mechanical devices is to help the individual gain voluntary control over them. This works by means of operant conditioning in that the individual is constantly reinforcing their relaxation—indicated by a change in the biofeedback signal. Biofeedback has been used for an enormous range of problems, from incontinence to anxiety. Its use in clinical treatment is well established (Glick & Greco 2010).

We actually use informal biofeedback when we regularly weigh ourselves or take our temperature. A mechanical device is used to give us information we need to change the result through voluntary behaviour. Biofeedback as a stress management technique provides increased voluntary control of the physical manifestations of stress, such as to relax tight forehead or neck muscles, to reduce sweaty hands, or even to lower blood pressure without medication. It is important to remember that operant conditioning can also take place when the organism is not aware that it is taking place. This principle is also true for biofeedback. It may work better for children than adults, possibly because children are more enthusiastic about the machines or have higher expectations of success.

Biofeedback: the control of internal processes through conditioning, using mechanical devices to make those internal processes perceptible.

CROSS-REFERENCE

For a reminder about operant conditioning and how it works, see Chapter 6.

MEDITATION

There are a large number of approaches to meditation, ranging from highly structured programs to general guidelines. Some, such as yoga or transcendental meditation, were originally based on a philosophy or religion, but can also be practised without this component and still produce benefits. Other meditation approaches did not derive from philosophy or religions, which gives an individual who is interested in the general approach of meditation the opportunity to choose a form that best suits their own needs and interests. In general, the idea of meditation is to rid the mind of worries and concerns so that a peaceful state is achieved.

The similarities between meditation and physical relaxation are many. Whatever suits the individual, makes sense to them, and makes them feel comfortable is the appropriate method for that individual. There is also no reason why the individual cannot create a personal method based on personal experience and the suggestions of others. Meditation approaches tend to fall into two categories: concentrative meditation, in which attention is concentrated on an image or sound to the exclusion of other stimuli; and mindfulness meditation, in which where the individual allows thoughts and stimuli to pass without reacting to them and becomes more mindful of the present moment.

Many guides to meditation are available, and with so many varieties it is hard to identify a single example that covers the range of issues. In general, the individual needs to find a physical setting or position that will not intrude into the meditation. In some approaches, particular postures are required; in others, the same guidelines as for progressive relaxation are appropriate.

Breathing is important to every meditation approach and usually forms the first step in the process. Slow, regular, deep breathing sets the tone for the mental side of meditation. From there, a variety of techniques is used to rid the mind of conscious thought. Concentrative meditation often uses images, such as: 'Imagine that you are in the middle of a cloud, nothing can be seen clearly and everything that comes to your mind is allowed to fade into the cloud.' It can involve repetitive actions, such as repeatedly chanting or saying a sound or phrase (known as a mantra). Eyes may be closed, but in some concentrative meditation approaches, the eyes are open and focused on an image, an object or a mandala (a geometric or pictorial design usually enclosed in a circle, representing the entire universe).

As with physical relaxation, techniques can be learnt from books, recordings and courses, or directly from experts. Studies looking at various meditation approaches have shown physical benefits, including lower levels of stress hormones, decreased blood pressure and easier breathing, along with psychological benefits, including decreases in negative emotions and improved learning ability and memory.

CASE STUDY

EDUARDO (CONT.)

As soon as Eduardo thinks about his work, he experiences a flash of panic, becomes tense and his symptoms return. It is the thoughts that he has about his situation that have now become the focus of his stress response. The only thing that seems to help him to 'switch off' these thoughts is alcohol. His drinking has increased, but now it is not to help him to sleep but to help him stop thinking. It also stops him thinking about other more appropriate stress management techniques. He has stopped exercising, eats too much and, combined with the alcohol, this has led him to putting on a lot of weight. He eats a lot of comfort food when he is drinking—chips, chocolate and pies. His wife has grown tired of his drinking and irritability, and particularly his level of anger. She forbids him from drinking at home, so he spends more time in pubs, and drives when he know he shouldn't because he does not think about the risks when he has been drinking. Through some of the people he has met in the pub, he has begun experimenting with illegal drugs.

1 How could a 'two-factor' theory about emotion explain the link between Eduardo's panicky feelings and his anger and irritability?

2 What can a biopsychsocial model of stress contribute to understanding why some techniques work for Eduardo, while others do not?

PHARMACOLOGICAL APPROACHES TO RELAXATION
PRESCRIPTION DRUGS

Another way to achieve lower levels of physical arousal involves the use of drugs of various sorts. Some of these are prescription drugs and some are freely available and often used for self-medication by people who are feeling tense or stressed.

Probably the most familiar prescription drugs for lowering arousal levels are benzodiazepines (Ativan, Xanax and Rohypnol are examples), which are minor tranquillisers that are usually prescribed for anxiety or sleep problems. Benzodiazepines can be very effective but have a number of negative effects, the worst of which is the risk of addiction or psychological dependence. Their use under a doctor's supervision for a short time for acute problems (such as reactions following a bereavement or trauma) is quite important, but because of the problem of dependence, abuse is common. Often, benzodiazepines are used to deal with anxiety until other, more permanent coping strategies can be learnt and become effective.

The other major class of drugs used for relaxation effects are beta-blockers. These drugs block the receptor sites for a neurotransmitter and interfere with the physical effects of sympathetic nervous system activation. As a result, they don't have an effect on anxiety of a purely psychological nature. While they have fewer negative effects than benzodiazepines, they still need to be used only under a doctor's supervision. Beta-blockers can produce physical dependence.

One problem shared by both of these classes of drugs is that when they are stopped, they can produce rebound effects; that is, higher levels of the very symptoms that they were used to treat, such as increased anxiety or tension. While prescription drugs have a place in short-term treatment of anxiety and depression, they also have risks (Ipser et al. 2010).

NON-PRESCRIPTION DRUGS

There are some more common drugs used to deal with stress and anxiety that don't need a doctor's prescription. At the top of the list is alcohol. Many people self-medicate their stress responses or anxiety with alcohol. In small amounts, it produces relaxation. As with the prescription drugs, however, it can result in addiction, and even death. It also disinhibits behaviour, which means it reduces the amount of control that the individual usually exercises over their behaviour and makes it more likely that they will do things that they wouldn't if they were sober. Because of its easy availability, its effect on motor control and its disinhibiting effect, alcohol is implicated in a large proportion of automobile and other accidents. It also is frequently found to have contributed to violence and suicide.

The other common over-the-counter drug is nicotine. Mostly administered using cigarettes, nicotine is actually a stimulant, but the way in which smokers use cigarettes results in the perception on their part that they are relaxing. As nicotine is extremely addictive, what is almost certainly being relieved is the craving for nicotine, rather than the stress itself.

ILLEGAL DRUGS

CROSS-REFERENCE

Opponent–process theories of motivation are discussed in Chapter 6.

There are many illegal (sometimes called recreational) drugs, such as marijuana, cocaine, ecstasy and heroin, that are used to produce strong physical and psychological effects that can include a reduction in stress or anxiety. Their use is not primarily for stress management, but for their other physical effects, such as changes in perception or a short rush of highly pleasurable sensation. All of these substances are prone to physical addiction and/or psychological dependence, and show the same kind of rebound effect as tranquillisers. Drugs' effects are best understood using opponent–process theories of motivation.

CROSS-REFERENCE

Risky behaviours are also discussed in Chapter 6.

PAUSE & REFLECT

Some substances that are stimulants, such as the caffeine in coffee or energy drinks, are often taken when people say that they are relaxing or taking a break. Why do you think this occurs? Do you use substances such as caffeine to regulate your levels of arousal?

COGNITIVE BEHAVIOURAL TECHNIQUES

The focus of the techniques that have been discussed so far is physical relaxation, but in meditation and progressive relaxation, emphasis is usually placed on thoughts as well and how to keep them from intruding into relaxation. Clearly, this is often easier said than done.

The contribution of thoughts, or cognitions, to the experience of stress is significant, and worrying thoughts are often the biggest barrier to coping with stress. A group of cognitive techniques based on this idea, broadly referred to as **cognitive behavioural therapy** (CBT), has been developed. Such techniques have been used in a wide range of mental health conditions, and have shown excellent therapeutic outcomes (Butler et al. 2006).

Cognitive behavioural therapy: a general category referring to talking therapies in which worrying or intrusive cognitions can be controlled or modified, thereby improving mental health.

If worrying or intrusive cognitions can be controlled or modified, stress can be avoided much more easily. Although some of these techniques are simple and can be used by the individual without professional support, they have been developed as therapeutic tools, and the expertise of the psychologist or other trained health professional is important to their proper use. There is some evidence accumulating that online interventions, with minimal direct therapist contact, can also be of significant value (Carlbring et al. 2005). This chapter only considers a few of these techniques and does not go into great detail about them.

SYSTEMATIC DESENSITISATION

Systematic desensitisation: a cognitive behavioural strategy for dealing with phobic anxiety by linking increasing exposure to the stimulus that produces anxiety with practice of relaxation.

Once the individual has learnt what relaxation feels like and has practised one of the techniques often enough to gain a sense of control over tension, strategies to deal with specific sources of stress can be utilised. One of the most commonly used of these techniques is **systematic desensitisation** (Wolpe 1973). This technique is typically used when the individual suffers from a simple phobia: an anxiety response to a specific stimulus that is out of proportion to the real risk (see Chapter 6 for a discussion of how phobias are learnt).

Common phobias include fear of spiders, flying, hypodermic needles and high places. A very common but seldom recognised phobia among students is examination anxiety. It is important to distinguish degrees of anxiety. A slight fear of spiders is probably a good idea as it sensitises us to a genuine environmental danger, and a slight fear of heights may keep us from doing dangerous things. Some anxiety about examinations motivates us to study and stimulates maximum levels of performance. When a phobia prevents an individual from carrying out normal activities, though, it needs attention. A severe phobia or a phobic reaction to a wide variety of stimuli (social situations, for instance) represents a more serious psychological condition, which is best dealt with by seeking professional help.

Systematic desensitisation involves linking exposure to the stimulus that produces anxiety with practice of relaxation. This begins with exposure to a very small dose of the stimulus and gradually works up to the desired level of desensitisation. The first step is to identify a hierarchy of exposure to the stimulus from a level that can almost be dealt with now, up to the highest level of exposure that the individual feels is desirable (Rimm & Masters 1979). For example, an individual with a fear of flying may wish to reach a level of no fear at all, so that they can fly in comfort, regardless of the length of the flight or the size of the aeroplane. For fear of spiders, the individual would probably be wise to stop short of being comfortable picking up venomous varieties.

PAUSE & REFLECT

Abel has a phobia about flying. Thinking about flying makes him feel so anxious that he cannot get onto an aeroplane. How could systematic desensitisation be used to help him to overcome this phobia?

It is possible to imagine a stimulus hierarchy that is made up of events; gradually increasing amounts of exposure to snakes, for example. However, often thoughts about events are enough to trigger anxiety. This means that steps in the hierarchy may include just thinking about events, such as thinking about snakes. To deal with fear of examinations, the hierarchy might look something like this:

1   thinking about examinations that are a long time away
2   studying for ones that are a long time away
3   thinking about exams that are closer in time
4   studying for them
5   practising exams
6   thinking about exams immediately before they happen
7   sitting minor exams
8   sitting major exams.

At each level in the hierarchy, the individual would carry out the activity while practising relaxation. They might start by holding an exam paper and, if they felt anxious, meditating or relaxing until they felt comfortable. When they were able to hold the paper without anxiety, they could move to the next level in the hierarchy. If they were to experience anxiety while studying, they would practise relaxing until they were comfortable, then resume studying. Gradually, they would become more comfortable with studying and could then move on to the next stage. If, at any time in the process, they felt anxiety at a lower level in the hierarchy again, they could return

CROSS-REFERENCE

Optimal level theories of motivation are discussed in Chapter 6.

to that level, and then resume progress to higher levels as they were ready to do so. Dropping down a level does not indicate failure, only that that stage was not yet complete.

The most important aspect of this approach is that it is systematic: there is a defined progression of steps, and at each of those steps the individual can gain a sense of self-efficacy with regard to their anxiety. Self-reinforcement should be given at every step. Whether a therapist is involved or not, positive reinforcement for progress is critical.

CASE STUDY

EDUARDO (CONT.)

All of the substance abuse has lead to a serious deterioration in Eduardo's performance at work. His employer insists that he work through his problems with professional help if he is to keep his job. His wife also threatens to throw him out of the house unless he gets some help. Eduardo and the psychologist the company sends him to spend the first session just talking about which elements of his life are actually most important to him. Eduardo realises that he is in danger of losing what he values most because he is using alcohol and drugs to try to cope with stress.

It is decided that he needs strategies to help him deal with the unrealistic anxiety caused by his negative thinking about his work. This includes developing skills that enable him to think about work only when it is useful to do so (that is, when he is preparing strategies for it) and not to think about it when he does not need to. They also include focusing his attention on positive thoughts. As he applies these techniques, and with ongoing practice, he finds that many of the other issues simply go away when he is not worrying about work. Being able to focus on positive and realistic thoughts means that he is less tempted to drink, which means that he is more able to control his irritability and comfort eating. Spending more time at home repairing his relationships with his wife and children provides him with additional positive experiences.

Of course, all of this takes time. Fear that he will lose the support of his wife and lose his children provides powerful motivation for him to stick to his treatment. Support from his employer is also vital, as it makes work issues less negative, and gives him a sense that his employer really wants him to succeed.

1 How important is unrealistic negative thinking to the experience of stress?
2 What are some of the techniques that might be used to reduce unrealistic negative thoughts in your own experience?

MENTAL IMAGERY

Mental imagery involves using positive images to counteract the negative thoughts that cause or accompany stress responses. Positive images are incompatible with feeling stressed; active images are incompatible with feelings of helplessness. The use of mental imagery goes far back into human history, but the modern origins may be in the school of positive thinking that arose during the middle of the twentieth century. A famous example from that era encouraged people to look at themselves in a mirror and repeat positive slogans over and over. While this is a somewhat naive approach, an extraordinary number of people benefited quite considerably from it.

Some theorists have offered physiological or biochemical theories for the effects of positive imagery and related techniques (Delmonte 1984), stating that they increase circulating endorphins, or that they interrupt positive feedback loops in adrenal functioning. Others have focused on psychological factors. Whatever the source of the effects, there is a considerable literature indicating that mental imagery can produce genuine benefit (Hirsch & Holmes 2007). It is often used to help patients with chronic or serious pain to feel more comfortable, frequently in conjunction with drugs, but it can also reduce the need for those drugs. Imagery can help to improve immune function, speed healing and slow the progression of illness. It is often used in conjunction with relaxation techniques or meditation as a way of enhancing the effects or of speeding the achievement of a relaxed state.

PAUSE & REFLECT

Think of a peaceful place that you have been in during your own life. Close your eyes and imagine that you are there again. Recall as much detail as you can about how it looked, felt and smelt, and how you felt while you were there. How did this exercise make you feel? How did it compare to the physical relaxation that followed clenching your fist very hard?

The range of benefits reported for imagery is very similar to those for placebos, for relaxation in general, for meditation and for other mind–body techniques. It is likely that the mechanism for all of these relates to preventing the wastage of resources on unproductive, ineffective or untimely coping strategies, and allowing the parasympathetic system to restore resources instead.

CROSS-REFERENCE
Placebo effects are discussed in Chapter 7.

Imagery is frequently combined with relaxation techniques—the individual is asked to fix on a specific mental image. As already mentioned, this happens as an integral part of some schools of meditation. It can also be used as an adjunct to physical relaxation. Many people find it useful to think of a specific image while they are relaxing to ease relaxation as well as to help block other thoughts that might interrupt relaxation. The image could be a particular place, person or object that helps to occupy the individual's attention. The image becomes conditioned to relaxation. This means that later on the individual may be able to induce relaxation by thinking about that image.

Rimm and Masters (1979) discuss a number of techniques in which the individual carries out reinforcement, non-reinforcement and punishment of behaviour in their imagination. These techniques lead to covert reinforcement or extinction of targeted behaviours.

COVERT SELF-CONTROL

Individuals who are feeling stressed frequently carry out internal discussions with themselves that are often dominated by negative thoughts or cognitive distortions. These might involve the person thinking that they are weak because of difficulty handling stressful situations, or thinking that terrible things will happen if they do not handle those situations.

Some cognitive distortions

1   All-or-nothing thinking—if your performance falls short of perfect, you see yourself as a total failure.
2   Overgeneralisation—you see a single negative event as a never-ending pattern of defeat.

3 Mental filter—you pick out a single negative detail and dwell exclusively on it.

4 Disqualifying the positive—you reject positive experiences by insisting that, for some reason, they don't count.

5 Jumping to conclusions—you make a negative interpretation even though there are no facts.

6 Magnification (catastrophising) or minimisation—you exaggerate the importance of things or shrink things so they appear tiny.

7 Emotional reasoning—you assume your negative feelings reflect the way things really are.

8 'Should' statements—you try to motivate yourself with 'should' and 'shouldn't' statements, as if you had to be whipped or punished before you do or stop doing anything.

9 Labelling and mislabelling—instead of describing your error as an event that occurred, you attach a negative label to yourself.

10 Personalisation—you see yourself as the cause of some negative external event (Burns 1980).

These thoughts serve as a form of punishment and share all the drawbacks of punishment. They cause the individual to avoid situations that cause them to have the distressing thoughts (avoidance learning) and produce negative emotions towards the punisher, in this case the self. And, most importantly, they give no information about the desired response.

Cognitive restructuring (Lazarus 1971; Clark & Beck 2011) is a technique aimed at interrupting these patterns of negative thinking. It involves training the individual to recognise that these patterns are occurring, and then replacing them with positive thoughts. This positive self-talk is used to define and increase the probability of adaptive behaviour; it is used as a positive reinforcer. A therapist may first model this kind of reinforcement by encouraging adaptive behaviour for a client, and then hand the task of reinforcement back to the client to carry out mentally, or covertly, for themselves.

Negative cognitions often serve as antecedents for undesirable behaviour; for example, thinking 'I'm a fat slob and I'll never lose weight' can trigger eating. Covert self-control— replacing these maladaptive thoughts with adaptive ones—attempts to trigger desirable behaviour instead. When a lapse occurs, it is then possible to minimise its importance.

Cognitive restructuring: a technique aimed at interrupting patterns of negative thinking by training the individual to recognise that they are occurring, and then replacing them with positive thoughts.

SOCIAL SUPPORT

Social support is a very important resource that has far-ranging effects on stress and coping (Cohen & Wills 1985). Support may exist in the form of instrumental support (money, labour, time or information support), advice and suggestions, appraisal support (affirmation, social comparison or emotional support), affection, concern or listening (Allen 1998: 166). Support may make it easier for an individual to deal with stress or illness when it occurs, but may also reduce the likelihood of occurrence by reducing the likelihood of adverse life events.

Social support has been linked to mental health among several populations, including university students (Hefner & Eisenberg 2009). There are indications that women are more likely to have good social supports than are men, possibly because they are better at maintaining and using the relationships they have with others. It has been suggested that this may be one of the factors contributing to women's longer lifespan. Particularly in the later years of life, when more support is required, greater access to social support becomes a key resource for facing demands. As with coping in general, the better the match between the types of social supports available and the demands of the situation, the more effective the support will be. In severe and uncontrollable situations, emotional support is seen to be the most helpful; however, when events are controllable but overwhelming due to lack of time or money, instrumental support may be far more helpful. It is important to recognise that social support is not always helpful. It may in fact do more harm than good if the help offered does not fit the individual's perceptions of what is needed; if it reduces the individual's self-esteem by suggesting that they are incapable; if it isn't perceived as support but as nosiness or interference; or if it encourages damaging behaviours, such as smoking or drinking heavily to relax.

MAHMOUD ALAWI AND HIGH BLOOD PRESSURE

CASE STUDY

Mahmoud Alawi is a 53-year-old chef. His job involves what are sometimes called 'unsociable hours'; that is, evenings and weekends are the busiest times. He finds it quite exciting, however, as his restaurant is popular and there is a long rush hour at dinner. The kitchen is hectic and hot, with his staff running around under his direction making sure that all the orders are dealt with promptly and correctly. Because this doesn't allow him regular meal breaks, he tends to eat on the run—whatever looks good to him at the time. Because his customers prefer food to be fairly high in salt content, he has grown used to his food tasting that way, and he also likes fried foods. Although he enjoys the stress of his work situation, he does find that he gets very wound up, and takes some time to wind down at the end of the day. By the time clean-up of the restaurant has finished, and all his jobs have been tied up, it is usually at least 1.00 a.m., and often later on the weekends. He has taken to having several glasses of wine with his staff to unwind, and to help him to sleep.

What he does find very stressful is the paperwork involved in running the restaurant. This involves everything from ordering supplies for the kitchen to organising workers' compensation for staff, paying taxes and getting insurance—the list seems endless to him. Even though he has an office assistant who is good at processing the paperwork, Mahmoud has to make all the decisions. He frequently finds that his heart is beating rapidly, and that he often has tension headaches during the day. Then one day, Mahmoud has a terrible headache that just gets worse. When he tries to stand, he collapses, and his office assistant—unable to get him to respond—calls an ambulance, and Mahmoud wakes in hospital several hours later. He is informed that he has had a stroke—fortunately a minor one—and will have to take time off work to recover. He is also told that his blood pressure (BP) is remaining disturbingly high, and that he has been given medication to bring it down to safe levels.

When Mahmoud visits his doctor after discharge from hospital, his BP remains elevated. In spite of the medication he has been given by the hospital, his systolic pressure is still 140mm/hg (when the preferred level would be around 120) and his diastolic pressure is 95mm/hg (when the preferred level would be around 80). The doctor has Mahmoud rest for 10 minutes lying down before measuring his blood pressure again. Mahmoud spends this 10 minutes worrying about the possible result, and also finds himself thinking about having another stroke, or not being able to work again. At the end of the 10 minutes, his BP has gone up to 200/100. The doctor decides that Mahmoud's BP responds quite quickly and strongly to stress, and that this needs to be part of his long-term management strategy.

This multifactor strategy involves continuing Mahmoud on medication, but also involves lifestyle changes. Mahmoud has to cut back on the amount of salt in his diet. Although the fattiness of his preferred food is not a direct issue, the extra salt that he always adds to that food is. So he begins to eat more fruit and vegetables instead. He is given an exercise program that he can manage to fit into his work schedule.

Mahmoud and his doctor then tackle the problems created by stress. After trying several relaxation techniques, Mahmoud reads about mindfulness meditation, and the particular approach appeals to him. He likes the idea of relaxing his muscle tension while also clearing his mind of worrying thoughts. He sets aside three regular times during the day to complete a 20-minute meditation exercise, and finds the results so helpful that he adds another at the end of each night's work. This makes it much easier for him to wind down, without the alcohol, and he gets to sleep more quickly and gets more restful sleep. He visits his doctor for regular reviews, and eventually his blood pressure has dropped enough that he is having occasional episodes of dizziness when he stands up after sitting for a while—especially after doing his relaxation. The doctor decides this is the result of sudden drops in his BP to lower than normal levels (postural hypotension), and the decision is taken to reduce his medication for a trial period. This becomes a permanent reduction.

As Mahmoud continues to practise his relaxation and meditation skills, he finds that he can use them for very short periods during stressful moments even while the restaurant is busy, without interfering with his efficiency. Eventually, the lifestyle changes combined with stress management allow Mahmoud to keep his blood pressure where it belongs.

1   Which of Mahmoud's behaviours prior to his stroke could be classified as problem-focused or emotion-focused?

2   What changes have taken place in Mahmoud's cognitions about his health and lifestyle as a result of this experience?

3   Can you identify the impact of stress on medical conditions of people you know?

4   Do you have stress management techniques that you use? Are these things that you do intentionally (perhaps yoga) or unintentionally (perhaps going to the movies to 'unwind')?

5   How common are inappropriate coping strategies among the people you know?

Points to consider

Hypertension, or high blood pressure, is not the only medical condition that does not produce obvious symptoms in many sufferers, but it is the most common. Because of the lack of obvious symptoms, the psychophysiological impact of stress may go unnoticed in these conditions, or be attributed to other causes. In other conditions (for example, asthma), the relationship between stress and symptoms may be immediately obvious, as the symptoms quickly worsen. The important issue is that all physical and psychological conditions are in fact psychophysiological to some degree. This indicates the importance of everyone—no matter how healthy—developing and practising some positive life skills. University students who suffer from examination anxiety (and almost all do) have been found to benefit most if they develop stress management skills early on, and practise them regularly, rather than waiting to use them until examinations have begun. As noted above, such skills can be a simple as regular exercise, getting enough sleep or improved time management. The key is that practice improves these skills, so that they become part of everyday life.

CHAPTER SUMMARY

- Coping strategies may be problem-focused—modifying the balance of demands and resources—or emotion-focused.
- Stress responses are emotional and, as a result, involve the interaction of physiological arousal and stress-related cognitive appraisals. Techniques aimed at stress management involve the modification of one or both of these components.
- Relaxation is central to stress management. Breathing, exercise and progressive muscle relaxation are techniques that are primarily effective in modifying the physiological arousal component of stress. Training and practice are required to enable the individual to develop these skills.
- Meditation is also targeted at reducing arousal, and includes techniques designed to affect cognitions as well.
- Cognitive behavioural techniques may be primarily aimed at changing cognitions—as in mental imagery and cognitive restructuring—but may incorporate relaxation as well, as in systematic desensitisation.
- Social support represents an important resource for coping, and may work in a variety of ways.

SELF TEST

1 Josie has experienced a panic attack for the first time. What is the most useful thing Josie could do immediately to alleviate her situation?

   a get her heart assessed to make sure she does not have a physical problem

   b consult her GP

   c breathe slowly and regularly

   d tell herself that it won't last forever and that she can deal with it.

2 The FITT principle looks at all of the following aspects of exercise except:

   a frequency

   b time

   c tradition

   d intensity.

3 Josie realises that she is anxious about things that have never happened to her and are very unlikely ever to happen to her. She decides to challenge these thoughts and take a more positive view of her life. This approach is most similar to:

   a the Jacobson method

   b yoga

   c covert self-control

   d systematic desensitisation.

4 An individual is most likely to use a stimulus hierarchy in:

   a psychoanalysis

   b systematic desensitisation

   c meditation

   d progressive relaxation.

5 Negative thoughts about the self:
   a may act as punishment for the individual
   b can be modified as a stress management technique
   c may lead to increased risk of health problems
   d all of the above.

FURTHER READING

Clark, D.A. & Beck, A.T. (2011) *The anxiety and worry workbook: the cognitive behavioral solution.* New York: Guilford Press.

Folkman, S. & Lazarus, R.S. (1985) If it changes it must be a process: Study of emotion and coping during three stages of a college examination. *Journal of Personality and Social Psychology*, 48(1), 150–70.

Hassed, C. (2002) *Know Thyself: The Stress Release Programme.* Melbourne: Michelle Anderson Publishing.

Linden, W. (2005) *Stress management: from basic science to better practice.* London: Sage.

USEFUL WEBSITES

Finding the relaxation exercises that work for you (Helpguide):
http://helpguide.org/mental/stress_relief_meditation_yoga_relaxation.htm

Self-help strategies for panic disorder (Anxiety BC):
www.anxietybc.com/sites/default/files/adult_hmpanic.pdf

Stress—learning to relax (Child and Youth Health, South Australia):
www.cyh.com/HealthTopics/HealthTopicDetails.aspx?p=243&np=293&id=2210

Worst stress relievers (Stress Hacker):
www.stresshacker.com/?s=worst+stress+relievers

PART 4

FACTORS AFFECTING HEALTH AND BEHAVIOUR

This book has explored the nature of agency and health. Part 1 examined how health, illness and diseases are defined, and explored ways in which people react to illness across the lifespan. Reactions to illness can be explained by the capabilities and vulnerabilities that an individual (as an agent of their own health) brings to the experience of having an acute illness or living with a chronic condition. Part 2 explored the effects of beliefs and attitudes on behaviour in order to understand how health behaviours develop and are maintained. Part 3 investigated the links between mind and body in response to illness. Our appraisal of symptoms (such as pain) and our capacity to meet these demands can be experienced as stressful. Fortunately stress can be managed and coping behaviours developed to enhance health and well-being. But an individual's cognitions alone cannot explain all that needs to be known about agency.

In this final part of the book we explore agents of health and behaviour that exist outside the individual, in the form of social, cultural and even physical or environmental influences. Ignoring the importance of these factors can lead to placing too much responsibility on the individual (known as blaming the victim). Social agents include family, friends, communities, organisations, cultures, many levels of government, and so on. It is a very long list and health professionals have an important place in it. These agents can have an effect on the individual in numerous ways. An alcohol company, for example, might try to subtly influence individuals' thoughts about their products through persuasion by portraying attractive (and healthy) sportsmen drinking alcohol in the media. At the other end of the scale of influence, other agents (such as government) may require or ban certain actions by introducing a law; for example, people who are involved in car accidents while under the influence of drugs or alcohol can be sent to prison. Often the influence is economic. Health insurance could be made more expensive for people who are obese. Although some agents would like people to eat healthy organic food, barriers exist because it is usually more expensive, either in terms of money or time (and time is money), than many unhealthy foods. Physical barriers can also serve as agents affecting behaviour for disability, or those who are outside the normal range of strength, agility and size. The variety of external agents is discussed in Chapter 14.

A person may not have the capabilities to be an agent of change. Recent studies suggest that limited health literacy in adults contributes to disparities in health, even though it is potentially modifiable. Chapter 15 defines health literacy, and explores possible ways to improve a person's capacity to obtain, process and understand information to assist them to make appropriate health decisions. The ultimate goal is to promote healthy behaviours and reduce the occurrence of harmful ones. Understanding how people learn and apply health messages to their lives can inform the development of communication strategies to promote healthy behaviour, along with better adherence to treatments for illness.

Chapter 16 examines some of the ways in which illness can be prevented and health promoted. Much of this is about empowering people to care for their own health, and about providing services to encourage that process to happen. The distribution of health care is not equal across any country or society in the world. As well, there are many different systems for supplying health care, each of which produces different patterns of inequity in health. As a result, there are many different ways to promote health, and some of them will require exactly those skills you are developing through your studies to become a health professional. Individuals can be helped to change, as can families, social systems, media, communities and governments.

14

SOCIAL INFLUENCES AND INEQUALITIES

CHAPTER OBJECTIVES

By the end of your study of this chapter, you should be able to:

- describe and compare the concepts of society, culture, ethnicity and race
- understand the impact of social factors on the individual's understanding and experience of health and illness
- know how equity in and access to health services influence health, and know how factors such as age, gender, socioeconomic status and location influence these variables
- understand how differences in treatment may arise from these factors.

KEYWORDS

culture
ethnicity
ethnocentrism
evidence-based medicine
explanatory model
medicalisation
social capital
socialisation

INTRODUCTION

In addition to the individual factors (such as stage of development, cognitions and behaviours) discussed so far in this book, there are many influences on health that arise outside of the individual. One observation, known as the Inverse Care Law (Hart 1971: 1) suggests: 'The availability of good medical care tends to vary inversely with the need for the population served.' This observation is true wherever you go in the world, whether the health system is organised on a public or private basis, and whether the nation is poor or rich. This inequality indicates the presence and importance of a number of social influences on health. This chapter looks at some of these influences, including culture, social class, gender and disability. It also looks at the ways in which health care systems can be organised and how this affects health. Each of these social factors can influence health by impacting on the individual's understanding and experience of the world, and on their access to health care, health knowledge and healthy environments, as well as on their treatment by others.

CULTURE

CROSS-REFERENCE

Health, illness and disease as social constructs are discussed in Chapter 1.

Culture: the total way of life shared by the members of a group.

Health and illness are social concepts. What is regarded as illness or health in one place, or by the members of one group, is not always regarded the same way in another. Even families can differ from one another in these concepts. A critical contributor to these understandings of health and illness is culture.

Culture refers to the total way of life shared by the members of a group. It is the totality of what the individual learns from the group about how the world operates. All cultures include information about what is appropriate behaviour for different age groups (for example, 'Children should be seen and not heard') and for males and females. They also tend to provide guidelines for body adornment, including clothing, and for cooking, education, music and art, housing, and a variety of other conditions of living. More importantly, but less obviously, culture teaches value systems (standards of good and bad), an understanding of time, and what constitutes health and illness.

> ## CASE STUDY
>
> ### MRS MECIR AND UNDIAGNOSED ABDOMINAL PAIN
>
> The aim of this case is to consider how the identification, experience and treatment of health issues can be influenced by cultural, social, family and gender issues.
>
> Mrs Mecir is a 65-year-old woman of Turkish ancestry. She moved to Australia from Albania to live with her recently widowed son in the small country town where he runs a mixed business. She cares for his children, aged 4 and 10, while he works long days in his shop. Mrs Mecir is suffering from abdominal pain, which has been going on for several weeks. It began as a minor irritation, but is gradually becoming more and more painful.
>
> In Albania, Mrs Mecir had lived in a world of extreme hardship and deprivation. She and her husband worked tirelessly to educate their son and give him the opportunity for a good life. She had witnessed the open conflict that broke out in 1997 between Kosovar Albanians and a hostile Serb regime in Belgrade. Fortunately her son had migrated to Australia two years earlier, but her husband was a civilian casualty during this conflict. For decades,

there was little on the market beyond basic staples, with little more to eat than bread, rice, yogurt and beans. She was overjoyed when her son was able to arrange for her to migrate to Australia. Albanian cuisine is meat-oriented, and since arriving in Australia Mrs Mecir has eaten meat twice a day. Mrs Mecir also likes to makes a custard dish made of flour, eggs and milk, or a special *ashura* (pudding) made of cracked wheat, sugar, dried fruit, crushed nuts and cinnamon. Her diet is high in red meat and sugar with little fresh fruit or fibre.

1   How might culture contribute to Mrs Mecir's physical and psychological health?
2   How might culture affect Mrs Mecir's experience of illness?

Groups of people differ quite a lot in size: from a few individuals to billions. They also differ in complexity and in homogeneity. Cultures also vary on these same dimensions. When we think of culture, we usually think of a national group—French culture, say, or an identifiable group within a nation, such as Torres Strait Islander culture. It is also perfectly legitimate to consider other kinds of groupings as having cultures. To take one extreme example, users of the internet number in the hundreds of millions, live in many countries and use many languages, but they share many common expectations and values. There are sites on the World Wide Web for older and younger users, along with men's sites and women's sites. There is a set of explicit behavioural rules, referred to as 'netiquette', to regulate behaviour in online discussions, while indiscriminate advertising mail-outs to users—called spam—are frowned on. At the other end of the spectrum, some tribal groups include only a small number of individuals—hardly more than an extended family group—and have little or no communication with outsiders.

PAUSE 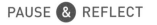 REFLECT

What do you consider to be your own cultural identity? Is it defined by where you or your ancestors were born, by what religious group you or your family belong to, or some other factors? How similar, or different, are your health beliefs to those of your grandparents?

Even in urbanised, technologically advanced countries, small isolated groups can continue to survive by cutting themselves off from the wider community. Such groups may isolate themselves for religious reasons, because of their political beliefs, or for motivations based on the dominance of an individual leader. Even if we describe such small and isolated groups as subcultures (the criminal subculture or a religious cult, say) rather than cultures, they share most of the same characteristics as bigger cultures.

It is worth emphasising the point that culture is learnt, because many people assume that there is something innate or divinely ordained about their own culture that should be obvious to everyone else. Encountering an individual who does not share those assumptions can be quite disturbing. Because we start learning about our culture from birth, it is often hard to recognise that our cultural concepts have been learnt; they seem to have always been there.

The result is, unfortunately, that all cultures seem prone to **ethnocentrism**: the belief that one's own culture is the natural, or the best, culture. Ethnocentrism can lead to arrogance, misunderstanding, conflict and even genocide. The key element in producing these negative

Ethnocentrism: the belief that one's own culture is the natural, or best, culture.

consequences of ethnocentrism is the conviction that others who do not share one's culture are inferior in some way; for example, ignorant, sinful or subhuman. Table 14.1 lists a small number of areas in which many industrialised Western cultures and other cultures have different values that can lead them to criticise one another.

Table 14.1   Some cultural differences between mainstream Western cultures and 'Others'

MAINSTREAM WESTERNERS MAY CRITICISE OTHERS FOR	OTHERS MAY CRITICISE WESTERNERS FOR
eating dog meat, insects or reptiles	eating pig meat or eating any meat
having more than one wife or husband at the same time	serial marriages or divorcing one spouse to marry another
exposing the dead to the elements	burying or burning the dead
superstition	lack of beliefs or lack of faith
laziness, or a lack of work ethic	materialism and aggression
being puritanical and restrictive	being promiscuous or drunk
ethnocentricity	ethnocentricity

Some elements of culture are fairly obvious and are consciously recognised as cultural. Values such as religion, ideology and morality are often easily recognised as being different from one culture to another. As soon as people from one culture encounter those from another, differences in these areas tend to be fairly apparent. The same is true of food choices, styles of dress and body decoration. Music, dance and celebrations are also quite overt. Obvious differences are often tolerated fairly well, and even those who dislike some elements of a culture may be fond of its food, music, religious ceremonies or dress styles.

Other cultural elements are less obvious but often just as important, or even more important. These more subtle differences include preferences for personal space, acceptable touching of one person by another, and small rituals such as taking off one's shoes before entering someone's house or not speaking about or showing pictures of recently deceased people. Because these differences may not be consciously recognised as cultural, individuals may find themselves made uncomfortable, even irritated, by them, without fully realising why.

PAUSE & REFLECT

What are some of the special problems that refugees can experience when seeking medical help in a strange culture? Think about language, culture and prior experience.

If someone from another culture refuses to make eye contact with a member of a European culture, they may seem to be rejecting them, or even may be labelled as shifty and untrustworthy. The fact that the failure to make eye contact is actually a sign of respect to members of many cultures may not be recognised by the Westerner. Someone who stands too close to you (as defined by your culture) may be regarded as pushy, while someone who stands too far away may be seen as distant or uninterested. In some cultures, the areas of the body that may be touched by others may be quite similar for all age groups, for family and non-family, and across genders. In other cultures, there may be striking differences in permissible touching across these categories, while what is acceptable touching of a particular individual within the first culture may be seen by a member of the second as insulting, provocative or even criminal.

RACE AND ETHNICITY

Race, although widely used as a way of categorising people, actually has no explanatory value as a biological concept. There is far more variability within each so-called racial group than there is between even the most different groups. The commonly understood racial characteristics of skin, hair and eye colour also have no major significance for health. While there may be a higher rate of occurrence of some diseases within races (for example, sickle-cell anaemia in those of African origin and skin cancer among blue-eyed blonds of Scandinavian origin), these are actually related to genetic characteristics of families rather than racial groups. Many of the health differences between groups have much more to do with behaviour than with genetics. In many places, other category systems—such as caste (India) or religion (Northern Ireland)—are far more important than race because they have more effect on the attitudes and behaviours that the individual learns from the group. Race only affects health and illness as it affects behaviour, or as it affects the treatment of the individual by others within society. Thus, for example, the very poor health status of Indigenous peoples in Australia is directly related to disadvantage, and social disadvantage is influenced historically by race.

How people define themselves and how they are defined by others can be quite important. This is roughly what is meant by the term '**ethnicity**'. Ethnicity may be determined by place of birth, historical roots, religious affiliation, skin or hair or eye colour, adherence to styles of dress and adornment, or any of a large variety of cues. It also can vary from place to place. The census forms in the USA do not ask whether the individual is Maori, but in New Zealand they do. Being a West Indian implies a great deal more about a person in the United Kingdom than it does in the Caribbean.

Ethnicity: how people define themselves, and how they are defined by others.

We often think about ethnicity in terms of disadvantages. Minority groups are often the victims of discrimination and stereotyping, and suffer poorer access to society's resources. But being a member of an ethnic group may also carry advantages. It can lead to special access to housing or education grants, land rights or preferential job opportunities, which may result in individuals claiming those rights when an objective classification of their ethnicity might deny them access to those advantages. Many countries recognise the phenomenon of an individual passing as a member of an advantaged group, and in some places this is accepted and even institutionalised. A person from Surinam may have obvious African racial features, a Dutch name and categorise themselves as being European. A blonde, blue-eyed English-speaker in Australia may be entitled to consider themselves Aboriginal because of past or current family relationships. Many Thais of Chinese descent take Thai names to help them integrate into the broader community in which they live, but still consider themselves to be Chinese.

Ethnicity is often statistically related to health, but this relationship is, like that of race, more related to social factors or behaviour than anything else. Ethnicity may lead to inequalities in access to healthy conditions of living, or even access to health services, which can have major consequences for health.

CULTURE AND HEALTH BELIEFS

Explanatory model:
the perceptions
and expectations
that members of a
culture have about
health and illness,
including causes
and mechanisms,
timing, future course
and outcome, and
appropriate treatment.

The understanding of health and illness is part of an individual's culture. Not all cultures agree on what health is, and there are wide variations in beliefs about the causes and treatments for illness. Kleinman (1988) proposed that all cultures provide members with **explanatory models** for illness. In his view, these models consist of a set of beliefs about a particular instance of illness and its treatment. Elements of these beliefs deal with:

1   the cause, and the mechanism by which that cause brought about the current symptoms
2   the prognosis, or the probable future course, nature and severity of the illness
3   the treatment.

There will be a need for the explanatory model to be logical within the context of the culture, but different cultures may produce quite different kinds of logic. In general, what every sick person will want to know is fairly well summed up by three questions: Why me? Why now? What now?

Within modern Western medicine, explanatory models tend to be based largely on biomedical science. Typical causes of illness are seen to include infections, injuries and problems within the body's systems. Mechanisms are usually at a biological level, although more attention is being given to the role of lifestyle and psychological factors as more is learnt about them. Predicting the future course of a disease once it has been diagnosed is expected to be relatively precise, and as knowledge about the biology of disease becomes more specific, the expectations that doctors will be able to predict the future accurately are rising. This can lead to problems when the sick person, or those close to the sick person, are led to expect a likely outcome and instead get one that is less likely. Treatment tends to fall into the categories of medicine (drugs), manipulation (including surgery) and rest. While most people in developed countries find this explanatory model satisfactory, many others do not, especially when the outcome is undesirable for the self or a loved one, or when no treatment is offered. When scientific medicine fails, people often seek alternative models that may promise a more positive outcome.

Outside of Western cultures, explanatory models may be based on philosophical systems other than biomedical science. Traditional Chinese medicine bases much of its explanatory model on balance within the person; for example, between hot and cold, and between motion and stability. In such a model, treatment must aim to restore balance. Some of the methods used to achieve that balance are very similar to science-based medicine. Herbal treatments parallel medicinal ones, for example, but it is not necessary for them to do so, because the explanatory model only happens coincidentally to provide a similar treatment using substances.

Other models view illness as the manifestation of witchcraft. In such a model, the first step in treatment is likely to be identification of the source of the curse, followed by intervention to remove it. This may include an apology to the witch so that the curse is removed or counter-magic to break it. It surprises some people to discover that models based on witchcraft can often easily accommodate modern medicine. Modern medicine may be seen as providing the explanation for the mechanism of illness, while witchcraft is still seen as providing the cause—the curse made you catch the infection now, for example. In this case, the treatment might be to placate the witch who applied the curse and to complete a course of antibiotics. As the recommendations provided by the two explanatory models do not actually contradict one another, both can be followed.

PAUSE 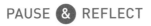 REFLECT

How is the meaning of symptoms influenced by culture? Think of some examples using common symptoms such as pain and tiredness.

As indicated, explanatory models can coexist but they can also conflict. It is important to understand that not all people share a common set of beliefs about health. This is particularly true within modern multicultural societies, creating a significant potential for misunderstanding and conflict. This issue is discussed more fully in a later section of this chapter.

THE FAMILY AS TRANSMITTER OF CULTURE

As a person grows up, their family provides the primary place for **socialisation**; that is, for the training of the child in its culture. It has been observed that babies start by making a very wide variety of sounds, but over the first year gradually stop making sounds that do not occur in languages spoken by the people around them. This means that, even before we begin to talk, our culture is having an impact on our speech.

Socialisation: the process of learning the culture of a society or group, its language and customs.

Child-rearing practices—such as how babies are held, fed, dressed and comforted—differ between cultures and have an effect from the earliest stages of life (Ainsworth 1993). The content and form of the language we learn to speak has an effect on how we regard the world around us. A language that has many terms for snow will be more useful in the Arctic than in the tropics. If we live on a tropical island, our understanding of what food means will be different from that of people living in a desert.

The family also provides much of our understanding of health and illness. Some families are relatively tolerant of complaints about feeling unwell, while others are intolerant. Children in the former may miss many days of school as a result, while children in the latter may attend school even when quite unwell. Each family will have knowledge about the health problems that have affected its members, and this may sensitise members of the family to certain symptoms. If a father suffered from asthma when he was a child, for example, he may be more watchful for the signs of breathlessness and wheezing in his own children. If several members have had a particular kind of cancer, others in the family may watch for its signs, or change diet or behaviour to try to prevent its occurrence.

This family explanatory model of health and illness works in much the same way as that of the broader culture (that is, explaining cause, prognosis and treatment), but it can differ quite considerably from it. There may, for instance, be family rituals that are based on habit or on traditions passed down from earlier generations. Individual members may have experiences of successful or unsuccessful treatments, which may add to the family's model. One elderly colleague of mine told of his father's belief that medicine that did not taste bad was probably a placebo. Whenever a member of the family brought home medicine, the father would taste it, and if it tasted good he would throw it out. The local doctor, who in those days mixed up most of the medications for the family himself, learnt about this quirk and would add a bit of turpentine to each medication just to make sure that it tasted so bad that the father would let the patient take it.

Families can regulate access of family members to outside health care. Parents decide when children are sick, when they are sick enough to see a health professional, and which health professional will be seen. They decide what—if any—kinds of insurance the family will have and what treatments are affordable. The norm in some families will be to allow each family member to decide when they are ill and what care to seek. Others will leave control in the hands of one person. In many families in developed countries, especially more traditional families, mothers are regarded as having responsibility for health matters. In other cultures, health may be a religious matter and regulation may fall to whoever is the family's religious authority, usually the father. All of these elements of family culture affect the behaviour and health of family members.

PAUSE 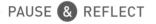 REFLECT

What are your family's health beliefs? Do any of them differ from those of health professionals or the broader society?

CASE STUDY

MRS MECIR (CONT.)

While it is extremely unlikely that race or ethnicity alone played any part in Mrs Mecir's health problem, cultural factors may have influenced her condition in a variety of ways. For example, culture may, for example, influence her diet, which could produce, encourage or worsen the disease process; alternatively, it might improve it over what it might otherwise have been. The fact that Mrs Mecir is a recent immigrant will influence the levels of stress that she experiences, which may affect her condition directly or indirectly. Culture will also affect her sense of responsibility to her family, her view of what are appropriate roles for females within her community, and her beliefs about health, which are all very important influences on her thinking about her abdominal pain.

Culture, and the ideas and values that Mrs Mecir has acquired from her own family, are likely to affect the kind of care that she seeks for her physical distress and whether she treats herself or seeks the help of expert others. She may see her pain as being within the acceptable range for health and simply tolerate it, or she may treat herself using traditional or medical techniques. She might even see her pain as a matter to be dealt with through faith, and use prayer. She may consider stomach and bowel problems as matters too intimate and embarrassing to discuss with others at all or she may regard her pain as a social issue to consult family and friends about. These consultations may be restricted to other women, or specific other individuals who are seen as having special knowledge in the area.

1   How might Mrs Mecir's perceptions of her abdominal pain affect her behaviour?
2   What factors might influence her ability to obtain care from a health professional?

MEDICINE AS A CULTURE

As immigration brings different groups and belief systems into contact, and electronic media expose us all to the same events and ideas, most countries around the world are becoming progressively more multicultural. Within this diverse mix of cultures, health care must provide for a variety of explanatory models and value systems, which leads to health care providers becoming another subculture within the larger community. Conflicts over what is acceptable health care practice inevitably arise between health professionals and other groups within society.

Some of these conflicts involve beliefs or behaviours of groups within society that are seen as medically bad—or at least medically unjustifiable—by the majority of health professionals. Dramatic examples include female genital mutilation, sex involving children or ritual drug use, all of which are frowned upon by most members of Western societies. They may also include widely practised behaviours, such as boxing, tattooing, body piercing and alternative medicine, which some health professionals believe are acceptable while others do not.

Other conflicts are over practices that are seen as acceptable by the health establishment but opposed by small or large groups within society. These may involve customs that are widely practised and accepted within the community at large but rejected by some groups, such as autopsies, blood transfusions, organ transplants, in vitro fertilisation, inoculation programs and fluoridation of the water supply. On the other hand, they may involve things that are opposed by sections of the community but regarded as good medical practice, such as birth control, safe sex, abortion, sterilisation procedures and heroic efforts to maintain life in the final stages of terminal illnesses.

As the world community has moved towards an acceptance of scientific evaluation as the dominant model for determining standards of good health care (that is, **evidence-based medicine**), there has also been a move towards allowing the experts in medical sciences to define the laws and regulations for provisions of care. Complementary treatments, whether they involve herbal medications, acupuncture, manipulative therapies or rituals, are now required to meet the same tests of validity as new medical treatments. As evidence-based medicine becomes the standard for evaluating treatments, many traditional procedures have been banned or regulated; many others have been accepted and incorporated into best professional practice.

Evidence-based medicine: the view that all clinical practice should be based on evidence from randomised clinical trials to ensure treatments are effective and better than a placebo.

INEQUALITIES IN HEALTH

SOCIOECONOMIC FACTORS

Socioeconomic status (SES) is one of the strongest predictors of health in industrial nations (Alder & Stewart 2010). Socioeconomic groups within society have different health patterns. Across a number of countries, and racial and cultural groupings, it has been observed that the higher one's income, the better one's health. This can be seen in areas as varied as infant mortality, heart disease, infections, cancers and respiratory problems. These socioeconomic differences could result from several causes, including behaviour, living conditions and social selection.

BEHAVIOUR

For whatever reason, health-related behaviours of individuals from different socioeconomic classes can, and do, differ. Smoking is more common the lower the individual's social class, which may be the result of attitudes and values—it may be seen as cool or tough to smoke among those with little money—or the result of a relative lack of awareness of the risks associated with smoking. Diet varies as well, with poorer individuals eating less fruit and fibre and more fried food. Inexpensive ways of making uninteresting but cheap food more palatable include frying it and adding salt. Although work activities of poorer paid jobs may involve more physical effort, this is usually not the healthier aerobic kind of exercise that produces the most health benefit. Work-associated risks are higher in poorer paid positions, and the work tends to be less interesting and repetitive. Poorer people also drive older, less maintained cars, resulting in an increased risk of accidents and injuries.

LIVING CONDITIONS

The lower the family's or individual's income, the poorer the physical and social conditions of living tend to be. Old or damp buildings, poor sanitation, high population density, urban fringe location and environmental pollution all tend to make housing cheaper, but also less healthy. The spread of infectious diseases is more likely in poor living conditions. Those conditions also make many healthy activities more difficult to achieve due to the increased effort and cost needed to carry them out. Educational, recreational and occupational quality and choice tend to be poorer in the same areas in which individuals on restricted incomes live, which contribute to more limited opportunities for people to leave these areas.

SOCIAL SELECTION

This explanation for socioeconomic differences in health is based on the assumption that society filters people on a variety of conditions, including health-related factors. The fittest, tallest, strongest individuals are thus more likely to gain access to better circumstances, including health. Sports, marrying above oneself, and careers in the military offer ways for strong, healthy men and women from lower socioeconomic classes to gain an improvement in status. Access to expensive education by means of scholarship or sponsorship also produces access to better health.

Conversely, disadvantaged groups—such as those who face discrimination on the basis of race or ethnicity, the disabled or those with psychiatric illnesses—tend to be 'selectively' downwardly mobile (Alder & Stewart 2010). Social selection works across the whole range of social classes, as demonstrated by the observation that medical students tend to be taller and healthier than other university students, in spite of the fact that most university students already come from advantaged backgrounds.

AN INTEGRATED VIEW OF DISADVANTAGE

The most likely explanation for social class differences in health is that these, and possibly other factors, cluster together. Each kind of disadvantage is likely to lead to others. No single factor explains all of the health disadvantages faced by the world's indigenous peoples (Commission on Social Determinants of Health 2008). Whatever the explanation, many of these disadvantages directly affect the individual's ability to access important resources related to health.

PAUSE & REFLECT

Many indigenous peoples, including Australian Aborigines, Maori in New Zealand, First Nations in Canada, Native Americans in the USA and black Africans, have poorer health than the non-indigenous people in those countries. What are some of the common factors that all of these indigenous peoples share that may help to explain this observation?

Most societies regard health as something to which everyone has an equal entitlement. The World Health Organization (WHO 1946) has long had a policy of 'Health for All' that is supported by all of its member countries. Ensuring equity in health may be very difficult to achieve, however. Health is not only affected by socioeconomic status, as discussed above, but many other factors as well.

SOCIAL ORGANISATION OF HEALTH

The ways in which health care, including public health and clinical care, is managed differ from place to place. This difference in the social organisation of health is most obvious when we compare one country with another. In some countries, the available resources for health care are simply insufficient to deal with the needs of the whole population. In parts of sub-Saharan Africa, for example, the number of people who are HIV positive is so large that all of the financial resources of the country could not possibly provide even minimal care for all. Unless richer countries contribute to care, there will inevitably be many who will receive nothing. In other places, health problems of segments of society may not be dealt with simply because they represent rare problems. Facilities for the management of sickle-cell anaemia, for instance, may simply not exist in many parts of the United Kingdom because only a small minority of the population is susceptible to the condition. Other locations within the United Kingdom, with larger at-risk populations, may have excellent and readily available facilities.

In general, countries with public funding of health care (such as Australia) do a better job of providing equitable health care to all of residents than those with private funding models (for example, the USA), but the overall quality of health care may actually be lower in the former than the latter. If the proportion of total economic resources of a country devoted to health care stays constant, the quality of care available to some may be higher in privately funded systems than the quality of care available to all in a public-funded system. The best health care in the USA is unmatched in the world, but even though the proportion of gross national product devoted to health is greater there than anywhere else in the world, many US citizens have extremely poor access to health care of any kind. Health care in the former Soviet Union was free to all, but because the overall resources available for care were limited, care was often poor for everyone, except for those who could gain access to special facilities or leave the country to find care elsewhere.

RATIONING OF HEALTH

Whether total resources are insufficient to provide adequate health care for everyone or resources are unequally distributed, there are a number of ways in which health care may be rationed (Taylor & Hawley 2004). People in certain groups may simply be denied treatment, or have limited access to treatment. For example, transplant organs are generally in short supply, so when decisions about transplants are made, the elderly, or patients with multiple health problems, may not be considered for treatment. People may be deterred from accessing a service by making it more expensive. The Pharmaceutical Benefits Scheme (PBS) in Australia, for example, has refused to list Viagra for benefit, not because impotence is not recognised as a health problem, but because listing it would result in a huge increase in the number of men being treated for it at public expense. A demonstration of what this is intended to avoid came with the listing of a new and highly effective class of medications (statins) to control cholesterol levels, resulting in better cardiovascular health for many. This has caused a significant blowout in the cost of the PBS, even though the outcome is likely to be lessened demand on medical services overall.

Services may be diluted by, say, requiring that patients be offered generic brand medications rather than proprietary brands in order to qualify for subsidies. Another way of diluting services is having them carried out by professionals with less training who are paid lower wages. Waiting lists for health care represent rationing by delay in providing services. Those procedures that are defined as less urgent are simply delayed until there are sufficient resources to provide them. One unfortunate outcome of this is that they may be delayed until they become urgent. The consequences of delay for the individual in this situation have become much more serious. It is not uncommon for the costs of managing an urgent condition to be greater than those of preventing it with care at an earlier point. As a result, waiting lists may not contain the cost of health care, but instead push that cost to a later point in time, thereby also increasing it.

CASE STUDY

MRS MECIR (CONT.)

Mrs Mecir's ability to obtain health care will depend on things such as money, time and whether her family believes that she needs care. After talking to her son, she is persuaded that she needs to seek a doctor's advice about her pain, and that time can be found for her to visit the doctor. The one doctor in her country town is willing to bulk bill—that is, accept the government-funded medical rebate as full payment for treatment—so money is not seen as an issue. An appointment is made for Mrs Mecir to see the doctor. As she speaks only a few words of English, and her son is too busy to go with her, she decides that she will have to take her 10-year-old granddaughter along to interpret for her. The doctor's surgery is on the other side of town and Mrs Mecir does not drive, so she and her grand-daughter will have to walk half an hour each way to get there. The doctor is a young man, recently arrived in the town.

Mrs Mecir was not able to speak to the doctor directly. Her granddaughter tried to help, but did not clearly understand what her grandmother was telling her; nor did she communicate all the symptoms clearly to the doctor. The doctor became aware that there were cultural differences in the terminology Mrs Mecir used to describe her pain, its causes or the treatment she had tried. The doctor performed a physical examination while Mrs Mecir remained fully clothed. The doctor thought he located two sites of abdominal pain and ordered a scan of Mrs Mecir's large bowel, which could be performed locally. He also asked the receptionist to make a follow-up appointment for Mrs Mecir and to coordinate with a telehealth translation service based in Sydney to provide assistance during that follow-up appointment.

1   How would the nature of the medical services in Mrs Mecir's town affect her access to health care?
2   Even though the telehealth translation service will be helpful, what will be some of the barriers to using this technology during the appointment?
3   How can Mrs Mecir's son be informed and involved in supporting her at this time?

MANAGING INEQUALITIES IN HEALTH

Alder and Stewart (2010) describe a number of ways in which inequalities in the provision of health care, particularly socioeconomic inequalities, can be addressed. Social policies can be changed to build up the physical assets (such as hospitals, schools and housing) or social assets (such as education and social security) of the society. Causes of socioeconomic disadvantage, such as unequal distribution of wealth and unemployment, can also be addressed by social policies. Living and working conditions can be improved, particularly in disadvantaged areas. Behavioural risk factors can be modified for disadvantaged groups through health education and behaviour change programs, and by removing barriers to change. A public-funded, universally available health care system can be maintained—one that is responsive to the needs of the disadvantaged and to the reasons for the existence of that disadvantage.

One common factor in all of these kinds of interventions is that they build **social capital** within the society. That is, they increase the trust that people have in one another, in the government institutions within their society, and in the health professions. This increase in trust is associated with an increased willingness to cooperate for the mutual benefit of all. Where social capital is low, cooperation is less likely; individuals will tend to fight for their own interests and hoard their own resources rather than work for the interests of the whole social group.

Social capital: the level of trust people have in one another, in government institutions and in the health professions.

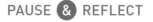

PAUSE & REFLECT

Could differences in social capital help in understanding the different reactions of people living in areas that suffered disasters such as the Victorian bushfires in 2009, the Queensland floods in 2011 or cyclone Yasi in 2011?

Clearly, there are many factors—some apparent and some subtle—that affect the equity of health in any society. Access and gender are two factors that have a significant, but often unrecognised, influence on equity. They are now considered in more detail.

ACCESS TO HEALTH

Even in developed countries—which provide significant advantages to most of their populations in transportation, technology and standards of living—access to health is highly variable. Access may be determined by financial factors: those on high incomes are able to purchase better food, more and better medical care, and better living conditions overall. Access may also be determined by cultural factors: those who speak the dominant language, who are more educated, and who are more confident and assertive are better able to find out what is available and to access it. Within some cultural groups, women's access to health care is controlled by fathers, brothers or husbands; women in those groups may be denied needed care for reasons of modesty, because they are seen as not worthy of the expenditure, or from fear that they may lose their value as workers.

Access may also simply be geographical. For the individual who lives in an isolated locality, almost all choices are relatively restricted. This means that there are fewer schools to choose from, less variety in the local shops, and transport costs may make uncommon items much more expensive than they are in heavily populated areas. Occupational choice will be less. Most importantly, travel time will affect access to anything specialised, including medical services.

Travel incurs costs in several ways. There is less frequent public transport in areas of lower population, and the varieties of public transport may be restricted. The greater the distance travelled, the more expensive travel on public transport will be. In order to deal with long distances (and possibly bad roads), private transportation needs to be of better quality, which will make it more expensive. Inevitably, travel to access health care will result in higher fuel costs, more expensive servicing for vehicles, and other higher costs for the rural dweller than for the urban dweller. In many cases, no public transport will exist, so the individual may have to walk or find transport with relatives, friends or neighbours.

Time must also be seen as a cost: not just the time spent in travel but also the fact that time will be lost from income-earning activities or from other social obligations. The efficiency of timing of treatment becomes a factor as well. An early-morning medical service may require a night spent in a hotel, not just for the individual receiving the service but also often for a parent, companion or driver. A delayed or cancelled appointment may lead to the loss of an entire day and the need to set aside another. Hospital stays may involve more than one person having to travel, and then to purchase meals and accommodation in the area of the hospital—or, in the case of children, within it.

Even in Australia where most of the population is concentrated on the southeastern fringe, isolation becomes a serious problem for patients and practitioners. Some residents are geographically so distant from facilities than only air transport will get health care to them—or get them to health care—quickly enough. Australia's Flying Doctor Service, a reaction to this kind of isolation, provides airborne emergency treatment and air ambulance services. Such services are expensive and they will be available only where government subsidies support them.

The problem of practitioners' geographical isolation is often overlooked, yet there is a whole range of issues that affect doctors, nurses and other health professionals who live in small communities or far from specialised services. These include not having other professionals around to compare notes with, not having easy access to continuing education programs or certification updates, and not having back-up or replacement staff for times of personal illness or for holidays. While weblinks with urban facilities can ease some of these problems, they cannot help with the problem of lack of back-up services or the sense of professional (and sometimes social) isolation that some practitioners feel. Programs to encourage health workers to practise in isolated areas are receiving a high priority in most countries, and most aim to increase the rewards of rural practice by attacking these problems.

GENDER AND HEALTH

Whether one is male or female has a complex effect on health and on the equity of care. This is indicated by the observation that at any age of life, women are more likely to be sick, but men are more likely to die (Verbrugge 1985). There are several factors that contribute to this imbalance, and these are partially related to the age of the individuals as well as their gender.

As discussed in Chapter 2, early in life, males are very slightly more prone than females to a variety of genetic and biological problems. Why this should be so is not clear, although it is known that some differences in the course and pattern of development are due to hormone differences. At this stage, the male death rate is only very slightly higher than the female death rate.

During childhood, and then on into adulthood, gender differences tend to be related more to differences in behaviour than to biology, as discussed in Chapter 3. Male children are more prone to accidents as a result of different preferences for activities or differences in the maturation of physical abilities. Later, males are more likely than females to be involved in risky behaviours, including working in riskier environments and playing dangerous sports. They also have a greater likelihood of indulging in dangerous habits: they tend to have poorer diet, a greater tendency to become overweight, and to have riskier drinking and smoking behaviours than females.

An area of gender difference relates to cigarette smoking. Cigarette smoking began as an activity of status among more affluent, culturally influential men and (later) women. As the adverse effects of smoking came to be recognised, the more educated and affluent people in Western societies largely quit or refrained from starting smoking; rather than denoting high social status, smoking has now come to represent socioeconomic disadvantage. Both men and women with lower levels of income, education and other indicators of low socio-economic status (SES) are more likely than those with higher SES to become smokers; they are also more likely to progress to heavy smoking and, once they become smokers, they are less likely to quit (Chilcoat 2009). As more women are smoking, we are now seeing the consequences of this behaviour in rates of respiratory disease and cancer (AIHW 2010).

As a generalisation, however, women appear to take better care of their health and are more likely to seek professional help when ill. One contributor to this may be that women are more likely to take children or elderly relatives to the doctor, which could lead to a greater feeling of comfort in the setting. It is possible that some women may take the opportunity offered by a visit to the doctor with someone else to seek care for themselves.

Pregnancy and childbirth can expose women to some health risks (such as high blood pressure and gestational diabetes), but also to greater interactions with health care professionals and probably to a better level of lifestyle advice than men receive during the equivalent young adult years of life. Increasingly, midwifery researchers and some women are questioning whether the **medicalisation** of normal birth is necessary or appropriate. Australia has one of the highest rates of Caesarean section in the world. In 2009 the rate of Caesarean section was 31.5 per cent (AIHW 2011b), which is double the recommended rate of 15 per cent by the World Health Organization. This high level of medical intervention in birth needs to be questioned, especially given the increasing prevalence of depression and anxiety symptoms following a distressing birth (Gamble & Creedy 2009). Home births with access to

Medicalisation: the process of defining non-medical issues or problems as medical issues, often because health professionals are the only (or the most easily accessible) resources for dealing with them.

birthing facilities if required, and the use of special birthing rooms in hospitals provide a more normalised birthing experience for many women where no complications are foreseen. Even though most pregnant women prefer to know that hospital support is readily available should it be needed, the overuse of medical intervention during childbirth should be reviewed.

PAUSE 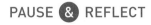 REFLECT

Consider the major factors that influence the differences in health and death rates between men and women. What can be done to change them? Should they be changed, or are there actually advantages to society in allowing some of these differences to exist?

The differences in male and female death rates lead to an increasing predominance of females over males as people get older. In middle age, there are slightly more females than males at each age (ABS 2009b). Among the very old—say, greater than 100 years of age—the proportion of males is only about 10 per cent. This longer survival for females means that they need a different kind and level of care than men. Hip fractures provide a good case in point. Most hip fractures occur among the elderly, and since most of the elderly are female, they are far more likely than males to have hip fractures. Elderly people—again mostly female—will also tend to have multiple health problems.

CROSS-REFERENCE
Lifespan development is addressed in Chapters 2 and 3.

Differences in treatment can also arise from a variety of factors. Health professionals may treat men and women differently because of their gender, even when the problem is the same. If women are experiencing the same health problems several years later than men, age may have an impact. Also, men may be less likely than women to seek and to accept social support, thereby missing out on an important contributor to health and well-being.

CASE STUDY

BELINDA AND SOCIAL DETERMINANTS OF SOCIAL AND EMOTIONAL WELL-BEING DURING PREGNANCY

The aim of this case study is to explore the social determinants that increase the likelihood of poor health outcomes for Aboriginal and Torres Strait Islander people. With a focus on maternal mental health during childbearing, the case study aims to identify how this mother's experience differs in important ways from the experiences of other Australian mothers.

Belinda is a 17-year-old woman of the Kalkadoon people who live in the area around Mount Isa in the Gulf region of Queensland. Officially she has completed Year 10, but her reading and numeracy skills are poor due to absenteeism from school. She has never been in paid employment and mainly does work round the house for her mother. Ten people live in the house. All the adult members of the family receive Centrelink payments. Her parents are heavy drinkers and two years ago her father was involved in a fight in town. He caused grievous bodily harm to the hotel owner and is currently serving three years in prison. Belinda had a boyfriend, but they broke up when she told him she was pregnant. He left and went to Mt Isa and she has not heard from him since. Belinda drinks every day and smokes around 20 cigarettes daily, but she has been trying to cut down since she became pregnant.

There is a health service near where Belinda lives. Belinda went to the clinic when she thought she was pregnant, but has not been back. She said, 'That nurse there, she was rude and told me I was stupid to get pregnant. She told me to stop smoking and don't come back until I do.' Belinda's grandmother talks to her about the growing baby, and one day they walked into the bush to find some bush bananas that are good for the mother and the baby.

At 32 weeks, Belinda was not feeling well. Her older brother drove her back to the clinic. Medical investigations identified that Belinda had a urinary tract infection, was anaemic (had a low red blood cell count) and had high blood pressure, all of which could threaten the safety of her baby. Flying Doctor service staff who were visiting the clinic that day wanted to take Belinda to Mt Isa and then to Townsville (the closest tertiary health provider) for care during her pregnancy. Belinda had never been away from her family and she wanted the baby to be born on her country. But she was told that if she did not go, the baby would not survive.

Belinda reluctantly decided to go to Townsville. All she had were the clothes she was wearing, $20 from her mother and a packet of cigarettes. Once she was admitted to the Townsville hospital, Belinda was restricted to bed most of the time because of her high blood pressure. Belinda used to sneak out for a smoke, but once these were gone she was craving for a cigarette. One nurse was kind, but the others ignored her. A social worker and Indigenous liaison officer spoke with her to arrange things so she could get money from the government when the baby was born. Her blood pressure continued to be high. At 36 weeks, her pregnancy was induced. After a long labour, a baby girl was born using forceps. The baby had low birth weight and difficulty breathing, so was transferred to the special care nursery. Belinda was frightened during labour. She was in pain, alone and unsupported. When her baby was taken away she burst into tears.

1   What are some of the stressors and predictors for serious psychological distress that Belinda may have been experiencing during the early part of her pregnancy?

2   At the time Belinda had to choose whether or not to go to Townsville, what were the immediate and long-term medical, social and psychological implications of her decision? Should Belinda have choices in where and how she gives birth to her baby? If not, why not?

3   What are some of the factors that contributed to the poor health and distress of Belinda and her baby?

4   Throughout this episode of Belinda's life, what could have been done to enhance her sense of well-being and resilience?

Points to consider

According to Zubrick and colleagues (2010), social and emotional well-being of Aboriginal and Torres Strait Islander people may be constrained by four factors: accumulating and overwhelming stress, chaos, social exclusion and social inequality. Belinda lives in a stressful and chaotic environment. Negative life events include trauma and abuse, violence, substance misuse, physical health problems, incarceration of her father, cultural dislocation and social disadvantage. Her grandmother provides some stability and nurturing. Belinda understands the land is central to the spiritual and emotional well-being of her people.

In Townsville, Belinda was experiencing an accumulation of stressors associated with being dislocated from her family and community. She was alone with no resources, and was dependent upon the health care staff. It is likely that staff in the birth suite were not sensitive to her needs and once again Belinda had no support. Women often experience a high level of anxiety associated with labour and can become fearful for the life of their baby. Development of the baby in utero would have been compromised due to Belinda's stress, alcohol intake, smoking, poor diet, anaemia, hypertension and lack of antenatal care.

CHAPTER SUMMARY

- Culture—the total way of life shared by members of a group—has a significant influence on the understanding and experience of health and illness.
- Much of the influence of culture on health arises from its impact on the behaviour of the individual. Groups have different health beliefs, only some of which are incompatible with modern medicine. Other traditional models of health are able to cooperate with modern medicine, although additions to it may be seen as necessary or desirable.
- The family serves as the main transmitter of cultural beliefs and values regarding health. Medicine needs to be understood as a culture with its own values and standards.
- Socioeconomic status has a strong impact on health, through behaviour, living standards and social selections, although these interact with one another.
- The process of ensuring equity in health involves more than ensuring equity in health care. It may include steps to increase the total pool of health resources available, or ensuring that there is equal access to resources. A number of factors—including location, travel, time and isolation—may have significant impacts on access.
- Gender influences health, as a result of biological and behavioural differences. The longer lifespan of women in developed countries may obscure some inequities in the distribution of health care.

SELF TEST

1 In Kleinman's view, the explanatory models of illness of all cultures include beliefs about:
   a spirits and how they can be appeased
   b what qualifications health professionals should have
   c what herbal medicines people should take
   d the causes, timing and likely outcomes of illness.
2 Culture:
   a is largely unlearned
   b helps to make life predictable
   c is usually easier to see in one's own life than in others'
   d refers to how much education people have.
3 Families influence the health of their members by:
   a regulating access to health services
   b providing health care
   c defining standards of health
   d all of the above.

4 Factors that contribute to women attending doctors more often than men include all of the following except:

   a Women are more likely than men to take children to see the doctor.

   b Women are more likely to have psychiatric illnesses.

   c Women have specific needs that men do not.

   d Women are more likely to seek advice for symptoms or concerns.

5 An individual who lives at a considerable distance from a big city in Australia will be least likely to be disadvantaged in terms of access by the:

   a cost of services available to them

   b time required to access health services

   c distance to services

   d diversity of services.

FURTHER READING

Adler, N.E., Stewart, J. & New York Academy of Sciences (2010) *The biology of disadvantage: Socioeconomic status and health.* Hoboken, NJ: WileyInterScience.

Dickinson, H., Freeman, T., Robinson, S. & Williams, I. (2011) Resource scarcity and priority-setting: From management to leadership in the rationing of health care? *Public Money & Management*, 31(5), 363–70.

Martin, C.R. (ed.) (2012) *Perinatal mental health: A clinical guide.* London: M&K Publishing.

Purdie, N., Dudgeon, P. & Walker, R. (eds) (2011) *Working together: Aboriginal and Torres Strait Islander Mental Health and Well-being Principles and Practices.* Australian Government Department of Health & Ageing. Canberra: Australian Government.

USEFUL WEBSITES

Bullying. No Way! (Australian School Communities):
www.bullyingnoway.com.au/issues/social-capital.shtml

Health and socioeconomic disadvantage (Australian Bureau of Statistics):
www.abs.gov.au/AUSSTATS/abs@.nsf/Lookup/4102.0Main+Features30Mar+2010

Social disadvantage (bgkllen):
http://bgkllen.org.au/research/external-research/71-social-disadvantage.html

HEALTH LITERACY

15

CHAPTER OBJECTIVES

By the end of your study of this chapter, you should be able to:

- define health literacy and it various components
- describe the cognitive, psychological and cultural factors associated with poor health literacy
- understand principles from cognitive psychology and learning theories to explain why some people have difficulty learning, remembering and applying health information in their lives
- appreciate health education strategies to enhance individuals' health literacy levels and promote behaviour change.

KEYWORDS

adult literacy and life skills
cognitive load
health literacy
learning
mastery learning
schema
teach-back
teach to goal
working memory

WHAT IS HEALTH LITERACY?

Health literacy is a relatively new concept in health promotion. Health literacy is the ability to read, comprehend and act on medical information, and effectively use health care services (World Health Organization 2009a). Health literacy comprises different skills beyond those of reading and writing; it also includes numeracy (such as everyday mathematical skills), speaking and listening, and is underpinned by cultural and conceptual knowledge (such as ideas from science and physiology). While low health literacy is often linked with low education level, along with ethnicity, age and the ability to understand and communicate in English, it is not a reflection of an individual's intellectual ability or motivation to learn. Chapter 14 addressed similar factors that may act as barriers to health care; however, this chapter draws on cognitive psychology and learning theories to explain why some people have difficulty learning, remembering and applying health information in their lives in order to make good decisions about their health.

There are different forms of literacy, which Zarcadoolas, Pleasant and Greer (2006) have categorised as fundamental, scientific, civic and cultural. Each type of literacy contributes to health. In order to have a good level of health literacy, individuals need to have fundamental skills of reading, writing, speaking and numeracy. Written and spoken health information can be complex and not easily understood. Adults with low literacy often have a reading ability equivalent of somewhere between a fifth to eighth grade education (that is, 10 to 13 years of age). Having limited reading ability means that many words or phrases will not make sense and as a result the person may take a long time to read a short passage, or may misunderstand the meaning. Using various forms of information technology (such the internet, mobile devices and email) is quickly becoming fundamental to communicating. Individuals who do not have the necessary skills to access and receive information are disadvantaged compared with others who do.

Scientific literacy refers to the ability to understand scientific concepts and comprehend technology, as well as to understand that science is continually evolving and changing. We simply know so much more and use more sophisticated tools and equipment than when our parents were young. It would be difficult for a person to understand their cardiac condition, for example, if they have no or limited understanding of what the heart looks like, how it functions and how fat can build up in the blood vessels feeding the heart muscle and cause a shortage of blood and, in some cases, the death of the muscle.

Civic literacy refers to the ability of individuals to be aware of public issues, participate in discussions and be involved in decisions that affect their lives. Individuals with civic literacy can use various forms of media (such as the internet, social media, newspapers and television) to be informed of health and social issues, and government systems and processes. This form of literacy is important because it allows a person to be aware of services in their area or to understand changes in government health policy that might affect the care or benefits they receive. Individuals who possess civic literacy understand that personal behaviours and choices affect others in their community. This may involve obeying laws that ban cigarette smoking in public places, or voluntarily contributing time and effort to organisations that raise awareness and promote health (such as the Asthma Foundation).

Finally, cultural literacy refers to individuals' abilities to identify, understand and respect the collective beliefs and customs of diverse groups in the community (Zarcadoolas, Pleasant & Greer 2006). For example, childbearing women of Chinese ethnicity commonly 'do the month' or *zuo yuezi* after the birth of the baby. It is common for these women to receive considerable

Health literacy: the ability to read, comprehend and act on medical information, and effectively interact with the health care system.

CROSS-REFERENCE

The role of culture in defining illness and reactions to illness is discussed in Chapters 1 and 4.

social support from their family such as the woman's mother, mother-in-law or other female relative. During this postnatal confinement period the woman is encouraged to rest, feed the baby and restore the lost 'yang' or heat to her body. Cultural literacy is particularly important in effective health communication and requires health professionals to understand the culture of patients. A Chinese woman living in Australia is not likely to accept health information that contravenes these traditional beliefs.

> **CASE STUDY**
>
> ## ANNE ELMORE AND UNDERSTANDING HEALTH RESEARCH ON HORMONE REPLACEMENT THERAPY
>
> Anne Elmore is a 52-year-old woman who experiences symptoms associated with menopause. Her doctor prescribed hormone replacement therapy (HRT) three years ago. At the time, Anne recalled that the doctor told her the tablets were to reduce symptoms such as hot flushes and to improve her mood so she would be less prone to tears and irritability. While driving to work one morning, she heard a report on the news: 'Researchers from the University of Queensland released a report that links HRT to ovarian cancer. Furthermore, recent trials that randomly assigned women to HRT or a placebo found that women on HRT were at increased risk for heart attack or stroke.'
>
> In order to understand this information, Anne drew on her scientific and health knowledge from her reading about health topics in magazines and searches on the internet. Let us imagine possible outcomes if Anne possessed different health literacy levels.
>
> *An example of limited health literacy.* Anne decides she is satisfied with her tablets. Her symptoms reduced in frequency and intensity, although they did not disappear. Her mother passed away from ovarian cancer, but she never had HRT. The news report annoys Anne, who thinks how scientists are always finding out that they did not know what they thought they knew. Consequently, she chooses to ignore the report and does not discuss it during her next appointment with her doctor to get a new prescription.
>
> *An example of adequate health literacy.* Anne knows that she has been on HRT for the past three years. Because her mother passed away from ovarian cancer six months ago, she knows that she has a higher risk of cancer herself. She is not sure what a placebo is, but because she has a scheduled appointment with her doctor next month, she decides to talk to her about the news report.
>
> *An example of good health literacy.* Anne knows that long-term HRT may have associated health risks. She recognises that the news report discussed the findings of a well-conducted study by reputable researchers. Given that the report linked HRT and ovarian cancer, and that her mother's recent death was from ovarian cancer, Anne believes that she may be at increased risk for this cancer. She sets out to find more information about HRT and ovarian cancer on the internet. She also makes an appointment to discuss her HRT protocol with her doctor in the next day or so with a view to discussing her risk and possibly stopping the medication.
>
> From the examples presented, it is easy to imagine different health outcomes for Anne based on her level of health literacy. In the third scenario, as an informed consumer of health care services, Anne proactively looks after her health, seeks to keep informed about

medical research and has a 'partnership' relationship with her GP. Her health outcomes are likely to be significantly better than if she had limited health literacy.

1   How could researchers better convey important findings in the media?

2   From your reading of social inequalities and health in the previous chapter, what might be some of the sociocultural factors that have positively influenced Anne's level of health literacy?

3   How common do you think it might be for health professionals to provide care for someone like Anne portrayed in the third scenario of good health literacy?

PREVALENCE OF POOR HEALTH LITERACY IN THE COMMUNITY

Governments in many developed countries have a vested interest in determining and improving the level of health literacy in the community. Adequate levels of health literacy in the population reduce health care costs, prevent illness and chronic disease, and reduce rates of accidents and death (ABS 2009a). In Australia, the **Adult Literacy and Life Skills Survey** (ALLS; ABS 2009a) aims to measure the literacy of adults aged 15 to 74 years. There are four sections in the ALLS: prose, document, numeracy and health literacy. Prose literacy is the ability to understand written information presented in newspapers and magazines. Document literacy is the knowledge and skills to use information presented in tables and charts. Numeracy involves the use of numbers across various situations (for example, measuring a dose of cough medicine).

Adult Literacy and Life Skills: a national survey to measure the literacy of adults aged 15 to 74 years.

Skill level on the ALLS is categorised from Level 1 (lowest) to Level 5 (highest). Skill Level 3 is regarded as the minimum required for individuals to meet the complex demands of everyday life. The most recent ALLS survey by the Australian Bureau of Statistics (2009a) identified that 19 per cent of adults had Level 1 health literacy skills and 40 per cent had Level 2. These people had difficulty with tasks such as reading information on a medicine bottle to find out the maximum number of days the medicine should be taken, or drawing a line on a container to indicate where one third would be. Only 41 per cent of adults had adequate or better health literacy skills, scoring Level 3 or above. At this level a person can combine information in text (such as understanding information on a brochure) and from a graph to correctly assess the safety of a product for them (such as the recommended dose of a drug for their weight).

The Australian ALLS survey results are similar to those in other countries. An ALLS survey of Canadians (aged 16–65 years) found that only 45 per cent of the population had adequate or better health literacy (Canadian Council on Learning 2008). Similarly, in the United States it is estimated that low health literacy affects over 36 per cent of people (Sheridan et al. 2011).

PAUSE & REFLECT

Think about when you began your program of study to become a health professional. What were some terms that were new to you? How did your lecturers help you to understand and remember these medical or scientific terms or concepts? What learning strategies were effective for you?

SOCIOCULTURAL FACTORS ASSOCIATED WITH LOW HEALTH LITERACY

There are several social and cultural factors associated with health literacy. These factors include age, education, income, self-assessed health status, employment status, occupation, being born overseas, first language and reading literacy. The prevalence of these factors in individuals with poor health literacy is summarised in Table 15.1. Unfortunately, relatively few health professionals are aware the rates of health literacy vary with age, or they may assume that young adults are well informed. In 2006 in Australia, around two-thirds of males and females aged 15–19 years had inadequate or low health literacy (ABS 2009a). The proportion of people with low health literacy decreased to around half of all people aged 20–49 years, before increasing once again in older age groups. Low health literacy in younger people may be because they are still completing their education and have fewer health-related experiences to draw upon. Low levels of health literacy in older age groups may be associated with the effects of age on information processing skills, and fewer years of formal education.

CROSS-REFERENCE

Social and cultural factors in defining and reacting to illness are discussed in Chapters 1 and 4.

Table 15.1   Prevalence of factors associated with poor health literacy

FACTOR	CATEGORY	PREVALENCE OF LOW HEALTH LITERACY (%)
Age	aged 15–19	65–70
	aged 20–49	50
	aged 50–74	60
Education	bachelor's degree or above	25
	completed their formal education	50
	Year 10 education or below	84
Income	high income	37
	middle income	57
	low income	74
Employment status	employed	53
	unemployed or not in labour force	75
Occupation	professionals	29
	labourers	76
Place of birth	born in a country other than Australia	66
	born in Australia	57
First language	English as a second language	75
	native English speaker	56
Assistance to read English	needing help to read information in English	81
	no assistance required	19
Self-assessed health status	who describe their health as poor or fair	75
	who describe their health as excellent or very good	52

Adapted from: *Australian Social Trends* (ABS 2009a).

The relationship between education and health is well recognised. People who complete higher levels of education are more likely to have higher rates of adequate health literacy (ABS 2009a). Around 75 per cent of people with a bachelor's degree or higher have adequate to good health literacy compared with only 16 per cent of people who finished their education at Year 10 (ABS 2009a). Generally, people with higher income have higher levels of education, as well as better health literacy skills. Like income, workforce status is influenced by educational attainment. Consequently, people employed in occupations requiring a high level of education and skill are more likely to have higher levels of health literacy.

People born overseas or whose first language is not English may have more difficulty understanding health information. In 2006, nearly three million Australians aged 15–74 years spoke English as a second language (ABS 2009a). Only a quarter of this group had adequate or better health literacy.

IMPLICATIONS OF LOW HEALTH LITERACY

There are several implications of low health literacy. Individuals with low health literacy may experience difficulty understanding what doctors, nurses, pharmacists and other health professionals tell them, as well as understanding written medical instructions. Even when individuals can access good health services, a lack of understanding of relevant information can make it challenging for them and their families to manage their illness or condition and make informed decisions (Bade et al. 2008). Individuals with low health literacy also have increased risk for hospitalisation (Baker et al. 2011). Importantly, people with low health literacy receive less preventive health care (such as screening for cancer and cardiovascular disease), and are likely to attend accident and emergency departments more often.

On a day-to-day basis, people with low health literacy may experience difficulty in a range of tasks that many of us consider routine. Challenges can include getting a prescription filled, understanding information about how to take medication and possible side effects, understanding appointment slips and reading a health promotion brochure. These routine skills are essential in order for a person to understand their condition and be able to act on certain information in order to improve their health. According to Parvanta and colleagues (2011), a person's health literacy influences their behaviour to:

- adopt healthier behaviours in their daily lives
- respond appropriately to health-related information
- share information with health-care providers
- manage their own health care
- be able to access services and how to learn what services are available.

People with limited health literacy also may feel ashamed about their lack of knowledge and skills, and may not voluntarily speak up if they do not understand information (Wolfe et al. 2007). Unfortunately, many health professionals seriously underestimate patients' health literacy levels. In one survey of 240 health professionals attending an education session on health literacy in the USA, fewer than 12 per cent correctly estimated the prevalence of adult health literacy (Jukkala, Dupree & Graham 2009). Those surveyed incorrectly believed that well-educated individuals were not at risk for low health literacy, and 16 per cent had no knowledge of what health literacy was prior to attending the session (Jukkala, Dupree & Graham 2009). Another study found that 80 per cent of nurses surveyed 'never' or 'rarely' formally assessed

CROSS-REFERENCE

The role of health professionals in promoting health is discussed further in Chapter 16.

health literacy; instead, 60 per cent reported using their 'gut feeling' to determine a patient's level of understanding. Just over half (56 per cent) of the nurses surveyed thought health literacy was a low priority compared with other patient problems (Macabasco-O'Connell & Fry Bowers 2011).

CASE STUDY

KAMALA SANJAY AND DIABETES SELF-MANAGEMENT

Kamala was born in Singapore to Indian parents. At the age of 32 she migrated to Australia to take up a senior position with a multinational accounting firm. She is married and has two adult children. Due to her long hours at work and sedentary lifestyle, Kamala had an incremental weight gain. Now at age 58 she weighs 86 kilograms and has a BMI (body mass index) of 30. Recently she felt very thirsty throughout the day and night, was urinating frequently and had extreme unexplained fatigue.

At the doctor's surgery, Kamala was given a brochure that contained the following information about diabetes: 'According to the Australian Diabetes Association, diabetes is a disease in which the body does not produce or properly use insulin. Insulin is a hormone that is needed to convert sugar, starches and other food into energy needed for life. The cause of diabetes is a mystery, although both genetics and environmental factors appear to play important roles.'

Kamala did not understand some of terminology or scientific concepts in the brochure, but agreed with her doctor's suggestion to run some tests to confirm the diagnosis of diabetes. She was referred to a diabetes clinic at the local hospital and made an appointment for the following day. That night Kamala searched the internet for more information. From personal experience she now knew some of the symptoms of diabetes, but didn't know what caused them. She decided to write down each symptom and learn about the related physiology, such as how the body produces insulin and the role of insulin in regulating the amount of sugar in the blood. Kamala had a medical dictionary and looked up every word that was unfamiliar to her. She also found that type 2 diabetes mellitus is a chronic disease associated with physical inactivity, poor diet and excess body weight. She was shocked to see that she had all the risk factors.

The next day at the clinic, Kamala had more tests and spoke with the endocrinologist about her condition. She was prescribed medication and was told to 'change her behaviour about eating and to exercise regularly'. She was also told to have her eyes checked and take good care of her feet by going to a podiatrist, although she had no idea why. She then had a session with the nurse in the clinic, who taught her how to measure her blood sugar (glucose) levels by pricking her finger (which hurt more than she thought it would) and testing the blood in a small device. Based on the reading, she then had to calculate how much insulin to inject. She was taught how do give herself an injection, which she found difficult. Five hours later, Kamala left the clinic to go to a chemist to purchase the blood glucose machine and have her prescription filled. By the end of the day she was exhausted, overwhelmed and burst into tears when her husband asked how the day went.

1   After initially reading the passage on diabetes, Kamala didn't understand several words (such as 'insulin', 'hormone' and 'properly convert'). Indeed, there are a number of key scientific concepts embedded in the passage. Can you identify these scientific concepts?

2   What can Kamala do to reduce the high level of stress she is experiencing?

3   What strategies could she have used to remember all the information she was given throughout the day?

4   How could the clinic change their process to reduce stress and information overload for patients?

Points to consider

Kamala, like many other in similar circumstances, has a great deal to learn about her condition. Although patient education is considered to be a key component of diabetes care, studies show that many patients who have attended a diabetes education program, especially those with low health literacy, still do not know the basis of their disease or the essential self-management skills (Funnell et al. 2010). For example, 50 per cent of people with low health literacy did not know that all people have some glucose (sugar) in their blood. One reason may be that most diabetes self-management education programs introduce too much information in a complex manner. Often that information is not linked to what a person needs to do on a day-to-day basis. Therefore a person receiving this education will not retain essential information because it's not seen as relevant or useful to them.

THEORETICAL CONSIDERATIONS TO ENHANCE HEALTH LITERACY

MEMORY AND COGNITIVE LOAD

Research in the field of cognitive psychology has demonstrated that a number of steps must occur in order for learning to take place. According to Wolfe et al. (2011), in order for learning to occur the person must:

1   accurately understand and make sense of new information in working memory

2   combine the new information with their existing background knowledge (things that are already known)

3   encode the information into long-term memory

4   retain that information until it is actually needed

5   retrieve that information at the correct time in order for the information to be used.

Learning can be defined as a change in long-term memory. When a person with a health condition successfully learns new information, it is understood in working memory, combined with existing knowledge and placed into long-term memory as part of a connected system of ideas. The act of combining new and existing knowledge fosters the formation of **schemas** (Clark, Nguyen & Sweller 2006). A schema is a map of ideas about a topic or issue. As the person

Learning: a change in behaviour that results from experience with the environment.

Schema: a map of ideas about a topic stored in long-term memory.

CROSS-REFERENCE
Memory and learning
are discussed in detail
in Chapters 6 and 7.

<u>**Working memory:**</u>
information that is
temporarily stored for
use in the short term.

<u>**Cognitive load:**</u> the
amount of information
kept in the working
memory.

encounters new information, they revise and update their existing schema. This new pattern of ideas is then encoded (stored) into long-term memory for retrieval at a later time when needed.

According to cognitive psychology, **working memory** allows us to temporarily store and use information in short-term memory (Baddeley 2003). Working memory is critical in almost all complex cognitive tasks (such as reading, reasoning and problem-solving). These tasks require the individual to hold information in memory while at the same time doing something else (or in the face of distractions). For example, when reading, working memory helps the reader to focus on certain elements of what they are reading, as well as keeping track of and monitor their understanding of information in the text. So if you were reading a novel, you will use your working memory to understand what you are reading in the third paragraph on the page, but also remember the key ideas in the previous paragraphs keep the overall plot in mind.

Working memory also allows individuals to ignore less essential information in order to avoid information overload. **Cognitive load** represents how much information a person can keep in the working memory. In the case of Kamala, she complained of 'information overload' when she was confronted with a lot of new information in a short space of time. The capacity of the working memory is relatively fixed. Miller (1956) first reported that the maximum number of elements that a person could remember and manipulate was around seven (plus or minus two). Clearly this proposal was made before the widespread use of ten-digit mobile phone numbers! However, the point is that the more a person has to learn in a short amount of time, the more difficult it is to process that information in working memory.

The amount of information that can be stored in memory is greater if the person is familiar with the content being presented. This is because related information has already been stored in long-term memory. This stored information can be retrieved and placed into the working memory, allowing the person to then focus on making links between what is known and the new information. So people who have less knowledge of a health topic will experience greater cognitive load when learning about the topic—because all the information is 'new'. Although Kamala spent time researching her diabetic condition, the concepts would have still been relatively unfamiliar to her. Looking up the information on the internet, and then discussing this same information at the diabetes clinic, would have assisted her understanding and retention of key points. However, it would not guarantee full understanding and recall. Key ideas or concepts may need to be revisited several times before learning occurs.

Working memory can be expanded if the information is stored in schemas that can be recalled as a large piece from the long-term memory (Clark, Nguyen & Sweller 2006). New information being discussed in a health education session, for example, should be designed to present blocks of information in order to build schemas of information that can be recalled and used later. People with low health literacy are less likely to use long-term memory because they have less background knowledge and no relevant schemas to draw on, compared with individuals who have higher literacy (Wolf et al. 2009). This does not mean that the person is less intelligent, but rather that they may have limited exposure to ideas about health, physiology and blood chemistry. Therefore, these new basic concepts need to be learnt and understood before further new knowledge is learnt and applied in day-to-day life to self-manage their condition. Teaching strategies to help Kamala form schemas could include having a plan or an overview of key topics to be learnt, using diagrams to explain concepts, taking notes and asking questions, and checking understanding before moving on to the next topic. Furthermore, Kamala could have been given printed materials to take home with her, as well as a written summary of key points to act on.

MASTERY LEARNING

Mastery learning theory (Ryan & Schmidt 1979) proposes that individuals learn at different rates, but can master material if given multiple opportunities (that is, practice makes perfect). Although the amount an individual can learn in a given time is relatively fixed, with repetition most can achieve mastery. To achieve mastery it is essential to: specify the learning objective or goal; present the content in tailored sequential blocks that builds on content; evaluate to determine whether the information has been mastered; and provide corrective, remedial teaching until mastery is attained.

The importance of **mastery learning** was demonstrated in a study that examined the number of times patients needed information repeated in order to understand informed consent (Sudore et al. 2006). Informed consent needs to be obtained by a health professional before conducting an invasive procedure. The patient indicates in writing that they have been informed about what the procedure involves and are aware of the risks. Although all participants mastered the material, 28 per cent achieved mastery on their first attempt, 52 per cent required two attempts and 20 per cent required three or more. Individuals with adequate literacy were more likely to pass on the first attempt.

INTERVENTIONS TO ENHANCE HEALTH LITERACY

Sheridan et al. (2011) undertook a systematic review of published research studies that tested the effectiveness of interventions for people with low health literacy. Of the thirty-eight studies that were reviewed, Sheridan et al. (2011) concluded that specific design features of an intervention improved comprehension. These features included:

- presenting essential information by itself or first
- presenting information so that the higher number is better
- adding icon arrays to numerical information (for example, a cartoon figure of a person where one figure represents 100 people)
- adding video/DVD to verbal discussions of topics.

The review also identified that interventions about self-care and disease management that were delivered in a short time frame (also called intensive mode) reduced the likelihood of the disease condition getting worse. People receiving health education in an intensive way also had fewer emergency department visits and hospitalisations. The extent to which the interventions were effective on changing other outcomes (such as adherence to health screening follow-up) was not clear. The reviewers concluded that interventions with multiple components showed promise for addressing low health literacy in clinical practice. Different components could include discussions, dvds, pictures, diagrams and practice sessions for skill development.

Common features of effective interventions to increase understanding included frequent sessions, using a framework (from learning theories) to inform the design of the intervention, doing a pilot test first to identify any problems, an emphasis on skill building, and delivery by an expert health professional (such as a pharmacist or a diabetes educator). Other features included using simplified text and teach-back approaches (see below). Findings of the systematic review also indicated the importance of first assessing a person's level of literacy and then deciding on the best approach for them rather than offering universal interventions (Sheridan et al. 2011). This means tailoring a health education session on the needs of the person rather than offering the same information and strategies to everyone and in the same way.

CROSS-REFERENCE
Mastery influences self-efficacy beliefs and behaviour, as discussed in Chapter 7.

Mastery learning: the repetition of a task until learning occurs.

CROSS-REFERENCE
Self-care is discussed in Chapter 5.

Teach-back: a learning cycle involving repetition and reinforcement of new learning.

Teach-back is a useful strategy for improving understanding and recall of health information by people with low literacy (Sudore & Schillinger 2009). Teach-back is a learning cycle. Firstly, the health care provider provides information or teaches a skill. They then check understanding by asking the patient to repeat, in their own words, what they know or need to do. If there is a gap in the person's understanding, the health care provider can review the information again and fill in the missing pieces or correct any errors in the skill. The person then repeats what they know or need to do. Teach-back may be an effective way to support long-term learning because it slows down the learning process and allows for repetition and reinforcement of new information. Teach-back approaches are effective because cognitive experiments have shown that repeating short sequences of information helps to activate the memory dedicated to storage and recall of information.

One research team found that while teach-back did assist in immediate recall of information, patients did not retain the information when tested two weeks later (Kandula et al. 2011). Indeed, all the participants, regardless of their literacy level, forgot approximately half the new information. Clearly further research is needed to identify the best way to encourage learning and long-term recall.

GUIDING PRINCIPLES FOR INTERVENTIONS TO ENHANCE HEALTH LITERACY

There is increasing amounts of research evaluating the effectiveness of strategies to promote health literacy. Some guiding principles for effective interventions were proposed by Baker and colleagues (2011) and are described below.

1 *Establish a defined set of learning goals and develop the curriculum(or learning program)*. There needs to be a limited set of learning goals for any educational program or set of materials. There is often a tendency to try to cover too much information. All information in a health education program should: explain a behaviour; provide background information to understand a recommended behaviour (that is, explain the underlying scientific concept); or promote attitude change about the behaviour (for example, explain how the behaviour helps the person). It may be helpful to work backwards in order to identify what information is necessary to understand the concept and change behaviour.

2 *Present information in discrete units*. A health education program should be divided into simple units of learning. The plan needs to logical, easily understood and remembered by participants. The program should start with behaviours that could prevent deterioration in the condition (that is, what the person needs to do to stay well) and finish with the most crucial behaviours for monitoring their condition and maintaining their their well-being. People are likely to remember information if only a few key points are presented rather than a lot of content. This approach reduces information overload.

3 *Determine the optimal order for each topic*. The order of content in the program needs to prepare learners for what is to follow.

4 *Use plain language and pictorial aids*. Using plain language to explain essential concepts is important, but there are other considerations as well. The plain language needs to be presented in an organised way (see point 1). Consideration needs to be given to the amount of information presented (point 2) and background information needs to be provided first (point 3).

5   Different forms of graphics (such as diagrams, pictures and cartoons) can be used to increase understanding and recall. Individuals with low health literacy may have limited reading fluency. They typically read slowly and struggle with individual words and phrases and may not grasp the meaning of a sentence or paragraph. Graphics can assist understanding by presenting complex concepts simply. There is a Chinese proverb attributed to Confucius that says 'a picture paints a thousand words'. In health education, a picture can be far more descriptive of something than words can ever be. Visual representations of ideas are understood and remembered more easily.

6   *Confirm mastery of learning goals.* Health professionals should confirm the person's understanding after each session, perform corrective or remedial instruction until mastery is attained, and review learned concepts until the person consistently masters the task. As discussed previously, learning could be checked through teach-back methods.

7   *Link information to behaviour change.* Knowledge, skills and behaviours need to be closely linked. This approach is known as '**teach to goal**' and involves the clear identification of content and skills to be learnt in order to change behaviour. All too often, health education interventions deliver information but do not teach the associated behaviour at the same time. Goals for specific behaviours should be established immediately after a person has understood the reasons for it and mastered the skills for performing it. The approach of linking education immediately to personal action plans has been used successfully in programs addressing chronic conditions such as diabetes (Wallace et al. 2009) and can also be applied to other chronic conditions such as cardiovascular disease.

Teach to goal: content and skills to be learnt in order to change behaviour.

GETTING THE MOST FROM EXISTING HEALTH SERVICES

In Australia, primary health care is most often provided through general practices. GPs are a valuable resource for information and health promotion. However, opportunities to enhance health literacy of people during a routine consultation are limited because of time constraints and lack of evidence-based health materials for GPs to give to patients. Research shows that most people find health information difficult to understand (Torpy, Burke & Golub 2011). This includes advice from doctors, nurses, pharmacists and other health professionals, along with written medical instructions and medical forms. Research is continuing to determine the best way to improve health literacy. The internet is a good source of health information if reliable sites are accessed. Government websites (such as the Australian Institute of Health & Welfare and the National Health & Medical Research Council) and not-for-profit organisations (such as the Cancer Council and the Heart Foundation) are trusted sources of information and are regularly updated. Increasing knowledge and empowering individuals to make informed decisions not only improves individuals' health status but also that of the family and community.

PAUSE 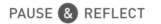 REFLECT

What advice would you give a family member with a chronic condition so they can make the most of a visit to their GP?

Torpy, Burke and Golub (2011) suggested that when visiting a GP, individuals could do the following:

- Write down their questions and concerns prior to the visit so nothing is forgotten.
- Take a trusted person, such as a family member or close friend.
- Always ask questions if they do not understanding something. The doctor or health professional wants to make sure patients know about their condition and how to follow medical instructions.
- Always bring an up-to-date list of all medications, including over the counter drugs and any natural or herbal preparations.
- Ask the doctor to write down information and instructions discussed during the visit.
- If the person has hearing or sight difficulties, ask the doctor to provide information in large print or use other resources.

CASE STUDY

PETER COSTA AND CARDIAC FAILURE

The aim of this case study is to explore how the learning principles for effective health education can be applied to assist a person who has heart failure.

Peter was born in 1948 and migrated to Australia from Italy in 1961 with his parents, three younger brothers and sister. He attended high school but struggled with English as a second language. At 15, he left school and commenced a carpentry apprenticeship with his uncle. Peter eventually established his own business. He married in 1974 and had three children. Because he did a lot of physical work, he was always able to eat and drink what he wanted without gaining a lot of weight. He smoked a pack of cigarettes a day and had beer in the afternoon after work and a glass of wine nearly every night. Two years ago, he suffered shortness of breath and after urging from his wife he went to see his GP. He was diagnosed with mild emphysema and hypertension (high blood pressure); he also had high cholesterol readings. Medication was prescribed, but Peter took this only when he experienced some symptoms. He subsequently suffered heart failure and after recovery in hospital was discharged home and referred to a cardiac rehabilitation clinic.

When Peter attended the cardiac rehabilitation clinic, he was asked to complete a short questionnaire to assess his level of health literacy. Peter read slowly and struggled with some words and phrases. He had relatively good numeracy skills due to his work as a carpenter.

The cardiac rehabilitation program was run by a team of nurses in consultation with specialist doctors, a pharmacist, physiotherapist, occupational therapist and exercise physiologist. As the program aimed to meet individual needs, the nurse educator met with Peter to discuss his learning goals. In order to help Peter manage his condition he needed to learn how to monitor his physical symptoms every day, take his medications as prescribed, have a low-salt diet, exercise regularly and adjust the dose of his diuretic medication if there were signs of fluid build-up in his body.

In line with the learning goals, Peter learnt about five topics: the nature of heart failure, medication, lowering salt intake, exercise and daily check-ups. Peter found this approach easy to understand and could remember the four things he needed to do. He needed to learn how to prevent deterioration of his heart condition (medication adherence and low-salt diet) and maintain health (daily check-up and exercise).

When he was discharged from hospital, Peter was told to weigh himself daily and was given an action plan if his weight changed by a certain amount (for example, to take two diuretic pills instead of one if his weight increased by more than two kilograms).

In order for Peter to maintain a low-salt diet (the goal), he was taught that salt is the same as sodium, that some foods are high in sodium even if salt is not added, and that foods labelled as low sodium have 140mg or less of sodium. Peter acknowledged that because his wife does all the shopping, he had little knowledge about the information on food labels. He needed this skill in order to calculate his daily sodium intake and therefore maintain a low-salt diet.

Addressing this learning goal highlighted to the team that certain skills they thought were well understood by the general public (such as reading a food label) did not apply to everyone. The team thought it might be useful to include Peter's wife in the education sessions.

For every topic there was an immediate behaviour that Peter had to practise. He learnt how heart failure occurs and so understood the importance of doing his daily check-up. He also knew why he had to change existing behaviours (such as giving up smoking and taking less salt). Six months later, Peter had lost eight kilograms, stopped smoking and was taking his medication regularly. He and his wife were looking forward to a more active and enjoyable life.

1   Based on his case history, what do you think Peter's level of health literacy would be?

2   What are Peter's likely strengths for learning and challenges for his learning?

3   Peter struggled to understand the need to weigh himself daily and vary his intake of diuretic pills accordingly. Why do you think this would be?

4   What were the benefits of including Peter's wife in his rehabilitation?

Points to consider

Cardiovascular disease (CVD) is the largest cause of premature death in Australia. CVD relates to the health of the heart, blood vessels and organs that depend on a strong blood supply (AIHW 2010). The major CVDs are coronary heart disease, stroke, heart failure and peripheral vascular disease. CVD is usually due to a build up of fat, cholesterol and other substances in the inner lining of arteries (known as atherosclerosis). Atherosclerosis accounted for over a third of all deaths in 2007. In that year an estimated 3.4 million Australians (16.5 per cent of the population) had one or more long-term diseases of the circulatory system (AIHW 2010). Around one in four people with CVD also report having a disability that restricted their self-care, mobility or communication. People with CVD are also more likely to report medium to high levels of psychological distress, fair or poor mental and physical health, and depression (AIHW 2010).

CHAPTER SUMMARY

- Health literacy is the ability of individuals to understand their health, medical care and overall wellness.
- Individuals with low literacy have difficulty reading and understanding written information, comprehending numerical information, performing calculations and understanding ranges of normal values (such as normal range for blood pressure). They tend to have poorer baseline knowledge, short-term memory and working memory compared with individuals with higher literacy.
- Inadequate health literacy is common among the elderly, individuals with chronic conditions or disability, individuals who do not speak English as a first language and people with a mental illness.
- Health professionals seriously underestimate the prevalence of low health literacy, and often fail to identify individuals with low health literacy.
- Improving health literacy through targeted education programs that provide information and motivate individuals to adopt healthy behaviours is important for illness prevention, reducing hospitalisations, improving quality of life and reducing health care costs. However, effective and efficient methods for self-management education remain unclear.
- Patient-provider communication plays an important role in care. Provider knowledge of patient characteristics associated with low health literacy influence these interactions.

SELF TEST

1 What are the elements of health literacy?
   a fundamental, civic and cultural
   b scientific, fundamental, cultural and civic
   c conceptual, scientific, cultural and civic
   d fundamental, numerical, civic and cultural.
2 Complete the following statement. Numeracy is an important aspect of literacy in order for individuals to understand:
   a the correct timing and dose of medications
   b risk and risk-benefit information
   c whether a measured value is within the recommended range
   d all of the above.
3 In order to successfully learn new information, an individual must do the following except:
   a process the information in working memory
   b integrate this with existing background knowledge
   c encode it into short-term memory
   d retain and retrieve it at the appropriate time.
4 The integration of new and background knowledge fosters the formation of schemas. A schema could be defined as the way in which:
   a a person thinks about a concept
   b a person organises ideas that can be revised and updated

    c new information is encountered, processed and encoded

    d new information is associated with existing knowledge.

5 Max is 64 years old and recovering from a recent heart attack. He needs to reduce his sodium intake but is unsure how to do this. The registered nurse at the cardiac rehabilitation clinic can use a variety of teaching strategies to assist Max. Which of the following would be most effective?

    a Confirm Max's understanding after each session.

    b Perform corrective instruction until mastery is attained.

    c Review learned concepts each time Max attends the clinic.

    d Use teach-back methods to ensure mastery.

FURTHER READING

Parvanta, C., Nelson, D.E., Parvanta, S.A. & Harner, R.N. (2011). *Essentials of Public Health Communication*. Sudbury, MA: Jones & Bartlett Learning.

Weiss, B.D., Mantz, W., De Walt, D.A., Pignone, M.P., Mockbee, J. & Hale, FA. (2005) Quick assessment of literacy in primary care: the newest vital sign. *Annals of Family Medicine*, 3, 514–22.

Wolf, M.S., Williams, M.V., Parker, R.M., Parikh, N.S., Nowlan, A.W. & Baker, D.W. (2007). Patients' shame and attitudes toward discussing the result of literacy screening. *Journal of Health Communication: International Perspectives*, 12(8), 721–32.

USEFUL WEBSITES

Cardiomyopathy is a disease of the heart which can affect anyone at any time (Cardiomyopathy Association of Australia):

www.cmaa.org.au/index.html

Coronary heart disease video:

www.youtube.com/watch?v=zfi5roAExMk&feature=relmfu

Heart disease support services:

www.healthinsite.gov.au/topics/Heart_Disease_Support_Services

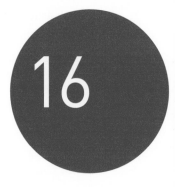

PROMOTING HEALTH AND PREVENTING ILLNESS

CHAPTER OBJECTIVES

By the end of your study of this chapter, you should be able to:

- describe and compare the concepts of illness prevention and health promotion
- understand the different types and levels of intervention and how these influence the behaviour and health of target groups
- be aware of the advantages and disadvantages of reactive treatment of illness and disease as compared with illness prevention and health promotion
- understand that access and equity issues may arise in illness prevention and health promotion, as well as in treatment of illness and disease.

KEYWORDS

health promotion
illness prevention
primary prevention
secondary prevention
teachable moments
tertiary prevention

INTRODUCTION

To this point in the text, the impression may have been given that illness is unavoidable: something that must be accepted and then coped with. It would be unfortunate not to challenge that impression. Much can be done to decrease the occurrence of illness and to increase the levels of health and well-being experienced by individuals and communities. This is a highly desirable outcome, not only because of the reduction in suffering and the improvement in quality and quantity of life that would follow, but also because of the reduction in expenditure necessary to treat illness. As a result, illness prevention and health promotion have become major growth areas in health care.

JULIE PERNFORS AND A YOUNG MOTHERS' PROGRAM

CASE STUDY

The aim of this case is to examine the role of illness prevention and health promotion in advancing the health of a group with special needs.

Julie Pernfors is a nurse who works with mothers and babies in the maternity unit of a general hospital. She believes that many of the youngest mothers, who are often in their early to mid teens, do not have enough knowledge and skills to successfully cope with their babies during the first days and weeks at home. Working together with other nurses in the unit, Julie would like to improve the health of babies and of their mothers during this critical time.

Young mothers are usually at high risk for parenting stress. Many will have dropped out of school, be unemployed and be in an unstable relationship with poor social support, meaning they are unlikely to receive the support they need to mother their baby successfully. Young mothers can potentially experience a great deal of difficulty if the baby suffers colic, cries for prolonged periods or cannot settle at night. Crying is a common trigger for child abuse. All infants cry; crying generally begins in the first month of life, and the duration of crying increases and peaks between two and four months of age. Understanding why the baby is crying and learning how to soothe the baby are important mothering skills.

1   What approaches could Julie and her colleagues use to prevent illness for the babies and mothers?
2   Some young mothers may have unrealistic expectations of motherhood and of their baby. What might be some common misconceptions held by young mothers?
3   How can Julie and her team engage with young mothers in order to provide information and support?

Illness prevention involves interventions by health care professionals or institutions to prevent the occurrence of illness. Two major examples—smoking and injury prevention—have been selected for particular attention here, as they represent at least partial success stories for illness prevention and health promotion.

STRATEGIES TO PREVENT SMOKING

Consider the advantages that would result for a community if it could manage to discourage young people from becoming smokers. The amount of day-to-day ill health that results from smoking—including reduced fitness, morning cough, breathing difficulties and irritation to non-smokers—would be drastically reduced. In the long term, less damage would be done to lung tissues, as a result of which the occurrence of emphysema and lung cancer would decrease. The largest gain would be in cardiovascular health, as smoking is a major risk factor for heart disease and stroke. What does smoking cost the community? Collins and Lapsley (2006) estimated that the total social cost of smoking in the Australian state of Victoria alone had reached over five billion dollars a year at the end of the twentieth century. This amount will no doubt have changed somewhat due to increases in costs, and decreases in the proportion of the population who are smokers.

However, the health damage caused by cigarette smoking increases over time. After World War II, the proportion of men who smoked was very much higher than the proportion of women, and in the decades following, the rates of lung cancer in men rose as well. Subsequently, however, the proportion of women who smoked increased at the same time that there was a great decline in the proportion of men who smoked—particularly after the link between smoking and lung cancer was publicised. This has led to a significant increase over time in the number of women developing lung cancer, just as the number of men with the condition decreased (Egelston et al. 2009). Given this time lag in the true health damage of smoking becoming apparent, it will be many years before there is a significant reduction in this social cost.

Many governments have launched campaigns to reduce the damage associated with smoking, using a variety of means such as higher taxes on tobacco products, elimination of subsidies to tobacco growers (to encourage them to change crops), bans on advertising and sponsorships, health warnings and graphic pictures on packets. In 2009, the Victorian state government added legal bans on smoking in a motor vehicle if a person under 18 is present, selling tobacco products from temporary outlets, and displaying products at point of sale (except for specific places); it also introduced ministerial power to ban particular tobacco products aimed at young people (Department of Health, Victoria 2009).

STRATEGIES TO PREVENT INJURY

The cost associated with preventable accidents is enormous. This includes road accidents, workplace accidents, sporting injuries, injuries to children in play settings, and even injuries in the home. Many of these injuries are not only preventable but also have easily identifiable causes.

An example of one of these causes that has received much attention is the use of mobile phones while driving—or even while walking near traffic (Tippet 2011). Strayer, Drews and Crouch (2006) estimated that the effects of using a mobile phone while driving were equivalent to having a blood alcohol level of 0.08, which is well over the legal limit in all Australian jurisdictions. The most likely drivers to phone, or even text, while driving turn out to be the youngest drivers, who already have the highest rates of injury and death on the roads. Improvement in cars—particularly the compulsory use of seatbelts, and better roads, traffic control and enforcement—have all contributed to decreasing rates of injury and death on the roads relative to the amount of miles that are driven, but there are still many improvements that can be made.

Workplace accidents leading to injury and death are also a significant cost to the community. Safe Work Australia (2009) estimated the total cost at 5.9 per cent (or $55.5 billion) of Gross Domestic Product. Many of the accidents are preventable, whether by improving workplaces, using safety equipment, changing work practices or educating workers.

Sporting injuries can seem entirely random, but they result from the combination of a predisposed athlete (perhaps with an internal risk factor to a particular kind of injury), external factors (such as equipment, facilities and even the weather) and a particular inciting event (Meeuwisse et al. 2007). Over the course of a sport's season, the likelihood that all of these factors will occur together increases. However, each of these factors can be changed. Prevention could include testing athletes for potential vulnerabilities and counselling them about risks, improving equipment and venues, avoiding dangerous conditions, and perhaps changing the rules of a sport to reduce the occurrence of inciting events. The Australian Football League and National Rugby League, for example, have modified their rules regarding players tackling late or high.

In young children, once the first year of life is passed, accidents become the major cause of illness and death (ABS 2005). The fact that boys are more liable to injury and death resulting from accidents than girls relates to the different activities each gender undertakes, along with the different socialisation experiences and attitudes each gender experiences. There are many programs aimed at reducing childhood injury (for example, Kidsafe) that emphasise the importance of supervision in particular, but also improvements in facilities and environments, and education of children about risks.

Injuries in the home account for about one-third of all injuries, and are particularly significant for children and those over 75 years of age (Turner et al. 2011). This indicates that much of the risk is related to individual vulnerabilities, such as vision and balance problems in the elderly, and lack of understanding of risks among children. Turner et al. were not able to demonstrate that programs aimed at modifying the home environment could significantly reduce the risk of injuries; however, the available data are limited.

PAUSE & REFLECT

What are some other major health issues that would make a major change in society if people changed their behaviour?

ILLNESS PREVENTION

Although it may appear that prevention of illness and promotion of health are the same thing, there are significant differences in the approaches that these two terms describe. The key element of **illness prevention** is that it refers to interventions by health care professionals or institutions to prevent the occurrence of illness. This means that it generally describes things that are done *to* or *for* people (that is, actions that may be carried out by health professionals), but it also includes actions by governments, companies, charities or other groups in society (Raczynski & DiClemente 1999).

There are as many ways to prevent illness as there are illnesses. Prevention could include preventing individuals from injuring and killing one another during attacks of road rage, decreasing the occurrence of dental caries by fluoridation of the water supply, draining pools of water where mosquitoes breed, and making it less likely that individuals confined to bed by

Illness prevention: interventions by health care professionals or institutions to prevent the occurrence of illness.

CROSS-REFERENCE

Epidemiology is
discussed in Chapter 1.

disability will develop bed sores. Clearly, each of these will require quite different interventions. The science of epidemiology provides necessary data about the nature, distribution and determinants of health issues (Yarnell 2006).

TYPES OF PREVENTION

It is helpful to look at two dimensions of prevention: type and level. Types of prevention are primary, secondary and tertiary, depending on who the intervention is intended to reach (Edelman & Mandle 2002). Level refers to the agent involved, which may be government, community or health professionals.

PRIMARY PREVENTION

Primary prevention:
interventions that
are aimed at well
individuals or groups,
with the intention
of keeping them in
that state.

Primary prevention describes interventions that are aimed at well individuals or groups with the intention of keeping them in that state. Examples are interventions aimed at stopping people from being injured or killed in automobile accidents, reducing the number of babies who acquire HIV from their mothers during the birth process, or reducing the number of young people who take up smoking. The first could be accomplished by legal requirements for fitting cars with seatbelts (made compulsory for the first time anywhere in the world in Victoria in 1971) and airbags, which prevent injury once an accident has occurred. It could also be accomplished by improving roads or brakes so that accidents are less likely to occur. In either case, the behaviour of the individual is not the target. The incidence of birth transmission of HIV from mothers to babies could be reduced by intervention to change the behaviour of doctors and nurses before (screening and antiretroviral drugs), during (Caesarean delivery) and after birth (not breastfeeding) (Chigwedere et al. 2008). The number of young people who smoke could be reduced by decreasing the availability of cigarettes and tobacco products, and perhaps by eliminating cigarette vending machines. Smoking could also be reduced by decreasing its desirability. Increasing the cost of cigarettes by raising taxes is a common approach.

Perhaps the most familiar example of primary prevention is immunisation. Immunising children against poliomyelitis has nearly eliminated a risk of a disease that most older people remember very well. The sight of friends in iron lungs or wearing leg braces occupies a place in the memories of people aged over 60 that is not shared to the same extent by the under 60s. Smallpox vaccinations are no longer required for most of the world's children because most of the world's adults had them in the past. The recent discovery of a vaccine for human papilloma virus (HPV) (Mahoney 2006) represents hope for an enormous reduction in the risk of genital warts and cervical cancer for girls who have not been exposed to HPV, and may even help those who have already been exposed.

Health education has an important role in primary prevention. It has been suggested that health promotion can also come under the general heading of primary prevention (Edelman & Mandle 2002), but because the agent is different—as will be described later—it is clearer to consider it under a heading of its own.

PAUSE & REFLECT

Consider a particular problem associated with primary prevention in which the individuals being targeted are not ill, and therefore may not be motivated to do anything. What would be the major difficulties in implementing a primary prevention program for HIV/AIDS?

SECONDARY PREVENTION

This type of prevention aims to reduce the prevalence of illness at a particular point in time by targeting at-risk individuals. Examples of **secondary prevention** include screening for signs of the early development of cancers, getting those who already smoke to quit before they develop significant disease, and reducing high blood pressure and cholesterol levels in individuals so that the pathological changes that result in heart disease do not occur. Screening for cancer includes a range of techniques, from blood tests that may indicate the presence of prostate cancer, to mammograms to look for early signs of breast cancer, to tissue samples or inspections to detect skin cancers. These are aimed at case finding, so that treatment can begin when it is most effective.

Smoking cessation programs are based on the prevention of damage to cells and tissues, or reversing these effects. After an individual quits smoking, some of their risks decrease rapidly, and others more slowly. Where pathological cell changes have already taken place, some risks may not decrease at all.

Limiting the amount of disability that the individual experiences from disease is also an element of secondary prevention (Edelman & Mandle 2002). Such limiting may involve treatment that arrests the effects of a condition (for example, the surgical removal of a tumour) or provision of facilities that limit the disability experienced (such as exercise and lifestyle change programs for victims of a heart attack in order to prevent the occurrence of another). A heart attack does a lot to focus attention on the need for change.

One of the most effective areas of secondary prevention has been in minimising the risk of premature illness and death from heart disease and stroke through reduction in blood pressure. The essential first step is identification; blood pressure testing in at-risk groups, such as the over 40s, has become a routine part of visits to the doctor. Intervention to reduce blood pressure is increasingly common, but because this includes daily medication for most people, there are some problems with compliance. The same is also true for high cholesterol. Compliance problems can arise with any secondary intervention because the process may involve inconvenience, cost, discomfort or side effects for an individual who does not experience any of those from the condition that puts them at risk. Healthy lifestyle programs for high blood pressure often combine medication with healthy diet (including losing weight and reducing salt, caffeine and alcohol intake), exercise and stress management.

> **Secondary prevention:** interventions aimed at reducing the prevalence of illness at a particular point in time by targeting 'at-risk' individuals.

TERTIARY PREVENTION

Tertiary prevention aims to decrease the adverse consequences experienced by people who already have a disease or condition. In many cases this involves rehabilitation, or the provision of treatment to manage disability arising from disease. Tertiary prevention could, for example, include the prevention of falls and subsequent broken bones in elderly people with osteoporosis. Such prevention could be achieved by the modification of buildings to make access easier for elderly people and others with limited mobility or strength, or by using surfaces that cushion falls when they do occur. Reducing the disability experienced by children with asthma could involve identifying appropriate medications to prevent asthma attacks occurring, or to treat

> **Tertiary prevention:** interventions aimed at decreasing the adverse consequences experienced by people who already have a disease or condition.

breathlessness when such attacks occur, or it could involve identifying situations that increase the risk of an attack so that they can be avoided.

CASE STUDY

JULIE (CONT.)

Julie has decided that teenage mothers are an at-risk group, so secondary prevention activities will aim to reduce the likelihood of this risk resulting in actual disease. One target may be to encourage breastfeeding among this group, as this has advantages in terms of ensuring that the babies get adequate nourishment, which helps with the development of their immune systems and encourages bonding between the mothers and babies. Another may be to ensure that the mothers attend health centres to get expert help with any problems that arise.

A common perception is that formula feeding is perfectly adequate and breastfeeding is 'a little bit better'. However, there is a great deal of scientific evidence about the benefits of breastfeeding and the potential health hazards of formula feeding (such as infections and higher level of fat intake). Successful breastfeeding is best fostered when mothers and babies are kept in close proximity and when infants are allowed to nurse in an unrestricted fashion. However, in our fast-paced, highly mobile society, many new mothers expect their babies to conveniently fit into a structured routine. They may be unprepared for the high frequency and unpredictability of breastfeeding and the fact that breastfeeding cannot be delegated to anyone else.

Julie and her team decide that mother-to-mother support groups may be a good way to support young mothers. They can observe other breastfeeding mothers and learn how they accommodate breastfeeding within their busy schedule. The group may also help the young mothers to view their breasts as a source of infant nutrition rather than a sensual organ, which causes many nursing mothers to feel self-conscious when they need to breastfeed in public and makes others feel uncomfortable in the presence of a breastfeeding woman. Breastfeeding mothers need to know how to nurse discreetly in public and they require frequent reassurance that breastfed babies are supported.

Another important issue for teenage mothers may be that they are less confident about what services are available to them and how to obtain those services. In addition to health education, programs can also be aimed at personal development. Programs offering assertiveness skills could be offered to young mothers to encourage them to take control of their own and their baby's health. Another approach might involve encouragement to share knowledge and skills, and to develop social networks through the development of a mothers' social group.

1   What strategies could be used to attract young mothers to the group?
2   What approaches could Julie and her colleagues use to promote health for the babies and mothers?
3   What problems may affect the access of this group of mothers and babies to health and health care?

LEVELS OF PREVENTION

Regardless of whether they are primary, secondary or tertiary, preventative interventions can occur at a variety of levels within society. Some highly effective primary preventive measures have been brought about by action at a governmental or legislative level. These include changes to laws or regulations that are aimed at reducing a health threat. Seatbelt laws have dramatically decreased injuries and deaths resulting from car crashes. Gun-control laws have reduced gunshot wounds. We have recently seen massive regulatory programs, including the slaughter of millions of birds, to prevent the spread avian influenza (bird flu), aimed at the eventual prevention of a potential epidemic spread of this illness in humans.

Governments may also provide funding or other resources to make a preventative program possible. Changing the funding patterns for doctors so that they receive money for prevention of illness as well as for its treatment is an important example of such an intervention. In Australia, a great deal of attention is being paid to encouraging health professionals to practise in rural areas and, once there, to stay. These programs involve providing better support for rural practitioners, and attempt to encourage more applicants from rural areas to apply for admission to training as health professionals.

Government programs may also be aimed at secondary prevention. Mandatory identification by health professionals of child abuse is aimed at preventing long-term consequences of such abuse. Regulatory change to prevent the consequences of behaviour for at-risk individuals—such as placing clocks on gambling devices so that gamblers do not lose track of time, or placing limits on alcohol consumption—are often controversial. Many people feel that it is not the role of government to protect individuals from the consequences of their own decisions. Considering the compliance problems that have been noted to occur in secondary prevention, this should not be surprising. Tertiary government programs can include things as varied as regulation of the quality of care provided by nursing homes and fortifying beer with vitamins to prevent dietary deficiencies among problem drinkers.

Closely related to governmental changes are changes that take place at a societal level. Such changes are not legal or regulatory, but often arise out of grassroots demand for change. If enough people demand foods with lower levels of salt, sugar or animal fats, that demand will eventually be met by the market. Often, the first step towards change is that health professionals recognise the consequences of a situation for the health of the society, and this is gradually picked up by other groups within the community. The process is occasionally reversed, as when patient groups demand changes to health care to reduce undesirable actions of health professionals. The mechanism for much of the change that takes place at the societal level is education.

An interesting example of such grassroots change is the move to drinking bottled water. What makes this particularly interesting is that there are actually very few health benefits, and some health risks, from bottled water where a good community water supply is available. In Australia, most community water supplies are fluoridated to protect against dental cavities; bottled water is not, and widespread consumption of bottled instead of tap water by children may expose them to unnecessary dental disease later in life. Recently, concerns have been expressed about the effects of the plastic bottles on the water they contain. This has been one of the most successful public change programs, but is totally unnecessary for most people.

Individual level interventions play an important part in illness prevention, most often through the influence of the health professional. Identification of health needs for the individual

CROSS-REFERENCE
Behavioural prescriptions are also discussed in Chapter 8.

patient or client is increasingly seen as part of the role of all health professionals. Some individuals—both patients and professionals—see this as an unwarranted interference with the rights of the patient, an attitude that is rapidly changing. It is much more common now for a patient to be disappointed if the health professional sees a risk and does nothing about it, which can also lead to legal action against the health professional.

The most basic barrier to individual level prevention is that the professional may not be aware of the risk that the individual patient faces. It is still common for doctors and nurses not to know that particular patients smoke, or that they have undesirable levels of alcohol consumption. Other health professionals may also not have information that bears on their professional activities. Consider the importance of a nurse or physiotherapist, for example, knowing whether a patient experiences dizzy spells or if they have brittle bones because of osteoporosis. Similarly, it is vital for a radiographer to know if a patient is pregnant before risking exposure of the foetus to radiation.

PAUSE & REFLECT

Parents often bring teenage children to see health professionals and stay with them during examinations. Imagine the situation in which a 15-year-old girl is pregnant but trying to conceal that fact from her parents. Because she has abdominal pain, she is sent for x-rays. Her mother insists on staying with her while the x-rays are taken. The radiographer asks the girl if she is pregnant because the x-rays could potentially harm the foetus. Consider the issues from the viewpoint of the girl and from that of the radiographer.

CROSS-REFERENCE
Behaviour change for the individual is discussed in Chapter 8.

Once the professional has knowledge about the health needs of the patient, modifications can be made to the behaviour of either. Sometimes illness prevention is the responsibility of the professional (such as providing shielding material when a patient is exposed to radiation, or support during a period of bereavement), and sometimes it is the responsibility of the patient or client. Responsibility usually involves changes in the patient's behaviour. Achieving this change generally involves health promotion as distinct from illness prevention.

HEALTH PROMOTION

Health promotion: the process of enabling people to increase their control over, and to improve, their health.

So far, we have discussed the influence of genetics, biological, psychological and environmental factors on health. **Health promotion** involves changing some of these factors. Health professionals, even governments, cannot always enforce such changes, but they can help by providing information, skills and resources to encourage change.

The World Health Organization's *Bangkok Charter for Health Promotion in a Globalized World* (WHO 2009b: 25) defines health promotion as 'the process of enabling people to increase control over their health and its determinants, and thereby improve their health'. Health promotion involves activities carried out by people for their own benefit, rather than done for them by experts or governments. These activities may involve individuals, groups, communities or entire societies, and comprise a number of components. The WHO's various charters identify a number of activities that contribute to the promotion of health. These are to build healthy policies, create supportive environments, strengthen community action, develop personal skills (a major focus of this book) and reorient health services (WHO 2009).

As with illness prevention, health promotion can be primary, secondary or tertiary. Primary health promotion involves changes made to promote health in a healthy population, secondary to promote health in an at-risk population, and tertiary to promote health for those who already have a disease or condition. Table 16.1 gives a grid of examples.

Table 16.1   Health promotion interventions

	INDIVIDUAL	GROUP	SOCIETY
Primary	Teaching a child how to brush their teeth properly	Stress management workshop for university students	Mass media campaign to encourage seatbelt use
Secondary	Individual coping skills training for siblings of addicts	Weight loss group for sedentary office workers	Meals on Wheels program to improve nutrition for the elderly
Tertiary	Developing a diabetes management plan for a patient	Self-help group for patients with schizophrenia	Lobbying for public transport with easy disabled access

Health promotion can be carried out in a variety of settings, such as schools, workplaces, health care settings or in the community (Richmond & Germov 2005). It may be more accurate to say 'communities' in the latter case, as there are often advantages in targeting specific groups within the larger society, such as the elderly, rural residents or Indigenous communities (Dew & Kirkman 2002; O'Connor-Fleming & Parker 2001).

Clearly, the potential scope of health promotion is enormous, and there are many groups in society that are involved in activities that could be seen as health promotion. One of the largest of these groups is health professionals.

HEALTH PROFESSIONALS AND HEALTH PROMOTION

Health professionals are in many ways ideally placed to involve themselves in health promotion as they are seen as having expertise, access to knowledge and resources, and prestige. More and more, health professionals see health promotion as part of their duties (Edelman & Mandle 2002). At the same time, it is often true that the approaches used by health professionals are not well thought out, and they can end up being ineffective or even counterproductive. Doctors who badger patients repeatedly to quit smoking, without at the same time giving adequate information on why and how, are likely to accomplish little in the way of behaviour change. They may even end up driving away people who need their help, and who would otherwise be perfectly willing to accept that help if it were delivered appropriately. Helping patients to gain control over their health outcomes is more effective than trying to exert that control for them. Techniques for encouraging behaviour change have been discussed at length in this book.

Many professionals become so focused on changing the behaviours of their patients that they overlook the gains that can be made by changing their own behaviours, or changing their practice procedures or settings. The environments in which health care is provided need, in the terms of the *Bangkok Charter*, to be made supportive environments. The easiest way to prevent falls for patients who are having x-rays (a not uncommon problem) is not to warn patients about falling but to make falls less likely to occur, or the consequences less serious, by changing the environment. This could involve taking x-rays of frail or physically unstable patients while they are seated, designing tables that are hard to roll off (or providing pads that prevent rolling) or carpeting floors so that slips are less likely and falls less damaging.

None of this should minimise the high level of impact that professionals can have in promoting health. Patients are generally keen to have information about what can be done to improve their health and well-being, and are often willing to devote large amounts of time and energy to the process. Well-designed and readable information pamphlets, contact information and plans that have reasonable and achievable goals are all well received by most patients.

SCHOOLS AND WORKPLACES

Teachable moments: particularly effective times for concepts to be learnt or behaviours to be developed.

These environments provide considerable opportunity for health promotion. In part, this is simply because children spend many of their waking hours in school and adults in workplaces. As a result, these environments provide a number of **teachable moments** (Taylor 2006). Teachable moments are particularly effective times for concepts to be learnt or behaviours to be developed. As an example, schools are able to require healthy behaviours on the part of children, such as wearing sunscreen and hats during outdoor activities. As a result, these behaviours can become habits that are carried over into life outside school. Provision of safe play areas and healthy food, health screening and inoculations, and education about hygiene and risky behaviours have long been seen as responsibilities of schools. Sex education, coping skills and conflict resolution are other areas in which schools have become involved in more recent times.

Workplaces, like schools, provide a range of teachable moments. Health risks within the workplace frequently place the employer in a situation of legal liability. If equipment or environments in the workplace are poorly designed, the employer is likely to be found at fault in the case of injury, and the costs can be significant. This liability can be avoided by improving these aspects of the workplace. In a similar way, employers can be encouraged to accept responsibility for other aspects of the health and well-being of workers. This could include the provision of exercise facilities for those workers with sedentary jobs, childcare facilities to reduce worry about the well-being of children, stress and conflict management courses, and a large variety of educational programs. Employers are beginning to recognise that provision of health promotion programs not only pays off in the form of reduced health costs that result from less absenteeism, but also in improved morale, both of which have a positive effect on profits.

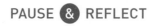

PAUSE & REFLECT

What are some examples of teachable moments for employees in a risky workplace such as a chemical factory? For university students, what might be a teachable moment about personal safety on campus?

COMMUNITIES

Communities also have a major role to play in promoting health. They can serve as focal points for education programs, provide facilities at low or no cost, and help to define an agenda for health promotion that fits community needs. Local communities often carry out this role on a geographical basis. Some activities, such as those requiring regulation or accreditation, can only realistically be carried out at local community level. The health needs of rural communities, even of outer suburban ones, are different from those of urban communities, and the appropriate programs need to be tailored to those needs (O'Connor-Fleming & Parker 2001).

Groups within the community may have their own special needs, and local institutions such as services or government can provide support for them. If the proportion of the local population that is elderly is increasing, resources may need to be directed away from programs aimed at children towards those aimed at older individuals. Ethnic groups may have different needs that require special programs, or at least alternative, culturally appropriate forms of programs that can meet those needs.

Access to health will probably be affected by financial issues (teenage mothers are unlikely to have the education or training to be in well-paid employment), by lack of education about health, by problems of transportation, and frequently by isolation. A variety of programs at all levels is needed to ensure the maximum level of health. These include not only health care programs but also financial aid, support and development programs. The youth of the individuals can be turned into an advantage through careful choice of interventions that capitalise on this resource.

ACCESS AND EQUITY

It is easy enough to see that health promotion and illness prevention produce win–win situations. The individual wins by having better health, and the community or society wins by having to devote less of its resources to the treatment of illness. Some commentators (for example, Richmond & Germov 2005) strongly criticise the focus of health promotion on the individual as the agent of change, partly because it places the responsibility on individuals who may not have the resources to change, and partly because it overlooks the structural or societal causes of ill health. Those who have the most to gain by avoiding illness and maximising their health are often those who are least able to do so. This may be because services are unevenly available within the community. For example, most programs are run in populated urban centres, causing rural dwellers to miss out. Some programs are dependent on access to facilities such as gyms, sports grounds, community centres or large medical practices, and access to these facilities is unequally distributed in the community. Programs that are provided only through health professionals in private practice are going to miss those individuals who do not use those practices as their source of primary health care. The homeless, the very poor and others on the margins of society are likely to spend larger proportions of whatever resources they have on cheap but unhealthy food and accommodation, or to self-medicate in unhealthy ways, such as with alcohol and tobacco use. They are less likely to have resources that can be invested in potential future benefits as these resources need to be used for survival today.

CROSS-REFERENCE
Access and equity issues are discussed in Chapter 14.

PAUSE & REFLECT

What are some of the costs to individuals when a society adopts a strongly preventative model of health? Consider what these costs may be with regard to the problem of obesity.

Environments are also inequitably distributed. Those who live in polluted areas or work in unhealthy workplaces are more likely to be financially less well off. High crime rates, community unrest and war are all relevant to health, and, again, it is the poor who are most vulnerable as they are least able to escape these problems.

It is imperative for societies to ensure that health is distributed equitably, which means more than just throwing money at health problems. In many cases, health resources are adequate, but the approach taken is not appropriate or is unacceptable to sections of the community. Many charitable schemes fail because the recipients do not wish to accept charity, particularly when the distributors of that charity sometimes restrict or deny what is provided if the recipients do not seem to be adequately grateful for it.

Health promotion schemes may be rejected by the target population because they are seen as labelling people as unhealthy, or because they have a moralistic tone: laying the blame for being sick or at risk on the individual. Management of relapse is a particular issue where this is a problem. Relapse must not be seen as a moral failure for the individual—a lack of willpower, for example—as this is likely to lower self-efficacy and drive participants out of health promotion activities. Unrealistic goals for participants often lead to failure and the abandonment of a perfectly viable program.

Symbols may also be critical. Some women with breast cancer object to the use of symbols such as pink ribbons and teddy bears because they are seen as infantilising them. Many people with chronic health problems feel that too much emphasis on positive outcomes, regardless of how unlikely they may be, diminishes the seriousness of their situation. They may feel closed out, as if their failure to gain benefit from a program is somehow a personal flaw. Involvement of the individual, the family and the community in controlling health programs is the principal way of avoiding these negative consequences.

CROSS-REFERENCE
The importance of cognitions about the illness and the self are discussed in Chapter 7.

HEALTH AND HUMAN BEHAVIOUR

Health promotion can be seen as the logical end point of the study of health and human behaviour. Because health relates in so many ways to behaviour, promotion of better health essentially means promotion of different behaviour. Such difference might involve habits, such as new approaches to diet, exercise or the use of substances such as alcohol and tobacco. It might involve changing emotional responses, such as coping with stress or reducing levels of arousal. It may involve changing broad societal approaches to health and illness, such as community development and support of the disadvantaged. Ultimately, it may involve changing our shared beliefs about what health is and where it comes from, and the provision of a new culture. Beliefs about the responsibility for health have been changing over recent decades, and will continue to change in response to new knowledge and technology. This book has aimed to increase understanding of some of these issues, and provide information about possible directions and methods to bring about this change.

CASE STUDY

ALFIE DAVIES AND HIS FALL

The aim of this case is to consider how an accident may occur, and what factors may influence the timing, nature and consequences of that accident.

Alfie is an 82-year-old Navy veteran. The local town hall is having a display of old photos of the history of the Navy—several of them contributed by Alfie—so he has walked down to see them. Although he wears glasses with bifocal lenses, and finds walking easier with the aid of a cane due to arthritis in one hip, Alfie does not think of himself as being disabled, and is proud of his general health and well-being. On his arrival at the town hall, Alfie enters the dark lobby from the sunshine outside, and finds it hard to see. As a result, he walks over the edge of a ramp installed for wheelchair access, and falls sideways, breaking the flimsy handrail in the process. He attempts to catch his balance with his cane, but the cane tip slips on the highly polished wooden floor of the lobby—a heritage feature of the century old hall—and Alfie falls. He braces his arm to catch himself, and feels something break in his forearm, and his hip begins to hurt badly. Several people in the lobby rush to help him, and one of them attempts to lift him into a seated position. This causes intense pain in his hip, and Alfie begs his helpers to let him lie flat.

An ambulance is called, and arrives within minutes. On reaching hospital, medical imaging shows that Alfie has broken a bone in his arm, and aggravated existing arthritic damage to his hip joint. At his age, healing is slow, so Alfie becomes an invalid for an extended period while healing takes place. Eventually, he requires a hip replacement to recover his mobility, but until that occurs he is largely confined to a wheelchair, and largely to staying inside his flat. As this is on the second floor, and the lift in the building is often out of order, his ability to participate in his usual activities is severely limited. As a result, Alfie becomes somewhat socially isolated, unhappy and less physically fit than before.

1   What environmental factors contributed to Alfie's injuries?
2   Are there characteristics of Alfie himself that contributed to this injury?
3   What other prevention and promotion strategies could be applied by the council to deal with the floor surface to reduce the risk of injuries?
4   What are the financial, social and other costs associated with this accident? To what extent could they have been prevented or lessened?

Points to consider

A city council staff member, responsible for health and safety, received the incident report about Alfie's fall. The next day he interviewed Alfie in his home and also did an inspection of the area. The staff member noted that the ramp, although designed to help one group of disabled people, had become a significant health risk in the absence of an adequate handrail. A high visibility strip marking the edge of the ramp might have prevented Alfie walking over the edge, as might have better lighting. Although it is an attractive heritage feature of the hall, the wooden floor has become a significant contributor to Alfie's injuries in this case. The slippery surface of the polished wood floor has made his cane useless as a balance aid in this situation, and the hard surface has worsened the impact of his fall. The separation of the ramp, with its non-slip surface, and the floor might have been adequate in this case if the handrail had been adequate. Other people, entering the lobby by other access, might still have problems with the floor's slickness; for example, women in high heels, people with ordinary plastic soles on wet days, or people with minor balance or mobility problems.

It would probably be unviable, and undesirable, to change the surface by coating it or covering it (primary prevention). The heritage value would be reduced or destroyed by too much change. However, at the simplest level, warning signs to let people know about the risks could be a help, or perhaps alternative access points could be provided for those at risk (secondary prevention).

CHAPTER SUMMARY

- Illness prevention and health promotion are major growth areas in health care.
- Illness prevention principally concerns programs that are done to or for people by health professionals, governments or other institutions.
- Primary prevention refers to programs aimed at keeping well individuals well. Secondary prevention is aimed at decreasing the prevalence of disease in at-risk groups. Tertiary prevention's goal is to reduce the negative consequences for those who already have an illness or disease.
- Prevention can take place at the legislative level by constraining behaviour, at the societal level by changing policy or procedures, and at the individual level.
- Health promotion enables people to exert more control over their own health. As for illness prevention, health promotion may be primary, secondary or tertiary.
- Groups involved in health promotion include health professionals, but schools and workplaces can provide additional teachable moments for influencing and encouraging change. Local communities and other groups with special needs can provide the opportunity and support for health promotion programs.
- Equity in the provision of health promotion is vitally important; it may involve helping disadvantaged groups to develop the necessary skills to take control of their own health.
- Health promotion is a logical endpoint for the consideration of the interactions between health and human behaviour that have been the focus of this book.

SELF TEST

1 Primary prevention is especially important in HIV/AIDS and cancer because:
   a   rehabilitation is very expensive in these diseases
   b   treatment is rarely curative in these diseases
   c   many people object to treating diseases that could be prevented
   d   neither of these diseases are inherited.

2 Of the following, the best example of secondary prevention is:
   a   requiring child restraint seats in cars
   b   increasing the tax on cigarettes to make them more expensive
   c   returning injured workers to different work activities in their companies
   d   subsidising the costs of stress management training for busy executives.

3 Screening programs are most useful when:
   a   there is no cure for the disease
   b   the disease has a large genetic component
   c   the screening method is reliable, acceptable and accessible
   d   people lose valuable resources if they choose not to be screened.

4 The main difference between illness prevention and health promotion is that the emphasis in:
   a   health promotion is on encouraging people to take control
   b   illness prevention is improving people's health outcomes
   c   health promotion is on services provided for patients by health professionals
   d   none of the above; there is no significant difference between them.

5 A rural health organisation wants to reduce the number of children who are injured in accidents involving farm machinery. It is likely that this program will be most effective if:

    a it involves advertisements on national television

    b better warnings are put into instruction manuals for the machinery

    c both children and parents are involved in the program

    d doctors are required to report children who are using farm machinery.

FURTHER READING

Fleming, M.L. & Parker, E. (2006) *Health Promotion: Principles and Practice in the Australian Context*. Allen & Unwin.

Keleher, H., MacDougall, C. & Murphy, B. (2007) *Understanding Health Promotion.* South Melbourne: Oxford University Press.

World Health Organization (2009) *Milestones in Health Promotion: Statements from Global Conferences*. WHO Press: Geneva.

Yarnell, J.W.G. (ed.) (2006) *Epidemiology and Prevention: A Systems Based Approach*. South Melbourne: Oxford University Press.

USEFUL WEBSITES

Injury Prevention in Children:
www.kidsafe.com.au

Lung cancer in women on the rise (Wall Street Journal):
http://online.wsj.com/article/SB10001424052748704764404575287081156194368.html

Preventing mother-to-child transmission of AIDS (UNICEF):
www.childinfo.org/hiv_aids_mother_to_child.html

The link between cervical cancer and HPV (human papillomavirus) (National cervical screening program):
www.cancerscreening.gov.au/internet/screening/publishing.nsf/Content/cv-hpv/$File/hpv.pdf

ANSWERS TO SELF-TEST QUESTIONS

CHAPTER 1

Answers are: b, c, d, c, a

CHAPTER 2

Answers are: b, c, c, d, a

CHAPTER 3

Answers are: d, a, a, c, b

CHAPTER 4

Answers are: c, b, c, b, a

CHAPTER 5

Answers are: c, b, d, a, d

CHAPTER 6

Answers are: d, d, c, c, b

CHAPTER 7

Answers are: d, a, a, c, c

CHAPTER 8

Answers are: c, a, c, b, c

CHAPTER 9

Answers are: c, b, c, d, a

CHAPTER 10

Answers are: d, c, d, c, d

CHAPTER 11

Answers are: a, d, a, b, d

CHAPTER 12

Answers are: a, d, c, b, a

CHAPTER 13

Answers are: c, c, c, b, d

CHAPTER 14

Answers are: d, b, d, b, a

CHAPTER 15

Answers are: b, d, c, b, d

CHAPTER 16

Answers are: b, d, c, a, c

GLOSSARY

abnormal illness behaviour
the persistence of inappropriate or maladaptive modes of perceiving, evaluating or acting in relation to health after the person has received an appropriate explanation of the nature and management of the illness from a professional

acceptance
a more neutral or middle-of-the-road reaction to a condition that diminishes the negative meaning of the condition and thus represents a decrease in negative thinking

accommodation
the modification of existing behaviours, or the development of entirely new behaviours, to allow an individual to deal with a new experience

acute illness
a single episode of illness (or disease), generally severe and over a limited period of time

acute pain
pain that is more intense and gains our immediate attention, but usually disappears within hours, days or weeks

Adult Literacy and Life Skills
a national survey to measure the literacy of adults aged 15 to 74 years

advanced health care directive (living will)
a statement—not legally binding on health professionals—signed by a patient about the treatment they would like to receive as they are dying

affective support
communicating positive feelings and providing constructive feedback and advice

agency
what or who is responsible for the modification of unhealthy behaviour

agent
the person who has control over the stimuli and/or reinforcements for change

algorithm
a mechanical routine or simple set of rules that can be used to solve all problems of a particular kind

allostasis
the process of maintaining balance in bodily systems, through physiological or behavioural means, in the face of a demand

allostatic load
the cumulative cost to the body of allostasis

Alzheimer's dementia
a significant loss of thinking, memory or problem-solving ability resulting from abnormalities of cells in the cerebral cortex

antecedents
stimuli that precede and lead to the occurrence of a behaviour

anticipatory grieving
grieving that takes place before an expected loss has actually occurred

appraisal
the cognitions that an individual has about the situation they are in at a given time

arousal
the activation of the sympathetic nervous system, which produces visceral changes and provides energy for behaviour

assimilation
the use of a reflex or an existing habit to allow the individual to deal with a new experience

attitudes
the thoughts, feelings and readiness to act that an individual has about any object, person or event

attribution theory of emotion
the idea that emotion results when physiological arousal and emotion-related cognitions about that arousal exist at the same time

automatisation
the carrying out patterns of behaviour or thinking that are so well learnt that they require no apparent thought

aversive conditioning
the use of punishment to decrease the occurrence of unwanted behaviour

avoidance learning
the learning of a response that will allow the individual to escape punishment, often fear; it is reinforced by a reduction in the level of fear experienced

balance theory
an approach that suggests that consistency is the organising principle of our cognitions

bariatric surgery
surgery aimed at weight loss in the obese that works by reducing the size of the stomach, either by mechanical devices (lap bands) or removal of part of the stomach

biofeedback
the control of internal processes through conditioning, using mechanical devices to make those internal processes perceptible

biopsychosocial model
a model of health that considers the individual as a whole person in a social setting, who may or may not be ill at any given moment

body mass index (BMI)

an approximate measure of the amount of body fat, frequently used by health professionals because it is easy to calculate

capability

a characteristic or behaviour of the individual that protects against a negative event

catastrophising

the appraisal by an individual that a situation is impossible for them to cope with when in fact it is not

chronic condition

a medical condition that is permanent, incurable and irreversible

chronic grief

unresolved grief characterised by an impaired ability to recall personal life details, imagine future events and plan for the future

chronic strain

the repeated or constant occurrence of a minor stressor

chronological age

the number of years that have passed sequentially since a person was born

classical conditioning

a learning process through experience where an already existing response to the presentation of food (salivating) becomes connected to a previously irrelevant stimulus (bell)

cognition

a general concept embracing all types of knowing, judging, thinking, reasoning and so on

cognitive behavioural therapy

a general category referring to talking therapies in which worrying or intrusive cognitions can be controlled or modified, thereby improving mental health

cognitive load

the amount of information kept in the working memory

cognitive responses

how a person views their condition

cognitive restructuring

a technique aimed at interrupting patterns of negative thinking by training the individual to recognise that they are occurring, and then replacing them with positive thoughts

collaborative model

a model in which patients are active participants, in partnership with health care providers, in regulating and managing their chronic condition

comfort food

food eaten primarily for positive emotional reasons rather than hunger—often with traditional or nostalgic connections

compassion fatigue
a deep physical, emotional and spiritual exhaustion related to repeated exposure to another's suffering

compliance
obeying another's instruction, or acting as they would like; it does not necessarily mean agreeing with the reasons behind the instructions

confabulation
the addition of plausible detail to a memory to make it seem more complete; this process takes place without the individual being aware of it

conservation withdrawal
an extreme pattern of withdrawal from interaction with a neglectful or abusive environment by a baby in order to save its life.

controllability
the level of control over a condition; it can be both actual and perceived

coping
any strategy by which an individual attempts to manage the perceived discrepancy between demands and resources

crystallised intelligence
the accumulation of knowledge that comes with experience and education

culture
the total way of life shared by the members of a group

cytokines
a group of proteins and peptides that work as signalling compounds, enabling cells to communicate with each other; they regulate the body's response to infection, inflammation and trauma

disability
a characteristic of the body, mind or senses that affects a person's ability to engage independently in some or all aspects of day-to-day life

disease
an abnormal state of the body or mind of a person as identified by a qualified observer

disengagement theory
the idea that aging individuals tend to modify the amount of interaction they have with the society around them to suit their capabilities

dysregulation of emotions
poor understanding or insight, negative reactivity, and ineffective or maladaptive coping intelligence

ecological model
a model proposing that overweight and obesity are based on biological, behavioural and environmental factors rather than just food intake

efficacy belief
the belief by a person that they can carry out required treatments

emotional intelligence
the ability to perceive, use, understand and regulate emotion

emotion-focused coping
behaviour, such as relaxation, distraction or prayer, aimed not at dealing with situational demands but with the way that the demands make an individual feel

emotions
positive or negative responses to external stimuli (situations, events, things and people) and/or internal mental representations (thoughts, dreams and ideas)

endogenous opioid peptides
opiate-like neurochemical substances, produced in the body, that act as an internal pain regulation system

endorphins
endogenous substances that are considered to be the body's own pain relievers, binding to the same receptor sites on neurons as morphine

epidemiology
the science of measuring the health status of a community

ethnicity
how people define themselves, and how they are defined by others

ethnocentrism
the belief that one's own culture is the natural, or the best, culture

evidence-based medicine
the view that all clinical practice should be based on evidence from randomised clinical trials to ensure treatments are effective and better than a placebo

expectancy–value theory
a model that suggests that rational choices between alternatives are based on the perceived probability of occurrence of each option and its value to the individual

expectations
the cognitions that individuals have about what is likely to happen in a given situation

explanatory model
the perceptions and expectations that member of a culture have about health and illness, including causes and mechanisms, timing, future course and outcome

extinction
the gradual diminution of a conditioned response when reinforcement is removed

fitness
a condition of health or physical soundness, which may be general or related to the ability to meet a specific demand ('fit for purpose')

FITT principle
the idea that four conditions determine the appropriateness of an exercise program for an individual at a specific time: **f**requency, **i**ntensity, **t**ime and **t**ype

flight or fight response
the release of catecholamines, which prepare the organism for action

fluid intelligence
using flexible reasoning to draw inferences, solve problems and understand the relationships between concepts

foetal alcohol syndrome
a syndrome, or group of symptoms, shown by the babies of mothers who drink excessive amounts of alcohol during pregnancy; babies of these mothers tend to be born prematurely, have low birth weight and an irritable temperament

food pyramid
a triangular-shaped figure divided into segments to indicate which food groups are more or less desirable as proportions of diet

gate-control theory
the idea that that the brain controls the experience of pain by influencing the amount of pain stimulation that is allowed to pass a sensory gate at the level of the spinal cord

gestalt
a meaningful grouping or whole that is perceived

good behaviour bond
a sum of money (or equivalent goods or services) that is set aside to be returned only if a behaviour change program is successfully completed

goodness of fit
the appropriateness of the specific resources of the individual to the specific demands that they face

habit
an activity that has become relatively automatic through prolonged practice

habituation
adapting to a stimulus so that it no longer arouses the same level of response that it originally aroused

hardiness
a behaviour pattern of commitment, a belief in ability to control events, and a willingness to tackle challenges as they occur that is associated with continued health in the face of high levels of stress

hassles
apparently minor events that can cause irritation, aggravate existing health problems or (in large numbers or over a prolonged period of time) affect an individual's health

Hawthorne effects
see validation

health
a concept that can vary over time, and can differ between social groups, cultures, countries, families and individuals

health behaviours
behaviours that are carried out specifically to promote the health of the individual

health literacy
the ability to read, comprehend and act on medical information, and effectively interact with the health care system

health (negative definition)
the absence of symptoms of illness and signs of disease

health (positive definition)
a state of complete physical, social, and mental well-being that is consistent with living a full and satisfying life

health promotion
the process of enabling people to increase their control over, and to improve, their health

helplessness
a negative, maladaptive response to a condition that has long-term, adverse implications for psychological and physical health

heuristics
problem-solving strategies that are based on general rules that usually or often work

holism
from the Greek, meaning entire or total

homeostasis
the tendency of the body to maintain internal constancy, and to try to restore equilibrium when that constancy is disturbed

hypnosis
a deep, trance-like state of relaxation

hypothalamus
a small structure in the midbrain that regulates behaviour to maintain homeostasis

illness
a subjective feeling on the part of a individual that something is not right with their health

illness behaviour
the process by which an individual goes from being a well person to being an ill patient

illness perceptions
personal views or theories that a person holds regarding their illness, made up from bodily experience such as symptoms, information from the external environment and previous experience with illness

illness prevention
interventions by health care professionals or institutions to prevent the occurrence of illness

incentive
an external object or stimulus that draws out behaviour or creates motivation in the absence of a need

incidence
the rate at which new cases of a specific disease occur in a population during a specified period

instincts
patterns of behaviour that are genetically programmed to occur in response to internal or external events

instrumental support
the act of giving physical assistance

in utero
the environment inside the uterus while the foetus is developing during pregnancy

learning
a change in behaviour that results from experience with the environment

learnt helplessness
distress to a point where behaviour is impaired or the individual gives up in the face of punishment that cannot be controlled

lifestyle disorders
diseases in which behaviours of the individual over a prolonged period of time influence the development or course, such as heart disease, cancer and stroke

locus of control
the degree to which an individual attributes the cause of events to either internal factors or external forces

low-awareness habits
habitual behaviours that the individual carries out without being particularly aware that they are doing so, such as nail-biting

mastery learning
the repetition of a task until learning occurs

medical model
a model of health that considers the individual as a case or patient, and primarily the host for a disease or malfunctioning organ

medical model for managing a chronic condition
a model that is prescriptive and focused on patients' compliance with or adherence to medical management instructions

medicalisation
the process of defining non-medical issues or problems as medical ones, often because health professionals are the only (or the most easily accessible) resources for dealing with them

memory
processes (including sensory, short-term and long-term memory) by which experience is retained within the organism

morbid grief
grieving that is too intense, or inappropriate to the loss

morbidity
the amount of disease observed within a group

mortality
the number of deaths observed within a group

motivation
factors that arouse, sustain and direct behaviour

multi-infarct dementia
a significant loss of thinking, memory or problem-solving ability resulting from small blockages of the blood supply that kill off localised groups of cortical cells

myelination
the development of a fatty insulation on nerve cells that helps them work faster

N type personality
see neuroticism

negative reinforcement
the termination of an unpleasant state that can serve to increase the likelihood of a behaviour

neuroplasticity
the brain's ability to reorganise itself by forming new neural connections throughout life

neuroticism (N type)
a tendency to develop neurotic symptoms under even relatively mild stress

nociceptors
nerve endings in the peripheral nerves that identify injury and release chemical messengers that pass to the spinal cord and into the cerebral cortex

obesity
a label for a range of weight that is significantly above that considered to be healthy, and regarded as presenting a serious risk to health

obesogenic environment
an environment (including culture, physical structures and other elements) that encourages overeating and/or inadequate physical activity

opponent–process theory
the idea that there are always two processes in motivation: the primary motivation or process, and a secondary and opposite one set up within the nervous system

optimal level theory
the idea that organisms have a preferred range of environmental stimulation, and that they will work to maintain themselves in that range

optimism
a tendency to expect that outcomes will generally be good

overweight
a label for a range of weight that is above that considered to be healthy

pain control
the ability to reduce the experience of pain, report of pain, emotional concern about pain, inability to tolerate pain or presence of pain-related behaviours

pain management programs
programs that address concerns associated with chronic pain, with strong emphasis on patient education

perceived benefit
a positive response to a condition that adds optimistic meaning through increased positive thinking

perception
the conscious experience of objects and events

perception explanations
the idea that placebos actually affect the perception of the symptom rather than the symptom itself

perceptual constancy
the tendency to see objects as unchanged in spite of changes in sensory input

perceptual set
the readiness to perceive something in a particular way or using a particular frame of reference

perinatal
refers to events occurring around the time of birth

persistent (chronic) pain syndrome
a subtype of abnormal illness behaviour that can occur if an individual experiences pain over a lengthy period of time

personal fable
the belief a person has that the world revolves around them

phi phenomenon
the generation of apparent movement by the successive appearance of two spatially separated stimuli, such as the flashing of two lights

phobia
a strong, persistent and irrational fear of some object, person or event

physical activity
bodily movement produced by skeletal muscles that requires energy expenditure

physical age
the state of a person's biological machine

placebo effects
the non-specific effects that a treatment produces

post traumatic stress disorder (PTSD)
a persistent pattern of symptoms, including preoccupation, dreams and flashbacks, that some individuals experience subsequent to a major stressful event

practical intelligence
common-sense thinking that enables a person to successfully negotiate their daily activities

prepubertal growth spurt
a period of dramatic physical growth that occurs just before puberty

prevalence
the number of existing and new cases of a specific disease present in a given population at a certain time

primary appraisal
the idea that in the presence of an environmental demand, individuals first assess or appraise the severity of the demand

primary drive
an unlearnt drive, for which there is an organic or physiological basis

primary prevention
interventions that are aimed at well individuals or groups, with the intention of keeping them in that state

problem-focused coping
behaviour, such as problem solving or increased effort, aimed at modifying the balance between demands and resources in a particular situation by reducing the demand or increasing resources

progressive relaxation
a stress management strategy involving relaxation of muscle groups one at a time so that the individual learns and remembers what relaxation feels like

psychoneuroimmunology
the study of the communications between the brain and the immune system

psychophysiology
the study of the interactions between the physiological and psychological aspects of a situation as experienced by an individual

psychosocial interventions
psychological, social and educational strategies that aim to minimise the adverse emotional and social impact of a condition on individuals and their families

psychosomatic illness
an outdated term reserved for a few specific conditions—such as bronchial asthma, neurodermatitis and gastric ulcers—that were regarded as being caused by worry

puberty

a developmental stage defined by the appearance of secondary sexual characteristics, such as body hair and deepening of the voice in males, and menstruation and breast development in females

punishment

a consequence or outcome that in conjunction with a behaviour makes that behaviour less likely in future

reaction range

the total range of outcomes that are possible for a particular individual as a result of their genetic potential

reflex

an unlearned response to stimulus

reinforcement

a consequence or outcome that in conjunction with a behaviour makes that behaviour more likely in future; this may be the beginning of a pleasant consequence (positive reinforcement) or the ending of an unpleasant consequence (negative reinforcement)

relaxation

the placing of one's body into a low state of arousal by progressively relaxing sections of the body and taking deeper and longer breaths

risk-reduction behaviours

the avoidance of unhealthy behaviours specifically to protect the health of the individual

risky behaviours

behaviours that increase the chance of ill health for the individual

rooting reflex

an automatic pattern of behaviour in newborn babies, where stimulation of the lips and tongue lead the newborn to turn towards the stimulus and initiate sucking activity

schedule of reinforcement

the pattern on which reinforcement is given; this may be continuous (every behaviour) or intermittent (less than every behaviour)

schema

a map of ideas about a topic stored in long-term memory

secondary appraisal

the appraisal that individuals make about their own resources

secondary gain

the gain or advantage an individual gets as a result of being ill

secondary prevention

interventions aimed at reducing the prevalence of illness at a particular point in time by targeting 'at-risk' individuals

self-agency model

a model in which individuals take charge of their condition, identify their responses and manage their lives accordingly

self-care

the management by health care practitioners of their own personal resources, including their time, energy and physical health

self-efficacy

the perception on the part of the individual that they can influence and control their own outcomes

self-esteem

the perception on the part of the individual that they are a good and worthy person

sensation

the response of receptor organs to stimuli from the environment

settling point theory

a theory that suggests that changes in energy balance become habitual, and remain at the new level

shaping

teaching a complex behaviour by reinforcing, one at a time, the series of steps that make up the behaviour

sick role

a social agreement involving a balance of rights and obligations granted to an individual who is regarded by others as sick

social age

the points at which an individual has reached milestones in their life

social capital

the increase of trust people have in one another, in government institutions and in the health professions

socialisation

the process of learning the culture of a society or group, its language and customs

stereotyping

the assumption that a member of a category of people will share all of the characteristics attributed to that category

stigma

a mark of disapproval that may be attached to an individual who differs from social or cultural norms

stimulus

any change in physical energy that activates a receptor, and activates or alerts an organism

stimulus control

changing behaviour by changing its antecedents

stimulus generalisation
the principle that a conditioned response will tend to occur in the presence of stimuli similar to the original conditioned stimulus

stress
a perceived imbalance between demands and resources

stress response
a pattern of physiological and cognitive reactions that an individual experiences to a situation

stressor
an event that appears likely to an observer to produce stress

synaptic cleft
the tiny space between two nerve cells, across which they communicate using neurotransmitters

systematic desensitisation
a cognitive behavioural strategy for dealing with phobic anxiety by linking increasing exposure to the stimulus that produces anxiety with practice of relaxation

task-focused coping
see problem-focused coping

teachable moments
particularly effective times for concepts to be learnt, or behaviours to be developed

teach-back
a learning cycle involving repetition and reinforcement of new learning

teach to goal
content and skills to be learnt in order to change behaviour

temporal extension
interpreting the past and future on a single or limited sample of behaviour

tend and befriend
a suggestion that women, when stressed, look after their children or seek out social support in order to deal with their stress

tertiary prevention
interventions aimed at decreasing the adverse consequences experienced by people who already have a disease or condition

type A (coronary prone) behaviour pattern
the idea that individuals who show a pattern of competitive achievement striving, an exaggerated sense of time urgency, and aggressiveness and hostility are at greatly increased risk of heart attack

type C (cancer prone) behaviour pattern
the idea that a passive and emotionally repressed personality style is associated with higher rates of cancer occurrence and death from cancer

type D (distressed) personality
a tendency to feel negative emotions combined with a reluctance to discuss these feelings with others that increases the probability of disease

unsafe sex
having sex without using contraceptive devices such as condoms, not finding out about a partner's sexual history and/or having multiple partners

validation
the idea that patients will assume that a health professional will not give them a diagnosis or a treatment unless they have valid reasons for seeking them (also known as Hawthorne effects)

vulnerability
a characteristic or behaviour of the individual that increases the impact of a negative event

well-being
a state of complete physical, social and mental health that is consistent with living a full and satisfying life

wonder drug effect
the observed tendency for a new treatment to work better while it is still new to the market

working memory
information that is temporarily stored for use in the short term

REFERENCES

Abel, M. (1998) Interaction of Humor and Gender in Moderating Relationships between Stress and Outcomes. *Journal of Psychology*, 132, 267–76.

ABS (2005) *Mortality and Morbidity: Children's Accidents and Injuries*. Cat. no. 4102.0 Australian Social Trends, www.abs.gov.au/ausstats/abs@.nsf/2f762f95845417aeca 25706c00834efa/1d72f5e5299decc5ca25703b0080ccbf!OpenDocument. Canberra: Australian Bureau of Statistics.

ABS (2008) *Overweight and Obesity in Adults, Australia, 2004-05*. Cat. no. 4719.0, www.abs .gov.au. Canberra: Australian Bureau of Statistics.

ABS (2009a) *Australian Social Trends*. Cat. no. 4102.0. Canberra: Australian Bureau of Statistics.

ABS (2009b) *The National Health Survey 2007–08*. Cat. no. 4363.0.55.001. Canberra: Australian Bureau of Statistics.

ABS (2010a) *Causes of Death*. Cat. no. 3303.0. Canberra: Australian Bureau of Statistics.

ABS (2010b) *Household and Family Projections, Australia, 2006 to 2031*. Cat. no. 3236.0. Canberra: Australian Bureau of Statistics.

ABS (2011) *Marriages and Divorces, Australia, 2010*. Cat. no. 3310.0. Canberra: Australian Bureau of Statistics.

Access Economics (2008) *The Growing Costs of Obesity in 2008: Three Years On*. Canberra: Diabetes Australia.

Access Economics (2009) *Keeping Dementia of Mind: Incidence and Prevalence 2009–2050*. Alzheimer's Australia.

Addison, R.G. (1984) Chronic Pain Syndrome. *American Journal of Medicine*, 77(3A), 54–8.

AIHW (2007) *Statistics on Drug Use in Australia 2006: Drug Statistics Series no. 18*. AIHW Cat. no. PHE 80. Canberra: Australian Institute of Health and Welfare.

—— (2008) *Australia's Health 2008*. Cat. no. AUS 99. Canberra: Australian Institute of Health and Welfare.

—— (2009) *Measuring the Social and Emotional Wellbeing of Aboriginal and Torres Strait Islander Peoples*. Cat. no. IHW 24. Canberra: Australian Institute of Health and Welfare.

—— (2010) *Australia's Health 2010*. Cat. no. AUS 122. Canberra: Australian Institute of Health and Welfare.

—— (2011a) *2010 National Drug Strategy Household Survey Report*. Cat. no. PHE 145, Canberra: Australian Institute of Health and Welfare.

—— (2011b) *Australia's Mothers and Babies 2009*. Cat. no. PER 52. Canberra: Australian Institute of Health and Welfare.

—— (2011c). *Headline Indicators for Children's Health, Development and Wellbeing*, 2011. Cat. no. PHE 144. Canberra: Australian Institute of Health and Welfare.

Ainsworth, M. (1993) Attachment as Related to Mother–Infant Interaction. In Rovee-Collier, C. & Lipsitt, L. (Eds) *Advances in Infancy Research*. 8, Norwood, NJ: Ablex.

Ajzen, I. & Madden, T. (1986) Prediction of Goal-directed Behavior: Attitudes, Intentions, and Perceived Behavioral Control. *Journal of Experimental Social Psychology*, 22, 453–74.

Akil, H. Watson, S.J., Young, E., Lewis, M.E., Khachaturian, H. & Walker, J.M. (1984) Endogenous Opioids: Biology and Function. *Annual Review of Neuroscience*, 7, 223–55.

Alder, N.E. & Stewart, J. (2010) *The Biology of Disadvantage: Socioeconomic Status and Health*. Hoboken, NJ: WileyInterScience.

Alexander, F. (1943) Fundamental Concepts of Psychosomatic Research: Psychogenesis, Conversion, Specificity. *Psychosomatic Medicine*, 5, 205–10.

Allen, F. (1998) *Health Psychology: Theory and Practice*. Sydney: Allen & Unwin.

Allport, G. W. (1954) *The Nature of Prejudice*. Cambridge, MA: Addison-Wesley.

American College of Sports Medicine (2009) *ACSM's Guidelines for Exercise Testing and Prescription* (8th edn). Lippinscott, Williams & Wilkins.

American Psychiatric Association (2000) *Diagnostic and Statistical Manual of Mental Disorders* (rev. 4th edn). Washington, DC: APA.

Andreassi, J.L. (2006) *Psychophysiology: Human Behaviour and Physiological Response* (5th edn). Mahwah, NJ: Lawrence Erlbaum.

Anisman, H. & Merali, Z. (2003) Cytokines, Stress and Depressive Illness: Brain-immune Interactions. *Annals of Medicine*, 35(1), 2–11.

Armstrong, D. (1980) *An Outline of Sociology as Applied to Medicine*. Bristol: John Wright & Sons.

Arnold, M. (1960) *Emotion and Personality*. New York: Columbia University Press.

Arria, A.M. & O'Brien, M.C. (2011) The 'High' Risk of Energy Drinks. *JAMA Online First*. Accessed 23 January 2012 at http://jama.ama-assn.org/content/early/2011/01/21/jama.2011.109.extract.

Australian Government National Drugs Campaign (2010) *GHB: Problems*. Accessed 23 January 2012 at www.drugs.health.gov.au/internet/drugs/publishing.nsf/Content/ghb4.

Aviv, A. (2004) Telomeres and Human Aging: Facts and Fibs. *Science*, 51, 43.

Baddeley, A. (1994) Working Memory: The Interface between Memory and Cognition.

Baddeley, A. (2003) Working Memory: Looking Back and Looking Forward. *National Review of Neuroscience*, 4 (10), 829–39.

Bade, E., Evertsen, J., Smiley, S. & Banerjee, I. (2008) Navigating the Health Care System: A View from the Urban Medically Underserved. *Wisconsin Medical Journal*, 107, 374–9.

Baker, D.W., DeWalt, D.A., Schillinger, D., Hawk, V., Ruo, B., Bibbins-Dimingo, K., Weinberger, M., Macabasco-O'Connell, A. & Pignone, M. (2011) 'Teach to Goal.' Theory and Design Principles of an Intervention to Improve Heart Failure Self Management Skills of Patients with Low Health Literacy. *Journal of Health Communication*, 16, 73–88.

Balcombe, J. (2010) Physicians Committee for Responsible Medicine, US (Letter). In M. O'Hare (Ed.) *Why Can't Elephants Jump?* London: (New Scientist) Profile Books.

Balis, G. (1978) Psychogenic Aspects of the Doctor–Patient Relationship. In Balis, G., Wurmser, L., McDaniel, E., & Grenell, R. (Eds) *The Behavioral and Social Sciences and the Practice of Medicine*. Boston, MA: Butterworth.

Bandura, A. (1977a) Self-efficacy: Toward a Unifying Theory of Behavioral Change. *Psychological Review*, 84(2), 191–215.

—— (1977b) *Social Learning Theory*. Engelwood Cliffs: Prentice-Hall.

—— (1986) *Social Foundations of Thought and Action: A Social Cognitive theory*. Engelwood Cliffs: Prentice-Hall.

—— (1998) Health Promotion from the Perspective of Social Cognitive Theory. *Psychology and Health*, 13, 623–49.

——, Ross, S. & Ross, D. (1963) Imitation of Film-mediated Aggressive Models. *Journal of Abnormal and Social Psychology*, 66, 3–11.

Banks, E., Byles, J.E., Gibson, R.E., Rodgers, B., Latz, I.K., Robinson, I.A., Williamson, A.B. & Jorm, L.R. (2010) Is Psychological Distress in People Living with Cancer Related to the Fact of Diagnosis, Current Treatment or Level of Disability? Findings from a Large Australian Study. *Medical Journal of Australia*, 193(5 Suppl.), S62–7.

Barlow, D.H. (2000) Unraveling the Mysteries of Anxiety and its Disorders from the Perspective of Emotion Theory. *American Psychologist*, 55(11), 1247–63.

Bell, E. (2006) Quali-quantitative Analysis (QQA): Why it Could Open New Frontiers for Holistic Health Practice. *Holistic Health & Medicine*, 321–31.

Benson, H. (1989) The Relaxation Response and Norepinephrine: A New Study Illuminates Mechanisms. *Australian Journal of Clinical Hypnotherapy and Hypnosis*, 10, 91–6.

Berger, K. (1998) *The Developing Person Through the Life Span*. (4th Edn). New York: Worth.

Berkel, L.A., Carlos Poston, W.S., Reeves, R.S. & Foreyt, J.P. (2005) Behavioral Interventions for Obesity. *Journal of the American Dietetic Association*, 105, S35–43.

Birkholtz, M., Aylwin, L. & Harman, R.M. (2004) Activity Pacing in Chronic Pain Management: One Aim, but which Method? Part One: Introduction and Literature Review. *British Journal of Occupational Therapy*, 67(10), 447–52.

Bodkin, J.A., Pope, H.G., Detke, M.J. & Hudson, J.I. (2007) Is PTSD Caused by Traumatic Stress? *Journal of Anxiety Disorders*, 21, 176–82.

Borigini, M. (2012) Chronic Pain's Parallel Universe: Congenital Analgesia. *Psychology Today* website. Accessed 22 February 2012 at: www.psychologytoday.com/blog/overcoming-pain/201201/chronic-pain-s-parallel-universe-congenital-analgesia.

Bradley, B., DeFife, J.A., Guarnaccia, C., Phifer, J., Fani, N., Ressler, K.J. & Westen, D. (2011) Emotion Dysregulation and Negative Affect: Association with Psychiatric Symptoms. *Journal of Clinical Psychiatry*, 72(5), 685–91.

Brodaty, H. & Cumming, A. (2010) Dementia Services in Australia. *International Journal of Geriatric Psychiatry*, 25(9), 887–95.

Brown, J. & Stoudemire, A. (1983) Normal and Pathological Grief. *Journal of the American Medical Association*, 250, 378–82.

Brown, W.J., Mummery, K., Eakin, E. & Schofield, G. (2006) 10,000 Steps Rockhampton: Evaluation of a Whole Community Approach to Improving Population Levels of Physical Activity. *Journal of Physical Activity and Health*, 3(1), 1–14.

Bunker, S.J., Tonkin, A.M., Colquhoun, D.M., Esler, M.D., Hickie, I.B., Hunt, D., Jelinek, V.M., Oldenburg, B.F., Peach, H.G., Ruth, D. & Tennant, C.C. (2003) 'Stress' and Coronary Heart Disease: Psychosocial Risk Factors. *Medical Journal of Australia*, 178(6), 272–6.

Burns, D. (1980) *Feeling Good: The New Mood Therapy*. New York: Avon Books.

Burns, M. & Seligman, M. (1989) Explanatory Style Across the Life Span: Evidence of Stability over 52 Years. *Journal of Personality and Social Psychology*, 56, 471–7.

Burroughs, S. & French, D. (2007) Depression and Anxiety: Role of Mitochondria. *Current Anaesthesia & Critical Care*.

Bussing A., Ostermann T. & Matthiessen P. F. (2005) Search for Meaningful Support and the Meaning of Illness in German Cancer Patients. *Anticancer Research*, 25(2B), 1449–55.

Butler, A.C., Chapman, J.E., Forman, E.M. & Beck, A.T. (2006) The Empirical Status of Cognitive Behavioral Therapy: A Review of Meta-analyses. *Clinical Psychology Review*, 26(1), 17–31.

Caltabiano, M. & Caltabiano, N. (1992) The Experience of Daily Hassles for University Young People. *Transitions*, 2(3), 46–50.

Canadian Council on Learning (2008) *Health Literacy in Canada, A Healthy Understanding 2008*. Ottawa.

Cannon, W. (1932) *The Wisdom of the Body*. New York: Norton.

Carey, S. (1985) *Conceptual Change in Childhood*. Cambridge, Mass: Bradford.

Carlbring, P., Nilsson-Ihrfelt, E., Waara, J., Kollenstam, C., Buhrman, M., Kaldo, V., Söderberg, M., Ekselius, L. & Andersson, G. (2005) Treatment of Panic Disorder: Live Therapy vs. Self-help via the Internet. *Behaviour Research and Therapy*, 43(10), 1321–33.

Carmelli, D., Cheney, M., Ward, M. & Rosenman, R. (1985) Twin Similarity in Cardiovascular Stress Response. *Health Psychology*, 4, 413–23.

Carver, C. S. (2005) Enhancing Adaptation during Treatment and the Role of Individual Differences. *Cancer*, 104(S11), 2602–07.

Carver, C.S. & Connor-Smith, J. (2010) Personality and Coping. *Annual Review of Psychology*, 61, 679–704.

Cattell, R. (1971) *Abilities: Their Structure, Growth and Action*. Boston: Houghton Miflin.

Centers for Disease Control and Prevention (2011) Health Weight: Assessing your Weight: BMI. Accessed 21 December 2011 at www.cdc.gov/healthyweight/assessing/bmi/ adult_bmi/index.html.

Chapman, B.P. & Hayslip, B. (2005) Incremental Validity of a Measure of Emotional Intelligence. *Journal of Personality Assessment*, 85(2):154–69.

Chigwedere, P., Seage, G.R., Lee, T. & Essex, M. (2008) Efficacy of Antiretroviral Drugs in Reducing Mother-to-child Transmission of HIV in Africa: A Meta-analysis of Published Clinical Trials. *AIDS Research and Human Retroviruses*, 24(6), 827–37.

Chou, R., Fanciullo, G.J., Fine, P.G., Adler, J.A., Ballantyne, J.C., Davies, P., Donovan, M.I., Fishbain, D.A., Foley, K.M., Fudin, J., Gilson, A.M., Kelter, A., Mauskop, A., O'Connor, P.G., Passik, S.D., Pasternak, G.W., Portenoy, R.K., Rich, B.A., Roberts, R.G., Todd, K.H. & Miaskowski, C. (2009) Clinical Guidelines for the Use of Chronic Opioid Therapy in Chronic Noncancer Pain. *Journal of Pain*, 10(2), 113–30.

Christian, L. M., Graham, J. E., Glaser, R., Loving, T. J., Malarkey, W. J. & Kiecolt-Glaser, J. K. (2006) Social Support Buffers Stress-induced Impairments in Wound Healing. *Brain, Behavior, and Immunity*, 20(3), 10–11.

Chummun, H. (2006) *Reductionism and Holism in Coronary Heart Disease and Cardiac Nursing*. British Journal of Nursing, 15(18), 1017–20.

Clark, A., Franklin, J., Pratt, I. & McGrice, M. (2010) Overweight and Obesity: Use of Portion Control in Management. *Australian Family Physician*, 39(6), 407–11.

Clark, D.A. & Beck, A.T. (2011) *The Anxiety and Worry Workbook: The Cognitive Behavioral Solution*. New York: Guilford Press.

Clark, R.C., Nguyen, F. & Sweller, J. (2006) *Efficiency of Learning: Evidence-based Guidelines to Manage Cognitive Load*. San Francisco: Jossey-Boss.

Clucas, C., Sibley, E., Harding, R., Liu, L., Catalan, J. & Sherr, L. (2011) A Systematic Review of Interventions for Anxiety in People with HIV. *Psychology, Health and Medicine*, 16(5), 528–47.

Cochrane Pain, Palliative and Supportive Care Group (2012). Accessed 22 February 2012 at http://papas.cochrane.org.

Cohen, S. & Wills, T.A. (1985) Stress, Social Support, and the Buffering Hypothesis. *Psychological Bulletin*, 98(2), 310–57.

Collins, D.J. & Lapsley, H.M. (2006) *Counting the Cost of Tobacco and the Benefits of Reducing Smoking Prevalence in Victoria*. Report prepared for the Victorian Department of Human Services. Accessed 16 January 2012 at www.health.vic.gov.au/tobaccore-forms/downloads/count.pdf.

Chilcoat, H.D. (2009) An Overview of the Emergence of Disparities in Smoking Prevalence, Cessation, and Adverse Consequences among Women. *Drug and Alcohol Dependence*, 104(S11), S17–23.

Colquitt, J.L., Picot, J., Loveman, E. & Clegg, A. (2009) Surgery for Obesity. *Cochrane Database of Systematic reviews*. Chicester: John Wiley & Sons. Accessed 2 December 2011 at www.mrw.interscience.wiley.com/cochrane/clsysrev/ articles/CD003641/frame.html.

Commission on Social Determinants of Health (2008). *Closing the Gap in a Generation: Health Equity through Action on the Social Determinants of Health*. Final Report of the Commission on Social Determinants of Health. Geneva: World Health Organization.

Consedine, N.S. & Moskowitz, J.T. (2007) The role of discrete emotions in health outcomes: A critical review. *Applied and Preventive Psychology*, 12(2), 59–75.

Coyne, E., Wollin, J. & Creedy, D. (2012) Exploration of the Family's Role and Strengths after a Young Woman is Diagnosed with Breast Cancer: Views of the women and their families. *European Journal of Oncology Nursing* (accepted 30/3/11) http://dx.doi.org/10.1016/j.ejon.2011.04.013.

Craig, A. D. (2005) Forebrain Emotional Asymmetry: A Neuroanatomical Basis?. *Trends in Cognitive Sciences*, 9(12), 566–71.

Creamer, M.C., Burgess, P. & McFarlane, A.C. (2001) Post-traumatic Stress Disorder: Findings from the Australian National Survey of Mental Health and Well-being. *Psychological Medicine*, 31(7), 1237–47.

Creedy, D., Collis, D., Ludlow, T., Cosgrove, S., Houston, K., Irvine, D., Fraser, J. & Maloney, S. (2005) The Impact of a Support Program for Children with a Chronic Condition on Psychosocial Indicators. *Contemporary Nurse*, 18(1), 46–56.

Cross, M. J., March, L. M., Lapsley, H. M., Byrne, E. & Brooks, P. M. (2006) Patient Self-efficacy and Health Locus of Control: Relationships with Health Status and Arthritis-related Expenditure. *Rheumatology*, 45, 92–6.

Cumming, E. & Henry, W. (1961) *Growing Old*. New York: Basic Books.

Dallman, M.F., Pecoraro, N.C. & la Fleur, S.E. (2005) Chronic Stress and Comfort Foods: Self-medication and Abdominal Obesity (Invited Minireview). *Brain, Behavior, and Immunity*, 19, 275–80. Accessed 17 October 2011 at http://chc.ucsf.edu/pdf/2005_article_Dallman_BBI.pdf.

Daniel, H.C. & Williams, A.C.D. (2010) Pain. In D. French, K. Vedhara & A.A. Kaptein & J. Weinman (Eds). *Health Psychology* (2nd edn). Chichester, UK: BPS Blackwell.

Daniels, H. (2008) *Vygotsky and Research*. London: Routledge.

Daniels, S.R., Arnett, D.K., Eckel, R.H., Gidding, S.S., Hayman, L.L., Kumanyika, S., Robinson, T.N., Scott, B.J., St. Jeor, S. & Williams C.L. (2005) Overweight in Children and Adolescents: Pathophysiology, Consequences, Prevention, and Treatment. *Circulation*, 111, 1999–2002.

Dantzer, R. (2005) Somatization: A Psychoneuroimmune Perspective. *Psychoneuroendocrinology*, 30(10), 947–52.

Day, J.R. & Anderson, R.A. (2012) Compassion Fatigue: An Application of the Concept to Informal Caregivers of Family Members with Dementia. *Nursing Research and Practice*, Article ID 408024, doi:10.1155/2011/408024.

De Leo D., Sveticic J. & Milner A. (2011). Suicide in Indigenous People in Queensland, Australia: Trends and Methods, 1994–2007. *Australian & New Zealand Journal of Psychiatry*, 45, 532–38.

DeLongis, A., Coyne, J., Dakof, G., Folkman, S. & Lazarus, R. (1982) Relationship of Daily Hassles, Uplifts and Major Events to Health Status. *Health Psychology*, 1, 119–36.

Delmonte, M. (1984) Physiological Responses During Meditation and Rest. *Biofeedback and Self-regulation*, 9, 181–200.

De Vaus, D., Qu L. & Weston, R. (2003) Changing Patterns of Partnership. *Family Matters*, 64, 10–15.

Denham, S.A. (2007). Dealing with Feelings: How Children Negotiate the Worlds of Emotions and Social Relationships. *Cognitions, Brain, Behaviour*, 11, 1–48.

Department of Health (2011) *Lifescripts*. Accessed 28 July 2011 at www.health.gov.au/lifescripts.

Department of Health, Victoria (2009) *Tobacco Reforms*. Accessed 18 January 2012 at www.health.vic.gov.au/tobaccoreforms/legislation.htm.

Dew, K. & Kirkman, A. (2002) *Sociology of Health in New Zealand*. Oxford: Oxford University Press.

Dimond, E., Kittle, C. & Crockett, J. (1960) Comparison of Internal Mammary Artery Ligation and Sham Surgery for Angina Pectoris. *American Journal of Cardiology*, 5, 483–6.

Dix, L. (1985) The Effects of Expectations on Outcomes. Unpublished thesis for the degree of Bachelor of Medical Science, Melbourne: Monash University.

Doidge, N. (2008) *The Brain that Changes Itself: Stories of Personal Triumph from the Frontiers of Brain Science*. Melbourne: Scribe.

Edelman, C. & Mandle, C. (2002) *Health Promotion Throughout the Lifespan*. (5th Edn). St Louis, MO: Mosby.

Egger, G. (2006) Are Meal Replacements an Effective Clinical Strategy for Weight Loss? (Editorial). *Medical Journal of Australia*, 184(2), 52–3.

Egleston, B.L., Meireles, S.I., Flieder, D.B. & Clapper, M.L. (2009) Population-based Trends in Lung Cancer Incidence in Women. *Seminars in Oncology*, 36(6), 506–15.

Ekman, P. (1980) *The Face of Man: Expressions of Universal Emotions in a New Guinea Village.* New York: Garland STM Press.

Engel, G. (1977) The Need for a New Medical Model: a Challenge for Biomedicine. *Science,* 196, 126–9.

Erikson, E. (1950) *Childhood and Society.* New York: Norton.

Eskelinen, M. & Ollonen, P. (2011) Assessment of 'Cancer-Prone Personality' Characteristics in Healthy Study Subjects and in Patients with Breast Disease and Breast Cancer using the Commitment Questionnaire: A Prospective Case-control Study in Finland. *Anticancer Research,* 31(11), 4013–17.

Espel, E., Blackburn, E., Lin, J., Dhabhar, F., Adler, N., Morrow, J. & Cawthorn, R. (2004) Accelerated Telomere Shortening in Response to Life Stress. *PNAS,* 101(49), 17312–15.

Evans, L. (1965) Preface. In Bloom, S.W. *The Doctor and His Patient: A Sociological Interpretation.* New York: The Free Press.

Evers, A.W.M., Kraaimaat, F.W., van Lankveld, W., Jongen, P.J., Jacobs, J.W.G. & Bijlsma, J.W.J. (2001) Beyond Unfavorable Thinking: The Illness Cognition Questionnaire for Chronic Disease. *Journal of Consulting and Clinical Psychology,* 69(6), 1026–36.

Eysenck, H. (1976) Neuroticism. In Krauss, S. (Ed.) *Encyclopaedic Handbook of Medical Psychology.* London: Butterworths.

Federal Trade Commission (2004) Weighing the Evidence in Diet Ads. Accessed 23 January 2012 at www.ftc.gov/bcp/edu/pubs/consumer/health/hea03.shtm.

Filoramo M. (2007) Improving Goal Setting and Goal Attainment in Patients with Chronic Noncancer Pain. *Pain Management Nursing,* 8(2): 96–101.

Finnegan, L., Marion, L. & Cox, C. (2005) Profiles of Self-rated Health in Midlife Adults with Chronic Illness. *Nursing Research,* 54(3), 167–77.

Fishbein, M. (2008) A Reasoned Action Approach to Health Promotion. *Medical Decision Making,* 28, 834–44.

Fishbein, M. & Ajzen, I. (1975) *Belief, Attitude, Intention and Behavior: An Introduction to Theory and Research.* Reading: Addison Wesley.

Fisher, S. (1986) *Stress and Strategy.* London: Lawrence Erlbaum.

Flanders Dunbar, H. (1947) *Mind and Body: Psychosomatic Medicine.* New York: Random House.

Flegal, K.M., Graubard, B.I., Williamson, D.F. & Gail, M.H. (2005) Excess Deaths Associated with Underweight, Overweight, and Obesity. *JAMA,* 293(15), 1861–7.

Fordyce, W.E. (1984) Behavioral Science and Chronic Pain. *Postgraduate Medical Journal,* 60, 865–8.

Fournier, M., Ridder, D. D. & Bensing, J. (2003) Is Optimism Sensitive to the Stressors of Chronic Disease? The Impact of Type 1 Diabetes Mellitus and Multiple Sclerosis on Optimistic Beliefs. *Psychology and Health,* 18(3), 277–94.

Frank, J. (1973) *Persuasion and Healing.* (Rev. Edn). Baltimore: Johns Hopkins University Press.

Frankenhaeuser, M. (1991) The Psychophysiology of Workload, Stress and Health: Comparison between the Sexes. *Annals of Behavioral Medicine,* 13, 197–201.

French, D., Vedhara, K., Kaptein, A.A. & Weinman, J. (eds) (2010) *Health Psychology* (2nd edn). Chichester, UK: BPS Blackwell.

Friedman, M. & Rosenman, R. (1974) *Type A Behavior and Your Heart.* New York: Knopf.

Gallien P., Nicolas B., Robineau, S., Petrilli, S., Houedakor, J. & Durufle, A. (2007) Phsyical Training and Multiple Sclerosis. *Annals of Rehabilitation and Physical Medicine*, 50, 373–6.

Gamble, J. & Creedy, D.K. (2009) A Counselling Model for Postpartum Women Following Distressing Birth Experiences. *Midwifery*, 25(2), e21.

Gibson, J.C., Smith, B. & Ward, C.D. (2011) Chronic Fatigue Syndrome. *InnovAiT*, 4(12), 691–6.

Gill, J.R. & Brown, C.A. (2009) A Structured Review of the Evidence for Pacing as a Chronic Pain Intervention. *European Journal of Pain*, 13(2), 214–16.

Glick, R.M. & Greco, C.M. (2010) Biofeedback and Primary Care. *Primary Care*, 37(1), 91–103.

Gould, F., Clarke, J., Heim, C., Harvey, P.D., Majer, M. & Nemeroff, C.B. (2012) The Effects of Child Abuse and Neglect on Cognitive Functioning in Adulthood. *Journal of Psychiatric Research*, 46, 500–6.

Graham, J. E., Robles, T. F., Kiecolt-Glaser, J. K., Malarkey, W. B. & Glaser, R. (2005) Hostility, CRP, and IL-6 in Older Adults: The Independent Role of Pain and Perceived Health. *Brain, Behavior, and Immunity*, 19(4), e26–7.

Gregory, R.L. (1971) Visual Illusions (ch. 20). In Atkinson, R. C. (Ed.), *Contemporary Psychology: Readings from Scientific American*, San Francisco, CA: W. H. Freeman & Co.

Grotmol, T., Weiderpass, E. & Tretli, S. (2006) Conditions in Utero and Cancer Risk. *European Journal of Epidemiology*, 21(8), 561–70.

Grundy, S.M., Blackburn, G. Higgins, M. Lauer, R. Perri, M. & Ryan, D. (1999) Roundtable Consensus Statement: Physical Activity in the Prevention and Treatment of Obesity and its Comorbidities. *Medicine and Science in Sports and Exercise*, 31, S502–8.

Gustafson, D. (2000) On the Supposed Utility of a Folk Theory of Pain. *Brain and Mind*, 1, 223–8.

Hall, C. (1979) *A Primer of Freudian Psychology.* (25th Anniversary Edn). New York: New American Library.

Hart, J. (1971) The Inverse Care Law. *Lancet*, 1, 405–12.

Haslam, D.W. & James, W.P. (2005) Obesity. *Lancet*, 366(9492), 1197–209.

Hassed, C. (2000) *New Frontiers in Medicine: The Body as the Shadow of the Soul.* Melbourne: Hill of Content.

Heath, R. (1964) *The Reasonable Adventurer.* Pittsburgh: University of Pittsburgh Press.

Hefner, J. & Eisenberg, D. (2009) Social Support and Mental Health among College Students. *American Journal of Orthopsychiatry*, 79, 491–9.

Heider, F. (1967) *The Psychology of Interpersonal Relations.* New York: John Wiley & Sons.

Hirsch, C.R. & Holmes, E.A. (2007) Mental Imagery in Anxiety Disorders. *Psychiatry*, 6(4), 161–5.

Hojsted, J. & Sjogren, P. (2007) Addiction to Opioids in Chronic Pain Patients: A Literature Review. *European Journal of Pain*, 11, 490–518.

Holmes, T. & Rahe, R. (1967) The Social Readjustment Rating Scale. *Journal of Psychosomatic Research*, 11, 213–18.

Hull, C. (1943) *Principles of Behavior.* New York: Appleton-Century-Crofts.

Imao, M. (2005) *The Mourning Process in Chronic Illness.* Nagoya: Nagoya University. Accessed 20 February 2007 at www.human.ritsumei.ac.jp/hsrc/resource/ series/01/pdf/01_96.pdf.

IASP (2011) *IASP Taxonomy*. International Association for the Sstudy of Pain. Accessed 22 January 2012 at www.iasp-pain.org/Content/NavigationMenu/General ResourceLinks/PainDefinitions/default.htm#Pain.

Ipser, J.C., Stein, D.J., Hawkridge, S. & Hoppe, L. (2010) A Systematic Review and Meta-analysis of Randomised Controlled Trials of Medication in Treating Anxiety Disorders in Children and Adolescents. *Cochrane Summaries*, 16 June. Accessed at http://summaries.cochrane.org/CD005170/a-systematic-review-and-meta-analysis-of-randomised-controlled-trials-of-medication-in-treating-anxiety-disorders-in-children-and-adolescents.

Jackson, K.M. & Nazar, A.M. (2006) Breastfeeding, the Immune Response, and Long-term Health. *Journal of the American Osteopathic Association*, 106(4), 203–7.

Jacobson, E. (1938) *Progressive Relaxation*. (2nd edn). Chicago: University of Chicago Press.

James, W. (1890) *Psychology*. New York: Holt.

Johnson, J. E. & Johnson, K. E. (2006) Ambiguous Chronic Illness in Women: A Community Health Nursing Concern. *Journal of Community Health Nursing*, 23(3), 159–67.

Jones, F. & Bright, J. (2001) *Stress: Myth, Theory and Research*. Harlow England: Prentice-Hall.

Jones, K. (1970) *Role Conflict: Perception and Experience*. PhD dissertation, Columbia, MO: University of Missouri.

—— (1985) The Thrill of Victory: Blood-pressure Variability and the Type A Behavior Pattern. *Journal of Behavioral Medicine*, 8, 277–85.

—— (1991) Type A Behavior as a Generally Available Strategy: Varying Activation by Tasks and Instructions. *Psychology and Health*, 5, 289–96.

—— (2001) Encouraging the Transition to Teamwork Learning Communities. *Communities of Learning: Who, Where, How*. Proceedings of the 2001 ANZAME Annual Conference, Nelson, NZ: Conferences & Events Ltd.

——, Copolov, D., & Outch, K. (1986) Type A, Test Performance and Salivary Cortisol. *Journal of Psychosomatic Research*, 30, 699–707.

Jones, K. & Lebnan, V. (1988) A 6-year Follow-up of the Type A Behaviour Pattern in Medical Students. *Medical Education*, 22, 211–13.

Jukkala, A., Dupree, J.P. & Graham, S. (2009) Knowledge of Limited Health Literacy at an Academic Health Centre. *Journal of Continuing Education in Nursing*, 40(7), 298–302.

Julliard, K., Klimenko, E. & Jacob M. S. (2006) Definitions of Health among Healthcare Providers. *Nursing Science Quarterly*, 19(3), 265–71.

Kalauokalani D., Franks, P., Oliver, J., Meyers, F. & Kravitz, R. (2007) Can Patient Coaching Reduce Racial/Ethnic Disparities in Cancer Pain Control? Secondary Analysis of a Randomised Controlled Trial. *Pain Medicine,* 8(1), 17–24.

Kandula, N., Malli, T., Zei, C., Larsen, E. & Baker, D. (2011) Literacy and Retention of Information after a Multimedia Diabetes Education Program and Teach-back. *Journal of Health Communication*, 16, 89–102.

Kanner, A., Coyne, J., Schaefer, C. & Lazarus, R. (1981) Comparison of Two Modes of Stress Measurement: Daily Hassles and Uplifts versus Major Life Events. *Journal of Behavioral Medicine*, 4, 1–39.

Karademas, E. C., Karvelis, S. & Argyropoulou, K. (2007) Stress-related Predictors of Optimism in Breast Cancer Survivors. *Stress and Health*, 23(1), 2–10.

Karasek, R., Baker, D., Marxer, F., Ahlbom, A. & Theorell, T. (1981) Job Decision Latitude, Job Demands and Cardiovascular Disease: A Prospective Study of Swedish Men. *American Journal of Public Health*, 71, 694–705.

Kastenbaum, R. (1992) *The Psychology of Death*. New York: Springer-Verlag.

Katon, W., Lin, E. H. B. & Kroenke, K. (2007) The Association of Depression and Anxiety with Medical Symptom Burden in Patients with Chronic Medical Illness. *General Hospital Psychiatry*, 29(2), 147–55.

Kearney, P. K. & Pryor, J. (2004) The International Classification of Functioning, Disability and Health (ICF) and nursing. *Journal of Advanced Nursing*, 46(2), 162–70.

Keating, C.L., Moodie, M.L. & Swinburn, B.A. (2011) The Health-related Quality of Life of Overweight and Obese Adolescents—A Study Measuring Body Mass Index and Adolescent-reported Perceptions. *International Journal of Pediatric Obesity*, 6, 434–1.

Kennedy, G.C. (1953) The Role of Depot Fat in the Hypothalamic Control of Food Intake in the Rat. *Proceedings of the Royal Society B: Biological Sciences*, 140, 578–92.

Keys, A., Fidanza, F., Karvonen, M.J., Kimura, N. & Taylor, H.L. (1972) Indices of Relative Weight and Obesity. *Journal of Chronic Disease*, 25(6), 329–43.

Kiecolt-Glaser, J., Dura, J., Speicher, C., Trask, O. & Glaser, R. (1991) Spousal Care-givers of Dementia Victims: Longitudinal Changes in Immunity and Health. *Psychosomatic Medicine*, 53, 345–62.

Kiecolt-Glaser, J., Glaser, R., Williger, D., Stout, J., Messick, G., Sheppard, S., Ricker, D., Romisher, S., Briner, W., Bonnell, G. & Donnerburg, R. (1985) Psychosocial Enhancement of Immunocompetence in a Geriatric Population. *Health Psychology*, 4, 24–41.

Kimble, D. (1992) *Biological Psychology* (2nd edn). Fort Worth: Harcourt Brace Jovanovich.

Kleinman, A. (1988) *The Illness Narratives*. New York: Basic Books.

Kugler, J., Seelbach, H. & Krüskemper, G.M. (1994) Effects of Rehabilitation Exercise Programmes on Anxiety and Depression in Coronary Patients: A Meta-analysis. *British Journal of Clinical Psychology*, 33(3), 401–10.

Kobasa, S. (1979) Stressful Life Events and Health: An Inquiry into Hardiness. *Journal of Personality and Social Psychology*, 37, 1–11.

Koch, T., Jenkin, P. & Kralik, D. (2004) Chronic Illness Self-management: Locating the Self. *Journal of Advanced Nursing*, 48(5), 484–92.

Kübler-Ross, E. (1969) *On Death and Dying*. New York: Macmillan.

Larson, H.J. & Ghinai, I. (2011) Lessons from Polio Eradication. *Nature*, 473(7348), 446–7.

Lawson, V. L., Lyne, P. A., Harvey, J. N. & Bundy, C. E. (2005) Understanding Why People with Type 1 Diabetes Do Not Attend for Specialist Advice: A Qualitative Analysis of the Views of People with Insulin-Dependent Diabetes who Do Not Attend Diabetes Clinic. *Journal of Health Psychology*, 10(3), 409–23.

Lazarus, A. (1971) *Behavior Therapy and Beyond*. McGraw-Hill, New York.

Lazarus, R. & Folkman, S. (1984) *Stress Appraisal and Coping*. New York: Springer.

Lazarus, R. & Alfert, E. (1964) The Short-circuiting of Threat by Experimentally Altering Cognitive Appraisal. *Journal of Abnormal and Social Psychology*, 69, 195–205.

Leventhal, H., Meyer, D. & Nerenz, D. (1980) The Common Sense Representation of Illness Behaviour. In Rachman, S. (Ed.) *Contributions to Medical Psychology* (Vol. 2), Oxford: Pergamon Press.

Levine, J, Gordon, N. & Fields, H. (1978) The Mechanism of Placebo Analgesia. *Lancet*, 23 Sept., 654–7.

LoCicero, J. (1991) *Grief Chart*. www.grief-chart.com.

Loftus, E. & Loftus, G. (1980) On the Permanence of Stored Information in the Brain. *American Psychologist*, 35, 409–20.

Lutgendorf, S.K. & Costanzo, E,S. (2003) Psychoneuroimmunology and Health Psychology: An Integrative Model. An Invited Review. *Brain, Behavior, and Immunity*, 17, 225–32.

Macabasco-O'Connell, A. & Fry Bowers, E. (2011) Knowledge and Perceptions of Health Literacy among Health Professionals. *Journal of Health Communication*, 16, 295–307.

Mahoney, M. (2006) Protecting our Patients from HPV and HPV-related Diseases: The Role of Vaccines. *Journal of Family Practice*, S10-7.

Manderscheid, R.W., Ryff, C.D., Freeman, E.J., McKnight-Eily, L.R., Dhingra, S. & Strine, T.W. (2010) Evolving Definitions of Mental Illness and Wellness. *Prev Chronic Dis*, 2010 January, 7(1), A19.

Marlatt, G. & Gordon, J. (1985) *Relapse Prevention: Maintenance Strategies in the Treatment of Addictive Behaviours*. New York: Guildford Press.

Masem, M. (2012) Benefits of Male Circumcision. *JAMA*, 307(5), 455.

Maslow, A. (1970) *Motivation and Personality*. (2nd Edn). New York: Harper & Row.

Matthews, D., McCullough, M., Larson, D., Koenig, H., Swyers, J. & Milano, M. (1998) Religious Commitment and Health Status: A Review of the Research and Implications for Family Medicine. *Archives of Family Medicine*, 7, 118–24.

Mayer, J.D. & Salovey P. (1997) What is emotional intelligence? In P. Salovey, & D.J. Sluyter (Eds.), *Emotional Development and Emotional Intelligence*. New York: Basic Books.

McClelland, D. (1961) *The Achieving Society*. Princeton: Van Nostrand.

McDonald, K. & Thompson, J.K. (1992), Eating Disturbance, Body Image Dissatisfaction, and Reasons for Exercising: Gender Differences and Correlational Findings. *International Journal of Eating Disorders*, 11, 289–92.

McEwen, B.S. (1998) Protective and Damaging Effects of Stress Mediators. *New England Journal of Medicine*, 338, 171–9.

McEwen, B.S. (2000) Allostasis and Allostatic Load: Implications for Neuropsychopharma-cology. *Neuropsychopharmacology*, 22, 108–24. Accessed 20 February 2012 at www .nature.com/?file=/npp/journal/v22/n2/full/1395453a.html.

Mechanic, D. (1968) *Medical Sociology: A Selective View*. New York: Free Press.

Medew, J. (2011) SensaSlim Banned for Advertising Breach. *The Age*, November 25. Accessed 12 January 2012 at www.theage.com.au/national/sensaslim-banned-for-advertising-breach-20111124-1nwxk.html.

Mennin, D. S., Holaway, R. M., Fresco, D. M., Moore, M. T. & Heimberg, R. G. (2007) Delineating Components of Emotion and its Dysregulation in Anxiety and Mood Psychopathology. *Behaviour Therapy*, 38, 284–302.

Maccallum, F. & Bryant, R. (2011) Imagining the Future in Complicated Grief. *Depression and Anxiety*, 28(8), 658–65.

Meeuwisse, W.H., Tyreman, H., Hagel, B. & Emery, C. (2007) A Dynamic Model of Etiology in Sport Injury: The Recursive Nature of Risk and Causation. *Clinical Journal of Sports Medicine*, 17(3), 215–19.

Melzack, R. & Wall, P. (2003) *Handbook of Pain Management*. Edinburgh: Churchill Livingstone.

Miller, G.A. (1956) The Magical Number Seven Plus or Minus Two: Some Limits on Our Capacity for Processing Information. *Psychological Review*, 63(2), 81–97.

Miller, W.R. & Rollnick, S. (2005) Motivational Interviewing: Preparing People for Change. New York: Guilford Press.

Mohlman, J., Carmin, C. N. & Price, R. B. (2007) Jumping to Interpretations: Social Anxiety Disorder and the Identification of Emotional Facial Expressions. *Behaviour Research and Therapy*, 45(3), 591–99.

Mols, F. & Denollet, J. (2010) Type D Personality in the General Population: A Systematic Review of Health Status, Mechanisms of Disease, and Work-related Problems. *Health and Quality of Life Outcomes*, 8, 9. Accessed 20 February 2012 at www.hqlo .com/content/8/1/9.

Multiple Risk Factor Intervention Trial Group (1982) Multiple Risk Factor Intervention Trial: Risk Factor Changes and Mortality Results. *JAMA*, 248(12), 1465–77.

Murray, H. (1938) *Explorations in Personality*. New York: Oxford University Press.

Nestoriuc, Y. & Martin, A. (2007) Efficacy of Biofeedback for Migraine: A Meta-analysis. *Pain*, 128, 111–27.

Nichter, M. & Nichter, M. (1991) Hype and Weight. *Medical Anthropology*, 13(3), 249–84.

Nisbett, R. & Ross, L. (1980) *Human Inference: Strategies and Shortcomings of Social Judgment*. Englewood Cliffs: Prentice-Hall.

Noar, S. & Zimmerman, R. (2005) Health Behavior Theory and Cumulative Knowledge Regarding Health Behaviors: Are we Moving in the Right Direction? *Health Education Research*, 20(3), 275–90.

Ochsner, K. N. & Gross, J. J. (2005) The Cognitive Control of Emotion. *Trends in Cognitive Science*, 9(5), 241–49.

O'Connor-Fleming, M. & Parker, E. (Eds) (2001) *Health Promotion: Principles and Practice in the Australian Context*. Sydney: Allen & Unwin.

Ogden, J (2003) Some Problems with Social Cognitive Models: A Pragmatic and Conceptual Analysis. *Health Psychology*, 22(4), 424–8.

—— (2007) *Health Psychology: A Textbook* (4th edn). Maidenhead, UK: Open University Press.

Olds, T.S., Tomkinson, R.S., Ferrar, K.E. & Maher, C.S. (2010) Trends in the Prevalence of Childhood Overweight and Obesity in Australia between 1985 and 2008. *International Journal of Obesity*, 34, 57–66, doi:10.1038/ijo.2009.211.

Ornish, D. (1990) *Dr. Dean Ornish's Program for Reversing Heart Disease: The Only System Scientifically Proven to Reverse Heart Disease without Drugs or Surgery*. New York: Random House.

Parsons, T. (1951) *The Social System*. New York: The Free Press.

Patterson C., Dahlquist G.G., Gyürüs, E., Green A., Soltesz G & EUROLAB (2009) Study Group Incidence Trends for Childhood Type 1 Diabetes in Europe During 1989–2003 and Predicted New Cases 2005–20: A Multicentre Prospective Registration Study. *Lancet*, 373, 2027–33.

Parvanta, C., Nelson, D.E., Parvanta, S.A. & Harner, R.N. (2011) *Essentials of Public Health Communication*. Sudbury, MA: Jones & Bartlett Learning.

Peck, C. (1982) *Controlling Chronic Pain: A Self Help Guide*. Sydney: Fontana Original.

Pedersen, S. S., Daemen, J., van de Sande, M., Sonnenschein, K., Serruys, P. W., Erdman, R. & van Domburg, R. T. (2007) Type-D Personality Exerts a Stable,

Adverse Effect on Vital Exhaustion in PCI Patients Treated with Paclitaxel-eluting Stents. *Journal of Psychosomatic Research*, 62(4), 447–53.

Penfield, W. (1969) Consciousness, Memory and Man's Conditioned Reflexes. In Pribram K. (Ed.) *On the Biology of Learning*. New York: Harcourt Brace Jovanovich.

Petrie, K., Broadbent, E. & Meechan, G. (2003) Self-regulatory Interventions for Improving the Management of Chronic Illness. In Cameron, L. D. & Leventhal, H. (Eds). *Self Regulation of Illness and Health Behaviour*, New York: Routledge. Accessed 12 February 2007 at www.health.auckland.ac.nz/psych-med/staff/keiths% 20papers.

Piaget, J. (1985). *The Equilibration of Cognitive Structures: The Central Problem of Intellectual Development*. Chicago: University of Chicago Press.

Pilovsky, I. (1978) A General Classification of Abnormal Illness Behaviours. *British Journal of Medical Psychology*, 51, 131–7.

Pincus, T., Santos, R. & Morley, S. (2007) Depressed Cognitions in Chronic Pain Patients are Focused on Health: Evidence from a Sentence Completion Task. *Pain*, 130(1–2), 84–92.

Piotrowski, K. & Snell, L. (2007) Health Needs of Women with Disabilities across the Lifespan. *Journal of Obstetric, Gynecologic, & Neonatal Nursing*, 36(1), 78–87.

Prochaska, J. & DiClemente, C. (1984) *The Transtheoretical Approach: Crossing Traditional Boundaries of Therapy*. Chicago: Dow Jones/Irwin.

Raczynski, J. & DiClemente, C. (eds) (1999) *Handbook of Health Promotion and Disease Control*. New York: Kluwer Academic.

Raphael, B., Schmolke, M. & Wooding, S. (2005) Links between Mental and Physical Health and Illness. In H. Herrman, S. Saxena & R. Moodie (Eds). *Promoting Mental Health, Concepts Emerging Evidence Practice*, A Report of the World Health Organization. Geneva: Department of Mental Health and Substance Abuse in collaboration with the Victorian Health Promotion Foundation and The University of Melbourne. Accessed 18 May 2007 at www.who.int/mental_health/evidence/MH_Promotion_ Book.pdf.

Rathus, S. (1997) *Essentials of Psychology*. (5th Edn). Fort Worth: Harcourt Brace.

Reinhardt, J. P., Boerner, K. & Horowitz, A. (2006) Good to Have But Not to Use: Differential Impact of Perceived and Received Support on Well-Being. *Journal of Social and Personal Relationships*, 23(1), 117–29.

Requena, C., Martínez, A.M. & Ortiz T. (2010) Vital Satisfaction as a Health Indicator in Elderly Women. *Journal of Women & Aging*, 22(1), 15–21.

Reynolds D. V. (1969) Surgery in the Rat during Electrical Analgesia Induced by Focal Brain Simulation. *Science*, 164, 444–5.

Richardson, G., Gravelle, H., Weatherly, H. & Ritchie, G. (2005) Cost-effectiveness of Interventions to Support Self-care: A Systematic Review. *International Journal of Technology Assessment in Health Care*, 21(4), 423–32.

Richman, L.S., Kubzansky, L., Maselko, J., Kawachi, I., Choo, P. & Bauer, M. (2005) Positive Emotion and Health: Going Beyond the Negative. *Health Psychology*, 24(4), 422–9.

Richmond, K & Germov, J. (2005) Health Promotion Dilemmas. (Ch. 11). In Germov, John (Ed.) *Second Opinion: An Introduction to Health Sociology*. Melbourne: Oxford University Press.

Rimm, D. & Masters, R. (1979) *Behavior Therapy Techniques and Imperical Findings*. New York: Academic Press.

Robinson, R.O. (2008) Fetal Alcohol Syndrome. *Developmental Medicine & Child Neurology*, 19(4), 538–40.

Rogers, R. (1985) Attitude Change and Information Integration in Fear Appeals. *Psychological Reports*, 56, 179–82.

Rosenkranz, M. A., Jackson, D. C., Dalton, K. M., Dolski, I., Ryff C. D., Singer B. H. et al. (2003) Affective Style and In Vivo Immune Response: Neurobehavioral Mechanisms. Proceedings of the National Academy of Science USA, 100. In Y. Borak (Ed.) (2006) The Immune System and Happiness. *Autoimmunity Reviews*, 5(8), 523–27.

Rosenstock, I. (1974) Historical Origins of the Health Belief Model. *Health Education Monographs*, 2, 328–35.

Rotter, J.B. (1996) Generalized Expectancies for Internal Versus External Control of Reinforcement. *Psychological Monographs*, 80, whole issue.

Royal Australasian College of Physicians (2010). Circumcision—RACP Position Statement. http://www.racp.edu.au/page/policy-and-advocacy/paediatrics-and-child-health .Accessed October 10 2011.

Rubak, S., Sandbaek, A., Lauritzen, T. & Christensen, B. (2005) Motivational Interviewing: A Systematic Review and Meta-analysis. *British Journal of General Practice*, 55, 305–12.

Ryan, D.W. & Schmidt, M. (1979) *Mastery Learning: Theory, Research, and Implementation*. Toronto: The Ontario Institute for Studies in Education.

Ryan, R. & Deci, E. (2000) Self-determination Theory and the Facilitation of Intrinsic Motivation, Social Development, and Well-being. *American Psychologist*, 55(1), 68–78.

Safe Work Australia (2009) The Cost of Work-related Injury & Illness for Australian Employers, Workers and the Community. Accessed 16 January 2012 at www .safeworkaustralia.gov.au.

Sawyer, S M., Drew S., Yeo, M.S. & Britto M. (2007) Adolescents with a Chronic Condition: Challenges Living, Challenges Treating. *The Lancet*, 369(9571), 1481–9.

Scarborough, P., Burg, M.R., Foster, C., Swinburn, B., Sacks, G., Rayner, M., Webster, P. & Allender, S. (2011) Increased Energy Intake Entirely Accounts for Increase in Body Weight in Women but not in Men in the UK between 1986 and 2000. *British Journal of Nutrition*, 105, 1399–1404.

Schachter, S. (1964) The Interaction of Cognitive and Physiological Determinants of Emotional State. In Berkowitz, L. (Ed.). *Advances in Experimental Social Psychology*, vol. 1. New York: Academic Press.

—— (1971) Some Extraordinary Facts about Obese Humans and Rats. *American Psychologist*, 26, 129–44.

—— & Singer, J. (1962) Cognitive, Social and Physiological Determinants of Emotional State. *Psychological Review*, 69, 379–99.

Scheier, M. & Carver, C. (1985) Optimism, Coping, and Health: Assessment and Implications of Generalized Outcome Expectancies. *Health Psychology*, 4, 219–47.

Scheier, M., Matthews, K., Owens, J., Magovern, G., Lefebvre, R., Abbott, R. & Carver, C. (1989) Dispositional Optimism and Recovery from Coronary Artery Bypass Surgery: The Beneficial Effects on Physical and Psychological Well-being. *Journal of Personality and Social Psychology*, 57, 1024–40.

Schwartz, V. (2007) Biopsychosocial Model: Helpful or Hindering? *Psychiatric Times*, 24(6), 47.

Secord, P. & Backman, C. (1964) *Social Psychology*. New York: McGraw-Hill.

Seligman, M. & Maier, S. (1967) Failure to Escape Traumatic Shock. *Journal of Experimental Psychology*, 74, 1–9.

Selye, H. (1978) *The Stress of Life* (rev. edn). New York: McGraw Hill.

Shapiro, A. & Morris, L. (1978) Placebo Effects in Medical and Psychological Therapies. In Bergin, A. & Garfield, S. (Eds). *Handbook of Psychotherapy and Behavior Change*. (2nd Edn). New York: Wiley.

Shaw, K.A., Gennat, H.C., O'Rourke, P. & Del Mar, C. (2006) Exercise for Overweight or Obesity. *Cochrane Database of Systematic Reviews*, 4. Art. no.: CD003817, doi 10.1002/14651858.CD003817.pub3.

Shelton, S. (1994) The Doctor–Patient Relationship. In Stoudemire, A. *Human Behavior: An Introduction for Medical Students*. (2nd Edn). Philadelphia: J. B. Lippincott.

Sheridan, S.L., Halpern, D.J., Viera, A.J., Berkman, N.D., Donahue, K.E. & Crotty, K. (2011) Interventions for Individuals with Low Health Literacy: A Systematic Review. *Journal of Health Communication*, 16, 30–54.

Silburn S., Glaskin B., Henry D. & Drew N. (2010) Preventing Suicide among Indigenous Australians. In N. Purdie, P. Dudgeon & R. Walker (Eds). *Working Together: Aboriginal and Torres Strait Islander Mental Health & Wellbeing Principles and Practice*. Canberra: Australian Government Department of Health & Ageing.

Skinner, B. F. (1938) *The Behavior of Organisms: An Experimental Analysis*. New York: Appleton.

Skodova, Z., Nagyova, I., van Dijk, J.P., Sudzinova, A., Vargova, H., Studencan, M. & Reijneveld, S.A. (2008) Socioeconomic Differences in Psychosocial Factors Contributing to Coronary Heart Disease: A Review. *Journal of Clinical Psychology in Medical Settings*. 15(3), 204–13.

Smart Richman, L., Kubzansky, L., Maselko, J., Kawachi, I., Choo, P. & Bauer, M. (2005) Positive Emotion and Health: Going Beyond the Negative. *Health Psychology*, 24(4), 422–29.

Smith, C., Hancock, H., Blake-Mortimer, J. & Eckert, K. (2007) A Randomised Comparative Trial of Yoga and Relaxation to Reduce Stress and Anxiety. *Complementary Therapies in Medicine*, 15(2), 77–83.

Smith, K., Flicker, L., Lautenschlager, N.T., Almeida, O.P., Atkinson, D.N., Dwyer, A. & Logiudice, D. (2008) High Prevalence of Dementia and Cognitive Impairment in Indigenous Australians. *Neurology*, 71, 1470–73.

Speakman, J.R., Levitsky, D.A., Allison, D.B., Bray, M.S., de Castro, J.M., Clegg, D.J., Clapham, J.C., Dulloo, A.G., Gruer, L., Haw, S., Hebebrand, J., Hetherington, M.M., Higgs, S., Jebb, S.A., Loos, R.J.F., Luckman, S., Luke, A., Mohammed-Ali, V., O'Rahilly, S., Pereira, M., Perusse, L., Robinson, T.N., Rolls, B., Symonds, M.E., Westerterp-Plantenga, M.S. (2011) Set Points, Settling Points and Some Alternative Models: Theoretical Options to Understand How Genes and Environments Combine to Regulate Body Adiposity. *Disease Models and Mechanisms*, 4(6), 733–45.

Spielberger, C.D. (1975) Anxiety: State-trait-process. In C.D. Spielberger & I.G. Sarason (eds) *Stress and Anxiety* (vol. 1). Washington, DC: Hemisphere/Wiley.

Spindler, H., Pedersen, S. S., Serruys, P. W., Erdman, R. & van Domburg, R. T. (2007) Type-D Personality Predicts Chronic Anxiety Following Percutaneous Coronary

Intervention in the Drug-eluting Stent Era. *Journal of Affective Disorders*, 99(1–3), 173–79.

Spiro, H. (1986) *Doctors, Patients, and Placebos*. New Haven: Yale University Press.

Stanton, A.L., Revenson, T.A. & Tennen, H. (2007) Health Psychology: Psychological Adjustment to Chronic Disease. *Annual Review of Psychology*, 58(1), 565–92.

Steptoe, A. (1981) *Psychological Factors in Cardiovascular Disorders*. London: Academic Press.

Steptoe, A. & Wardle, J. (2001) Locus of Control and Health Behaviour Revisited: A Multivariate Analysis of Young Adults from 18 Countries. *British Journal of Psychology*, 92(24), 659–72.

Sternberg, R., Wagner, R., Williams, W. & Horvath, J. (1995) Testing Common Sense. *American Psychologist*, 50, 912–27.

Storms, M. & Nisbett, R. (1970) Insomnia and the Attribution Process. *Journal of Personality and Social Psychology*, 16, 319–28.

Strayer, D.L., Drews, F.A. & Crouch, D.A. (2006) A Comparison of the Cell Phone Driver and the Drunk Driver. *Human Factors*, 48(2), 381–91.

Sudore, R.L., Landefeld, C.S., Williams, B.A., Barnes, D.E., Lindquist, K. & Schillinger, D. (2006) Use of a Modified Informed Consent Process among Vulnerable Patients: A Descriptive Study. *Journal of General Internal Medicine*, 21(8), 867–73.

Sudore, R.L. & Schillinger, D. (2009) Interventions to Improve Care for Patients with Limited Health Literacy. *Journal of Clinical Outcomes Management*, 16, 83–90.

Sullivan, T., Weinert, C. & Cudney, S. (2003) Management of Chronic Illness: Voices of Rural Women. *Journal of Advanced Nursing*, 44(6), 566–74.

Swinburn, B., Egger, G. & Raza F. (1999) Dissecting Obesogenic Environments: The Development and Application of a Framework for Identifying and Prioritising Environmental Interventions for Obesity. *Preventive Medicine*, 29, 563–70.

Taylor, C., Graham, J., Potts, H., Candy, J., Richards, M. & Ramirez, A. (2007) Impact of Hospital Consultants Poor Mental Health on Patient Care. *British Journal of Psychiatry*, 190, 268–9.

Taylor, G. & Hawley, H. (2004) The Construction of Arguments over the Rationing of Health Care. *Social Policy Journal*, 3(3), 45–61.

Taylor, S. (2006) *Health Psychology*. (6th Edn). Boston: McGraw Hill.

——, Klein, L., Lewis, B., Gruenewald, T., Gurung, R., & Updegraff, J. (2000) Female Responses to Stress: Tend-and-Befriend, not Fight-or-Flight. *Psychological Review*, 107, 411–29.

Thomas, S. & McLeod, C. (2011) Obesity Myths and one Inconvenient Truth. *Monash News* www.monash.edu.au/news/show/obesity-myths-and-one-inconvenient-truth.

Thompson, J.K. & Heinberg, L.J. (1999) The Media's Influence on Body Image Disturbance and Eating Disorders: We've Reviled Them, Now Can We Rehabilitate Them? *Journal of Social Issues*, 55, 339–53.

Tippett, G. (2011) Driving under the Influence. The *Age*, 30 October. Accessed 16 January 2012 at www.theage.com.au/victoria/driving-under-the-influence-20111029-1mpbh.html.

Tolman, E. (1932) *Purposive Behavior in Animals and Men*. New York: Appleton-Century-Crofts.

Torpy, J.M., Burke, A.E. & Golub, R.M. (2011) Health Literacy. *Journal of the American Medical Association*, 306(10), 1158.

Torpy, J.M., Lynm, C. & Glass, R.M. (2008) Premature Infants. *Journal of the American Medical Association*, 299(12), 1500.

Trentini, C. Wagner, G., Chachamovich, E., Figueredo, M, da Silva, L., Hirakat, V. & Fleck, M. (2011) Subjective Perception of Health in Elderly Inpatients. *International Journal of Psychology*. DOI 10.1080/00207594.2011.626046.

Turner, S., Arthur, G., Lyons, R.A., Weightman, A.L., Mann, M.K., Jones, S.J., John, A. & Lannon, S. (2011) Modification of the Home Environment for the Reduction of Injuries. *Cochrane Database of Systematic Reviews*, 2. Art. no. CD003600. Accessed 12 January 2012, DOI 10.1002/14651858.CD003600.pub3.

van Achterberg, T., Huisman-de Waal, G.G.J., Ketelaar, N.A.B.M., Oostendorp, R.A., Jacobs, J.E. & Wollersheim, H.C.H. (2011) How to Promote Healthy Behaviours in Patients? An Overview of Evidence for Behaviour Change Techniques. *Health Promotion International*, 26(2), 148–62.

Verbrugge, L. (1985) Gender and Health: An Update on Hypothesis and Evidence. *Journal of Health and Social Behavior*, 26, 156–82.

Vicary, D, Westerman, T. (2004) 'That's Just the Way He Is': Some Implications of Aboriginal Mental Health Beliefs. *Australian e-Journal for the Advancement of Mental Health*, 3(3), 1–10. Accessed 15 February 2012 at www.gtp.com.au/ips/inewsfiles/ P22.pdf.

Vitaliano, P.P., Maiuro, R.D., Russo, J., Katon, W., De Wolfe, D. & Hall, G. (1990) Coping Profiles Associated with Psychiatric, Physical Health, Work and Family Problems. *Health Psychology*, 9, 348–76.

Wallace, A.S., Seligman, H.K., Davis, T.C., Schillinger, D., Arnold, C.L., Bryant-Shilliday, B. et al. (2009). Literacy Appropriate Educational Materials and Brief Counselling Improve Diabetes Self Management. *Patient Education and Counselling*, 75(3), 867–73.

Walters, G. & Grusec, J. (1977) *Punishment*. San Francisco: Freeman.

Weinstein, N. (1984) Why it won't Happen to Me: Perceptions of Risk Factors and Susceptibility. *Health Psychology*, 3, 431–57.

Weinstein, N. (2007) Misleading Tests of Health Behavior Theories. *Annals of Behavioral Medicine*, 33(1), 1–10.

WHO (1946) *Constitution*. World Health Organization, Geneva.

—— (1986). *The Ottawa Charter for Health Promotion*. Copenhagen: WHO, Health Canada, CPHA.

—— (2009a) *Health Literacy and Public Health*. Paper prepared by M. Kanj & W. Mitic for discussion at the 7th Global Conference on Health Promotion, 'Promoting Health and Development: Closing the Implementation Gap', Nairobi, Kenya, 26–30 October.

—— (2009b) *Milestones in Health Promotion: Statements from Global Conferences*. WHO Press: Geneva.

Wicksell, R, Melin, L. & Olsson, G. (2007) Exposure and Acceptance in the Rehabilitation of Adolescents with Idiopathic Chronic Pain: A Pilot Study. *European Journal of Pain*, 11(3), 267–274.

Wilkie, D.J. & Keefe ,F.J. (1991) Coping Strategies of Patients with Lung Cancer-related Pain. *Clinical Journal of Pain*, 7(4), 292–9.

Wilson, D. & Barglow, P. (2009) PTSD Has Unreliable Diagnostic Criteria. *Psychiatric Times*, 26(7). Accessed 20 February 2012 at www.psychiatrictimes.com/print/ article/10168/1426942.

Wilson, P. M. & Mayor, B. D. (2006) Long Term Conditions. 2: Supporting and Enabling self-care. *British Journal of Community Nursing*, 11(1), 6–10.

Wolfe, M.S., Williams, M.V., Parker, R.M., Parikh, N.S., Nowlan, A.W. & Baker, D.W. (2007) Patients' Shame and Attitudes Toward Discussing the Result of Literacy Screening. *Journal of Health Communication: International Perspectives*, 12(8), 721–32.

Wolfe, M.S., Wilson, E.A., Rapp, D.N., Waite, K., Bocchini, M.V., Davis, T.C. et al. (2009) Learning and Literacy in Health Care. *Pediatrics*, 124(S3), S275–81.

Wolfe, M.S., Davis, T.C., Curtis, L.M., Webb, J.A., Bailey, S.C. Shrank, W.H. et al. (2011) Effect of Standardised Patient-centred Label Instructions to Improve Comprehension of Prescription Drug Use. *Medical Care*, 49(1), 96–100.

Wolpe, J. (1973) *The Practice of Behavior Therapy*. (2nd Edn). Oxford: Pergamon.

Yarnell, J.W.G. (ed.) (2006) *Epidemiology and Prevention: A Systems Based Approach*. South Melbourne: Oxford University Press.

Yerkes, R.M. & Dodson, J.D. (1908) The Relation of Strength of Stimulus to Rapidity of Habit-formation. *Journal of Comparative Neurology and Psychology*, 18, 459–82.

Zarcadoolas, C., Pleasant, A.F. & Greer, D.S. (2006) *Advancing Health Literacy*. San Francisco: John Wiley & Sons.

Zimmet, P.T. & James, W.P.T. (2006) The Unstoppable Australian Obesity and Diabetes Juggernaut: What Should Politicians Do? (Editorial). *Medical Journal of Australia*, 185(4), 187–8.

Zubrick, S.R., Dudgeon, P., Gee, G., Glaskin, B., Kelly, K., Paradies, Y., Scrine, C. & Walker R. (2010) Social Determinants of Aboriginal and Torres Strait Islander Social and Emotional Well-being. In N. Purdie, P. Dudgeon & R. Walker (eds) *Working Together: Aboriginal and Torres Strait Islander Mental Health and Well-being Principles and Practices*. Australian Government Department of Health & Ageing. Canberra: Australian Government.

INDEX